It's Only Natural

This famous health classic
is now completely revised
and enlarged so as to take
its place as the twenty-first
century's premier text on
natural treatment methods

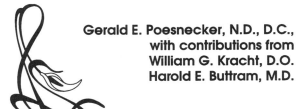

**Gerald E. Poesnecker, N.D., D.C.,
with contributions from
William G. Kracht, D.O.
Harold E. Buttram, M.D.**

Humanitarian Publishing Company
Quakertown, PA 18951

Other titles available from the Humanitarian Publishing Company
P.O. Box 220, Quakertown, PA 18951

Age of Treason
R.S. Clymer, M.D.
ISBN 0-916285-34-0

Chronic Fatigue Unmasked
G.E. Poesnecker, N.D., D.C.
ISBN 0-916285-39-1

Creative Sex
G.E. Poesnecker, N.D., D.C.
ISBN 0-916285-26-X

Dangers of Immunization
Harold E. Buttram, M.D.
ISBN 0-916285-27-8

Freedom of Choice in the Healing Arts
Harold E. Bunram, M.D.
ISBN 0-916285-28-6

Hidden Influences of Love, Touch and Affection
Harold E. Bunram, M.D.
ISBN 0-916285-29-4

How to Legally Avoid Immunizations of All Kinds
Grace Girdwain
ISBN 0-916285-36-7

Love, Sex and Marriage
Harold E. Butuam, M.D.
ISBN 0-685-10307-2

Today's Health Movment & the Future of America
Harold E. Buttram, M.D.
ISBN 0-916285-31-6

Vaccinations and Immune Malfunction
Harold E. Bunram, M.D.
ISBN 0-916285-37-5

Your Health & Sanity in the Age of Treason
R.S. Clymer, M.D.
ISBN 0-916285-32-4

CONTENTS

To all our respected readers: The diagnosis and treatment of
the conditions decribed in this book must be based on a
complete interrelationship and rapport between doctor and
patient. It is not possible to accurately diagnose or treat these
conditions from reading this book or any book. However,
included in this work are the efforts of a doctor with over
forty years of clinical experience treating thousands of patients
by natural healing. Nothing in this book should be necessarily
taken as a consensus of present medical opinion. In general
there is no such consensus on many of the treatments
described. We do not claim that the described procedures cure
anyone, but it is amazing how many patients seem to improve
"spontaneously" while they are under such treatments.

Advancements in natural healing are taking place constantly,
therefore if you feel that you or someone you love may have
be helped by natural methods of treament, you may call Dr.
Poesnecker direct at 1-800-779-3796 to receive the latest
information regarding the conditions described.

Introduction

An event occurred in August 1969 that was to change the face of healing and medicine forever. This was the opening of the Clymer Health Clinic on the outskirts of the pre-revolutionary village of Quakertown, Pennsylvania. While the opening itself was without fanfare, the results of this event have been far reaching and permanent. While there had been other non-allopathic clinics over the years, this was the first valid attempt to offer ailing humanity a center where they could be assured of receiving the best of all the known methods of healing under one roof. From its inception the Clymer Health Clinic was devoted to the interests of the patient first and foremost. The healing methods used had but one criteria: are they the best known way (irrespective of where they came from) to heal the patient. All other considerations were secondary.

The pundits all assured us that a center built on such Golden Rule principles could not succeed, but they soon had to eat their words as the Clymer Health Clinic succeeded beyond everyone's wildest early dreams. By the mid 1970's the Clymer Health Clinic had become internationally famous and was selected by one of the most respected health authorities as one of the two best natural healing centers in the entire world.

In 1983, Emerson Clymer, the man responsible for the establishment of the Clymer Health Clinic, passed on and the Director of the Clinic was selected to replace him as the head of the Beverly Hall Corporation, the Clinic's philosophical parent. This forced the Director to give up his Clinic position to assume new more comprehensive duties. He felt the success of the Clymer Health Clinic was such that its future could safely be turned over to those who had worked closely with him to create this boon to mankind. Unfortunately, his assumption was incorrect. Without his steadying hand, those left in charge began to quarrel and finally they departed one by one to enter more lucrative private practice. In 1989 the Clymer Health Clinic entered bankruptcy and the building was eventually sold by the widow of Emerson Clymer.

This is not the end of our story, however. That portion of the original healing effort, that was established by Harold Buttram, M.D. in a building adjacent to the original Clymer Health Clinic, survived. Once the main clinic closed its doors, the former Director, Dr. Gerald Poesnecker, knew he could not allow this needed concept to die so he returned to private practice with Dr. Buttram and together they kept the flame and spirit of the Clymer Health Clinic alive during several very difficult years. At what is now known as Woodlands Medical Center, they practiced with the same principles and spirit as animated those at

i

the Clymer Health Clinic and, thus, preserved the many treatments that were unique to this famous Clinic. Meanwhile, new young doctors, who had been inspired by the Clymer Health Clinic, were preparing themselves to come and help resurrect this much missed healing center.

In the summer of 1995 the first representative of this "new blood" began his practice at Woodlands. Shortly thereafter, Dr. Poesnecker decided that it was time to bring about a full rebirth of the Clymer Health Clinic concept and, so, on July 1, 1995 the Beverly Hall Corporation Healing Research Center was established. This new Center, close by the old clinic structure, was enthusiastically welcomed by new patients as well as by those who remembered the older Clymer Health Clinic.

This new Healing Research Center not only carries on the successful treatment methods of the Clymer Health Clinic but, like it, also has facilities for patients to be housed and cared for while being treated. From our many years with the Clymer Health Clinic, we learned what is needed to "get people well." With this experience we expect to be able to make our new Healing Centers even more effective in helping humanity than their predecessor.

As this introduction is written, we are in the planning stages of an even more advanced healing addition to be added to Woodlands and the new Healing Research Center. In recent years the most rapidly increasing disease conditions in America are those related to the environment. This is especially true if we include (as we do) the Chronic Fatigue Syndrome in this category. At the beginning of their healing process, these patients need to be isolated from the toxic and stressful world and accommodated in a Center where every factor that enters their life is designed to aid and not hinder their recovery. Such a sanctuary is essential if they are to get back on their feet with sufficient vitality to face the rigors of modern life without succumbing to its challenges.

We have long realized that while such a Healing Sanctuary would be beneficial to many of our patients, it is absolutely vital to other patient's healing process if they are to ever feel the joy of real life surging in their veins once again. We trust that by the time many of you are reading these words, this Sanctuary will not only be operational but will have a long list of grateful alumni to its credit.

It is said that if you build a better mousetrap the world will beat a path to your door. The Clymer Health Clinic was such a "better mousetrap" and the world did beat such a path. Our new Healing Centers are even better mousetraps and we expect more and wider paths to be built to them. You have an opportunity to follow these paths. Come with us; our paths leads to health, contentment and happiness.

Chapter I
What Is A Healing Research Center?

A Healing Research Center, at least the Beverly Hall Corporation Healing Research Center and the philosophically harmonious organization, Woodlands Medical Center, are places where the establishment of the greatest possible health and stability of body, mind and Soul is attempted. We don't consider a person healthy just because he is not afflicted with a named disorder or disease. We believe there is a difference between not being sick and being filled with the vibrancy of true physical health, a positive creative mind and a contented, guiltless Soul.

As we know it is possible for an automobile to move even though its cylinders are scored and passing oil, its valves burnt, its exhaust leaking noxious vapors, its brakes worn, its steering loose, and its body nearly rusted through. It may still run, but would we really want to drive such a car if we had any other choice? We'd probably either trade it in or do what must be done to put it in reasonable working condition.

The human machine is susceptible to pressures and stresses similar to those in an automobile. At our Centers, we are experts at detecting and correcting these signs of distress and imbalance in early stages so they can be more easily corrected long before the system stops working altogether. While most medical practitioners and facilities consider themselves to be a "safety net" at the bottom waiting to catch you after you fall off the edge of the plateau of health, we look upon our responsibility to be on that plateau to guide and help you to keep from falling in the first place.

In theory, unlike the automobile, the human machine is a selfrepairing mechanism. And, in truth, some persons are so blessed with natural vitality that despite all the pressures and strains of modern life, they are able to retain near optimum health to the end of their days. Such persons do not need the help of our Center; unfortunately, as our environment becomes ever more toxic, such people have become all too rare in recent years. Most of us do not pass through life without a variety of indispositions; it is in preventing and correcting these problems, before they reach major dimensions, that our Healing Research Centers can best serve their unique purpose.

I do not wish to imply that we don't treat named diseases at our Centers. We accept for treatment nearly every disease known to mankind. Over the many years that I have been the Center's Director, I can count on the fingers of one hand the patients we have turned away. I merely wish to stress that one of the major purposes of our work is to aid the patient in establishing a chemical, mechanical, mental and emotional

1

balance within his body, thereby helping him to a truly healthful and creative existence. This can and should be done before symptoms of actual specific diseases appear; for if such imbalances are allowed to exist long enough to produce a disease, the treatment is much more lengthy and complicated than if such needed corrections had been made earlier. With proper attention and sufficient dedication on the part of the physician many, if not most, so called diseases can be nipped in the bud before the patient experiences real distress.

The Health Status Evaluation Versus the Medical Examination

Most physicians suggest an annual or semi-annual physical check-up. What, you may ask, is the difference between this type of check-up and the type of health care that I am describing? To the uninformed observer, there may appear to be little difference, but in the purpose and, particularly, in the extent of the methods used, there is a great deal of difference. By nature and tradition the orthodox medical profession is disease oriented.

The standard medical examination, no matter how thorough, is therefore designed to ascertain if the body harbors any known disease entity. If no disease entity, discernible by their methods, can be found, the medical practitioner considers his patient healthy. We consider such a procedure to be valid up to a point, but basically negative and woefully inadequate to meet today's health needs.

To our way of thinking, the absence of demonstrable disease is not tantamount to physical health. A truly satisfactory state of physical health can only be assured, in our estimation, if the various mechanical, nutritional, hormonal, and enzymatic functions of the body are examined and found to be nearly optimal. In order to accomplish this, examinations far more sophisticated than those usually encountered in the orthodox medical examination must be utilized. Such methods are not designed to supplant orthodox medical diagnostic measures but only to supplement them. We feel that it is impossible to have too much information on a patient's health status. Therefore, in our Centers, whenever required and practical, we try to utilize every known effective diagnostic method available to ascertain the true state of health of our patients.

The Basic Health Examination

I know of no better way to illustrate what we mean by "The Health Examination" than to give in detail the method of examination and investigation used at our Centers.

2

The first prerequisite to any true health examination is a complete and carefully detailed medical history. I had a wise old professor in medical school who used to say, "Always listen well to your patients. They have *inside information*." The homeopath has always considered the patient's medical history by far the most important of the physical examination. Over the years, it has been our experience that more mistakes are made by physicians who simply have not listened carefully to what their patient had to tell them, than by all the other defects of the medical examination combined.

To aid our physicians in their evaluation of their patient's homeopathic history, we have recently installed a very complete and comprehensive computer program that helps them to detect and correctly evaluate even the most complex patient symptom patterns.

Once the medical history is completed, an extensive examination is made to discover any known pathologic conditions. All the generally known and accepted diagnostic procedures may be utilized where considered relevant. Those that entail some danger to the patient, however, are suggested only after extensive consultation has assured us that they are absolute necessities. Therefore, techniques in which dyes or other opaque substances are injected into the veins, arteries or spinal fluid are suggested by our Centers only after great deliberation and then only when we believe that the patient's condition is serious enough to warrant it and less dangerous methods would not suffice.

Modern blood chemistry is one of the physician's most useful tools. We have constantly expanded the extent of the blood, saliva and urine tests made at the Center. In almost every instance, with each new testing method utilized, we have been able to find problems that might previously have been missed. We therefore have felt it our obligation to make every effort to obtain as complete a laboratory picture of our patients as is possible in light of the current state of medical technology.

At the present time (Winter 1995/96) more and more specialized tests are being done by the use of saliva. These tests are not only noninvasive but they often much more accurately depict the true nature of the patient's internal functioning than the traditional blood tests since they are designed to measure the levels of vital factors in the tissues where the real body functioning takes place.

X-Ray Examination

Because of the possible adverse effects of radiation, we are extremely cautious in our use of X-rays. No X-ray examination is ordered without very carefully weighing its value in relation to the possible damage that

3

the attendant radiation might cause. While we do not shy away from X-rays we believe necessary, we don't use X-ray examination as a substitute for other less harmful diagnostic skills.

Diagnostic Ultra-Sound and Thermography

New methods are now being developed to investigate the internal functioning of the body without the use of X-ray examination. Two of the first of these are the use of ultrasound as a diagnostic device and the newer thermographic units which, by means of television camera and infrared radiation, measure various temperature changes of the skin. Records of the temperature changes can be used to detect possible pathologic conditions. These latter units were popular several years ago and the Clymer Health Clinic was one of the first to investigate them. They are still being used by some Chiropractors but the MRI seems to have stolen most of their thunder in the medical world.

The MRI (Magnetic Resonance Imagery)

The MRI has revolutionized the examination of internal soft tissue. Its main advantages over the X-Ray is that it is able to visualize soft tissue pathology that eludes X-Ray and the fact that, unlike X-Rays, it has no known detrimental effect to the body. Its main disadvantages are the time needed for its completion, the unavoidable constriction of the patient for this time period (up to one hour) and its very high cost. (A thousand dollars for a single body part is not unusual.) Where the cost, time involved and possible claustrophobia are not a deterrent, the MRI can give us information not possible to obtain in any other way.

As suggested earlier, the possible value of certain diagnostic tests is undeniable, but we believe that some of them, such as X-rays, must be carefully evaluated before they are used extensively. In this category I place such examinations as spinal myelography, the various types of angiography, heart catheterization and all other tests in which foreign objects are introduced into the bloodstream or other vital parts of the system, or in which instruments are placed in extremely delicate areas where damage is difficult to prevent and even more difficult to assess until it is too late. When the patient's ultimate welfare is considered, such tests may be bypassed, for ethical reasons, even in a most extensive examination, if the physician feels that the risks exceed the possible gains.

We also place some cancer biopsies in this category. Although at times nothing can take the place of a biopsy for a positive diagnosis of cancer, with some types of tumors any interference may encourage runaway growth of the tumor. It does seem that at times a biopsy is sug-

4

gested to satisfy the medical curiosity of the physician (or to guard against a possible law suit) and not necessarily for the ultimate benefit of the patient. I realize this is a controversial subject and each case must be judged on its own merits. We do not mean in any way to condemn the judgment of other physicians. However, we at the Healing Research Centers do not think it imperative that each case of suspected carcinoma automatically requires a biopsy, though we are quick to recommend a biopsy whenever we determine that it is in the patient's best interest.

The Health Status Examination

At the same time that the basic physical examination is being given our patients, we also take steps to ascertain their health status. Although great strides have been made to this end in recent years, we are not yet capable of giving a health status examination as complete or as extensive as we would like.

When I was a young doctor just out of medical school I dreamed of the day when we would have a machine that we could connect to the patient, push a button, and in a few seconds have a complete computer read-out of his body nutritional, hormonal and enzymatic chemistry. While every day that passes brings us closer to such a reality the full technology for such a machine is still not with us. But, you can be certain that when it does become available, we at the Beverly Hall Corporation Healing Research Center will be one of the first to have it installed.

Although we may not, as yet, have such a simple all inclusive diagnostic tool, you should not surmise from the foregoing that we are not without resources or methods to ascertain the health balance of our patients. In recent years great strides have been made in discovering methods by which the health status and nutritional balances of our patients can be known. However, instead of having a single source to check these balances properly, it is necessary for us to combine a great variety of methods and then to interrelate and correlate these findings, to give us a precise health quotient that we may utilize to help patients obtain their optimum functional status, which they desire and which they expect us to help them achieve.

Besides the new methods of chemical analysis, mentioned above, a variety of unique diagnostic methods have been developed over the years for use of the natural healer. The more useful of these special diagnostic tools are utilized at our Centers to give us a view of our patients' health status that is one step beyond that usually available.

Since we have been the nation's most advanced natural healing centers since 1969, we are one of the first to be given an opportunity to try out the newer and more revolutionary forms of health investigation in this field. If it is helpful in ascertaining the health status of an individual you can expect to find it at our Centers first.

Nutritional Balances

Nutritional balances can be ascertained by two methods. First, they can be detected from the symptom patterns resulting from their specific deficiencies. Unfortunately, nowadays single nutrient deficiencies seldom occur, and so it is difficult to diagnose deficiency diseases from the symptom pattern alone. However, a knowledgeable and dedicated practitioner can still obtain much useful information about the health status of his patient from a careful exploration of their symptoms.

Second, nutritional deficiencies and imbalances can be diagnosed by actual analysis of the substance present in the body fluids or tissues. Although this method might seem to be most direct and advantageous, such determinations are not simple or uncomplicated, although the newer technologies have provided us with some real breakthroughs in this area. In the following discussions, we will attempt to clarify this situation.

The Detection of Specific Nutritional Imbalances

Tissue and Hair Analysis

A revolutionary form of tissue examination was developed several years ago and, although this test has recently become much better known, we mention it here because it is used consistently in our Centers on practically every patient with metabolic problems.

This examination—the hair test—is used to detect the balance of the various minerals in the body. Today, it is possible to take a material, reduce it to an ash, and analyze that ash, in sensitive laboratory instruments, for its mineral content. It matters very little what organic material is used, as long as there is sufficient mineral matter in its makeup to be detected. When all organic matter is burned, three things are left: carbon dioxide, water and indivisible mineral elements. The carbon dioxide is given off as a gas, the water is or can be evaporated and from the combustion process we are left only with elemental mineral ash. Because these minerals are elements, they can not be broken down further, nor can they be altered or destroyed by ordinary chemical means. Thus, it is possible to take any piece of human tissue, to burn it, then to collect the ash and by a very sensitive method of analysis to analyze this ash to determine the exact number and amount of mineral elements present.

Frequently, patients with hair problems come to us for a hair test, assume that by analyzing the hair we can find out what is the cause of their hair problem. This is not the basic purpose of the hair test, although the correction of the mineral deficiencies that may be discovered could also correct their hair problem. Actually, any representative tissue of the body could be used for the test. Hair, however, is about the only tissue that most people are readily willing to part with. We could just as easily cut off a finger and send it in to be tested. In fact, in many ways it would probably be more representative of general body structure. But it is not common to find patients so dedicated to their health that they are willing to sacrifice a finger to this cause.

About the only other readily available body tissue patients are willing to surrender are fingernail and toenail clippings. But because a certain amount of bulk is needed in the representative tissue for proper analysis, it might take several months of collecting to acquire a sufficient supply of these tissues.

How do we make an analysis from a bald man? It is usually possible to use chest or pubic hair. The hormonal balances present in bald or balding men are usually such that while their head hair is thin, their chest and pubic hair may be profuse.

The hair test can prove to be invaluable. Through it, we can not only get an understanding of the balance of the basic minerals essential to human life, but we can also detect possible toxicity due to such metals as cadmium, lithium, cobalt, lead, and mercury. Time and again, problems that seemed almost unsolvable have been resolved through the agency of the hair test. However, the Healer who uses such a test must be aware that there can be many sources of contamination and he must always take this into consideration in his evaluation of this valuable test.

Another matter to consider is the fact that the amount of mineral in the hair does not necessarily parallel the amount of mineral in the body. At times, if the body cannot properly metabolize a mineral, it will distribute it in the hair. In this instance the mineral in the hair test may be much elevated while, in reality, there is a deficiency in the body. How can the Healer know which is which? That is where his long and dedicated experience comes into play. Sometimes, experience alone is the true guide that leads to correcting a patient's health problem.

The hair test is not an automatic road map to health though in some instances it may be one of the most important guide posts on this road. For example, one of the most difficult problems ever presented to our Centers was that of a lovely young lady from Georgia who came to us at her wit's end. She was filled with strange sensations and pains from head to foot. She had been in several institutions and had been examined by several medical specialists without any apparent solution for her problem. We gave her every test and examination we knew of at that time. We lavished on her our most dedicated care and yet nothing seemed to help.

This was in the early days of the Centers and we were just beginning to use the hair test (We were one of the first Centers anywhere to use this test). Results from her hair test were unexceptional, except for mercury, which showed an extremely high level. Re-evaluation of her symptoms suggested that they might come from some form of mercury poisoning, though we couldn't find its source. Before suggesting treatment for such a rather uncommon condition, however, we decided to confirm our work by running a second hair test using a different laboratory. The second laboratory was told nothing of what we suspected, and the second report was eagerly awaited by our physicians. When the report was finally received, it also showed a very high mercury level. With this confirmation, we hospitalized the patient for further tests. These also demonstrated a higher than normal level of mercury in the blood. Unfortunately, neither the hospital nor we could find the cause of the toxicity. We did, however, give her certain nutrients and dietary suggestions that we thought would help overcome this metal toxicity and, with these, the patient was sent back home. We did suggest however that she carefully go over all the items she used each day to see if they might be a source of the mercury.

A short time later, she wrote me that at last she had found the answer to her problem. For almost twenty years, she had nightly used a certain cream that she would religiously rub into her hands and wrists to keep them soft and supple. On our advice, she wrote the company and they admitted to her that this cream had a high percentage of ammoniated mercury. Since discontinuing this so-called cosmetic, the patient's symptoms have gradually improved, although we all believe it will still take some time for her to recover completely. Mercury poisoning can be very deep-seated and tenacious.

I have described this case for two reasons. First, it shows the type of problem that can really be readily diagnosed by the hair test. Second, it shows the insidiousness of some of the so called harmless agents we use on and in our bodies each day.

Hair analysis is now being offered by several laboratories. It is hoped that the ever-growing interest in this procedure will lead to more and more information about its usefulness and that it will help us in further guiding our patients to the state of health we strive for.

Tests for Vitamins and Blood Minerals

Since I wrote my first edition of this book, the methods of testing for vitamins and minerals in the blood has been revolutionized. The development of more sensitive laboratory equipment along with the use of advanced computer technologies have made it possible to approach my dream of a machine to detect the imbalances in our bodies. While these tests are not as inexpensive yet as we would hope, they are available and insurance will pay for them in some instances.

In order to make testing as available as possible we have incorporated it into our various nutritional testing programs.

To make these tests available to as many patients as possible we have designed three different levels of tests: The Basic Nutritional Profile, The Advanced Nutritional Profile and The Ultimate Nutritional Profile. Feel free to discuss these different profiles with your Center physician. He will help guide you to the profile that best meets your needs and pocketbook.

Function Tests for and Symptoms of Vitamin Deficiency

Frequently your Center physician will be able to determine your nutritional needs by function tests and his experience rather than by the more expensive, though very accurate computer blood and tissue analysis. Some of the methods and rationales for this type of investigation are given below.

Function Test for Vitamin A.

While most vitamins require laboratory procedures for determination, it is possible to determine the adequateness of vitamin A by a function test. This ability is due to the nature of this vitamin's effect on the eye.

There is a substance in the eye called *rhodopsin*, that is generated when little or no light reaches the retina. The production of rhodopsin sensitizes the eye so that twilight or low light vision is possible.

The human eye is blessed with two distinct types of vision. The common daylight, or colored, vision is mediated through nerve endings in back of the retina of the eye called *cones*. Night, or twilight, vision is mediated through nerve endings in the retinal field called *rods*. The rods are far more sensitive to light than are the cones, but it is not possible for the rods to detect color. They are strictly a black-and-white sensing agent. The rods can only function as long as rhodopsin is present in the retina. Because rhodopsin is rapidly made inoperative by strong light, the rods are not functional during most day light or bright light activities. However, once the light reaching the retina is reduced below a certain brightness level, the rhodopsin regenerates and the rods begin to function to give us our second form of vision. This is truly one of our Creator's most elegant mechanisms.

Rhodopsin production and regeneration are under the control of vitamin A, and it has been demonstrated that vitamin A deficiency affects the degree of rhodopsin production. Therefore, theoretically, if we had an instrument that could measure the speed with which rhodopsin is formed after it is first bleached out by light, then we would be able to measure vitamin A activity in the body.

Several years ago, the *American Optical Company* developed an instrument to do exactly this—the *Feldman Adaptometer*. With this device, an intense light is shown into the patient's eyes for a very short time in an otherwise dark room. This is done to bleach out all the rhodopsin that might be present in the retina. Next, the intense light is turned off and simultaneously an exceedingly weak light is turned on. At this time, the technician begins his stopwatch. The time from when the bright light is turned off and the moment the patient is first able to discern the glow of the weak light is determined. This time is the *rhodopsin regeneration time* for that patient. Normals have been calculated. If it takes longer for the patient to discern the weakened light than is considered within the normal range, it is assumed the patient's vitamin A activity is proportionally deficient.

In our Centers we have found this test to be extremely effective and accurate. Surprisingly, we have found that deficiencies occur much more commonly than we had assumed. Apparently, many of our patients do not absorb vitamin A properly, for definite slow rhodopsin regeneration times have been discovered in many patients taking vitamin A preparations at dosages well above the daily requirement. In most of these patients, normal rhodopsin regeneration times could be established once we changed the form of the vitamin A to one more adaptive for their body, or we gave nutritional substances to help these patients better assimilate and metabolize the vitamin A they were already taking.

In recent years we have been using a sublingual form of Beta-Carotene for these conditions and find that it can be tolerated even when the usual oral forms of this vitamin do not seem to be of value. Since it is assimilated directly into the blood stream it does not have to go through the liver and therefore there is much less chance of toxicity. We have found this form of vitamin A to be helpful in many conditions not helped by others. The difficult condition of dry eyes and throat called Shogren's Disease has been helped with this treatment.

Vitamin B Deficiencies

Many vitamin B deficiencies or imbalances are diagnosed at our Center by observation of specific symptomatology. Tuttle and Schottelius, in their Textbook of Physiology,* have this to say about B complex deficiencies: "Because the various B vitamins are found intermingled in many foods, it is difficult to differentiate positively between the disturbances created by the absence of each individual member of the group. Deficiency diseases attributed to a particular vitamin have in some instances been found to be multiple deficiencies, e.g. beriberi. Their absence may lead to a decrease in general well-being of the individual showing itself in reduced work output, increased fatigue and emotional disturbances, irritability and depression."

To any practicing physician, patients who complain of fatigue, irritability, and/or depression are legion. And although not all such patients are deficient in B complex vitamins, this is the basic symptomatology of such deficiencies. As you will see in Chapter II, these symptoms are also those of what is now called Chronic Fatigue Syndrome. Obviously, our physicians are alert to possible Vitamin B complex deficiencies in this condition which we treat so frequently.

A shortage of vitamin B should be suspected whenever the patient tends to show muscular weakness and a loss of coordinating power. The nerves of the skin, arms, and legs may be inflamed and degenerate, sometimes with great pain. The patient loses his appetite and may tend to lose weight or may not make the proper weight gains in childhood. Again, in all such symptom patterns, one may suspect vitamin B. deficiency.

To confirm such a diagnosis for this or any of the B complex vitamins, the most practical measure is to use a test known as therapeutic diagnosis, which merely consists of giving the patient a reasonably large dose of the vitamin(s) suspected of being deficient and observing the patient for symptom improvement over a short period. If the patient's problems are caused by vitamin B deficiency, dramatic improvement should occur within this period. If no improvement occurs, the physician should then look further for other unsuspected causes.

Vitamin B2 Deficiency

Vitamin B2 (riboflavin) deficiency causes skin lesions, especially fissures at the corners of the mouth—a disorder known as cheilosis. In these patients, the cornea (transparent part of the eye) becomes bloodshot and may even ulcerate in severe cases. In animals, cataracts are formed

---

*Tuttle, W. W., and Schottelius, B. A.: Textbook of Physiology, St. Louise Mosby 14th Ed. 1961.

11

in the lenses of the eye, possibly causing blindness. Although riboflavin has been used to treat cataracts in man, there is no specific evidence that its deficiency causes human cataracts. In our Center we have used a natural form of vitamin B2 with its various synergists to treat cataract with satisfying success for many years. Though not a cure-all we can honestly recommend this product to all who suffer from this condition.

Niacin Deficiency

Niacin (nicotinic acid) deficiency gives rise to pellagra, a disease characterized by want of strength and vitality, loss of appetite, indigestion, diarrhea, skin eruptions, pain, and sometimes great mental disturbances. Pellagra is not caused by niacin deficiency alone: for the full manifestations of this disease, deficiencies of thiamin (B1), riboflavin (B2), and perhaps other B vitamins are necessary.

A diet lacking the essential amino acid tryptophan also produces effects very similar to those due to niacin deficiency. Tryptophan apparently can replace niacin in abolishing many of the pellagra symptoms. Recent research has shown that tryptophan is probably the precursor of niacin and can be used to produce niacin in many animals.

Interestingly, the symptomatology of pellagra parallels, though in a much more severe degree, many of the more common chronic complaints of Americans. Many investigators think the great demand for tranquilizers today is a sign of subclinical pellagra caused by a deficiency of the vital B vitamins and perhaps tryptophan. In our own practice, we have found time and again that we can frequently wean patients off tranquilizers and have them lead nearly normal lives by substituting these nutritional factors in supplemental form. We have used a product called "Hi-G" to this end for many decades and find it as useful today as it was when we first began its use.

Vitamin B6 Deficiencies

Whenever we think of vitamin B6 deficiencies, we generally think of swelling (edema) in the arms and legs that seems to occur without specific cause—that is, where there are no heart, kidney, or other organic defects. Tingling of the hands and arms particularly is also a symptom due to B6 deficiency. There are many contradictory statements and opinions about the symptoms of B6 deficiency. We believe further research will shed more light on this useful vitamin.

Because a high-protein diet demands a greater than normal intake of vitamin B6, our patients put on high-protein diets to lose weight or for hypoglycemia are also given adequate amounts of B6 to ward off possible future deficiencies.

12

Some patients are not able to take B6 in its usual form. For these patients it is necessary to use a partially metabolized form known as Pyridoxal 5-Phosphate. This nutrient has been a great boon to those patients who require the benefits of B6 but who previously were not able to take it.

Vitamin B12 Deficiency

The only real sign of B12 deficiency is pernicious anemia. This condition is due not so much to a lack of B12 but to the body's inability to utilize the B12 from food intake. Because this is caused by a deficiency of a certain stomach compound, B12 must be injected directly into the muscle or bloodstream to effect a cure. Recently sublingual B12 has become available and, while we would not recommend that it be substituted for the injectable form for the treatment of pernicious anemia, we do find that many patients with other weakening conditions assure us that they feel better using it.

Undiscovered B vitamins

One of the main problems we encounter in attempting to ascertain the patient's need for B complex vitamins is that there seem to be several important factors that haven't yet been isolated. Therefore, even if we had simple adequate tests for determining the amounts and balance of the currently known factors, a patient could be deficient in some of the unknown factors and therefore be below optimum levels in these elements, even though our tests made it appear otherwise. Owing to this possibility, it has become routine, in our Centers, to recommend a balanced B complex formula obtained from a variety of specially processed natural sources to all of our patients in whom deficiencies of any of these elements may be suspected. This practice has proven most successful in controlling such possible deficiencies.

We don't advise patients to take large doses of the individual B complex vitamins unless they are specifically recommended to do so by a physician. Such dosing can cause definite relative deficiencies of some other members of this vitamin family. Even if an attempt is made to take large amounts of all the B complex factors so that a balance is established, one must remember that several factors of the B complex necessary for human nutrition have not yet been isolated. Even if a balance of all the known B complex vitamins is given, a relative imbalance in relationship to these unknown factors may be produced, and no one can say for sure what disorders may thereby be created.

Vitamin C Deficiencies

Because most of our patients are health-oriented, most of them are already taking adequate amounts of vitamin C, and it is only rarely that we find a patient deficient in this factor. However, some patients seemingly require much more than the accepted dosage, and sometimes it is necessary to raise the patient's daily intake up to one hundred times the normal amount before adequate levels are excreted in the urine.

Many authorities consider vitamin C to be a complex similar to vitamin B complex, and they hold that what we call ascorbic acid is but one component of this complex. They also suggest placing in this grouping such compounds as rutin, hesperidin, bioflavinoids and other related but as yet unnamed substances. There are to my knowledge no practical ways of ascertaining whether the body has adequate levels of all these related compounds, although the new blood testing methods are attempting to take these factors into consideration.

Years of practice have demonstrated to me that pains due to varicose veins can often be relieved by vitamin C and rutin and that the bioflavinoids are extremely useful in viral and bacterial infections. Chemical results also seem to demonstrate that certain of these factors present in specific commercial products are successful in preventing chronically bleeding gums and allied vascular difficulties.

Some patients have trouble with the acidic nature of this vitamin and so many buffered forms have been created. If you have such a problem please us let know and we will suggest the best form of this vital nutrient for you.

Vitamin D Deficiencies

Blood levels of vitamin D can be accurately measured by chemical analysis. In this instance, such a test could prove useful, especially in patients who may be using large amounts of synthetic D2 for some specific purpose. Vitamin D2—the synthetic vitamin D—is particularly toxic; if we fear that the patient is nearing toxic levels, we do such blood testing. In our more normal examinations, however, we test the functioning activity of this vitamin by measuring the urinary calcium level.

Vitamin D brings calcium from the digestive system into the blood, maintaining the blood level of calcium. Unfortunately, vitamin D does not take this calcium out of the blood and place it in the tissues where it may belong. If too much vitamin D is ingested, too much calcium may be drawn into the blood, producing toxic levels. On the other hand, if too little vitamin D or calcium is ingested, blood calcium levels may be low, in extreme cases causing cramps or even tetany.

The urinary calcium test commonly used is called the *Sulkowitch test,* in which a specific reagent is mixed with an equal amount of the patient's urine. In a normal patient, a small white cloud (precipitate) forms when these two are mixed, indicating that the calcium levels of the blood are within a reasonably normal range. If no precipitate forms, the blood calcium level is low, indicating that the kidneys are not able to eliminate calcium from the blood as they should. If the precipitate is very heavy or almost milky, the urinary calcium is high, indicating the possibility of vitamin D toxicity.

When a urinary calcium reading is discovered to be abnormal by our lab, we run a concurrent blood calcium test. If the urinary reading is low but the blood calcium normal, the vitamin D levels are probably adequate, indicating some abnormality with the excretory function of the kidneys. A careful search is then made to discover this possible kidney malfunction.

At our Centers we have found that this last situation often occurs in children who have a condition that simulates epilepsy. The children have seizures very similar to those of epilepsy, but their brain wave patterns are generally normal, and their physicians are at a loss to explain their difficulties. Most of these patients respond fairly well to the use of unsaturated fatty acids, previously called vitamin F. which helps to transport calcium from the blood into the tissues. This nutrient, plus the indicated herbal remedies and mild cervical manipulation, has proven of definite use in these cases. Our own number of patients, however, has been too few to make any positive statements about a direct connection between the condition and low urinary calcium. I mention it here only for those physicians who may encounter a similar case and may find a similar therapeutic trial worthwhile.

High urinary calcium levels are found in hyperparathyroidism, hyperthyroidism and acidosis, but the most common cause in our practice has been the overuse of vitamin D. Calcium levels usually return to normal within a reasonable time once the patient restricts his use of vitamin D, or at least switches to a lower dosage of the natural or D3 form of this vitamin, instead of the D2 or irradiated ergosterol type, which is so commonly used in the so-called natural or organic vitamin compounds.

Vitamin D can prove useful in a variety of disorders in relatively large doses, but such doses should only be prescribed by a physician and they should be controlled by the physician with fairly frequent urinary calcium determinations. We rarely recommend that the lay person take more than two or three times the daily minimum of vitamin D and this amount should be in the natural D3 form.

Vitamin E Deficiency

As popular as vitamin E has become, I know of no simple way of ascertaining the amount present in the body. If we could ascertain such levels, there would still be great dispute over what would be adequate. Even now, few authorities agree on the optimum amount of this vitamin for best body function.

To ensure an adequate supply, we usually recommend that a patient take 300 to 600 units of vitamin E daily in the natural, or alphatocopherol, form. In our Basic Health Maintenance Diet, we specifically recommend certain manufacturers of this product. Experience has taught us that with vitamin E particularly, "all that glitters is not gold." An inferior type of vitamin E can easily be produced by using inferior and/rancid oils or poor manufacturing procedures. We therefore only recommend vitamin E from sources whose integrity is well known to us. Unfortunately this varies from time to time as manufacturers are purchased by profit seeking conglomerates or are not able to meet the competition from less conscientious producers. Therefore, it is best that you always contact us for the best form of vitamin E available when you need it.

In specific conditions of circulatory insufficiency and certain heart problems, we may recommend, as do the Schute brothers, much higher doses of this vitamin than our general suggested dosage. We cannot, however, recommend that any patient take more than the prescribed 300 to 600 units a day unless he is under a physician's care.

Much has been written about not taking vitamin E at the same time that iron salts or female hormones are taken. Some authorities believe that iron salts particularly are capable of neutralizing the beneficial effects of vitamin E. In such instances, they are usually referring to inorganic iron salts such as ferrous sulfate. We don't use such compounds in our Centers, and the natural forms of iron we do use seem to combine with vitamin E without difficulty. One should always remember, that in many natural foods, vitamin E and iron are found dwelling happily along side one another. If this were such an inimical combination, surely the all-wise Creator would not have made them such common bedfellows. However, if you so desire, you can take vitamin E and iron at separate times. Because vitamin E is fat-soluble, it is stored in the body, thus making once-a-day vitamin E dosages acceptable.

The Lesser Known Nutrient Elements

Many other nutrient elemental compounds, such as bioflavinoids, vitamin F (unsaturated fatty acids, Co-enzyme 10, choline, inositol and the various amino acids, are useful, and some even essential to the human body, but only recently have practical tests been discovered to ascertain their proper levels in the body. Since these tests are very expensive they are used only on those patients who remain resistant to all our other healing efforts.

Many years devoted to nutritional research have given the physicians at our Healing Centers the ability to discern deficiencies of certain of these elements from a careful review of the medical history and investigation of certain specific symptomatology.

Structural Examination

The integrity of the structural system of the body is often ignored in most general physical examinations. At our Healing Centers, we consider it to be of paramount importance.

One of my medical school professors (a different one) used to say, "Your patients will usually have two things wrong with them. One will be chemical and the other mechanical. You'd better keep looking until you find both." The passing years have proven all too well the value of his words. We find in general that more mistakes have been made in evaluating structural difficulties than with any other single part of the diagnosis. It is not at all uncommon for us to treat patients who have been suffering for up to twenty years from undiscovered structural distortions that we are able to correct within a few weeks through proper diagnosis and treatment.

We analyze the structural stability of our patients by the use of the most modern methods available. However, we still find that the experienced eye of a well trained Chiropractor or Osteopath is one of the best tools for such an evaluation.

Before entering active practice, I always considered such postural examinations as more or less academic and clinically of little value. Years of clinical experience have proven this assumption to be unfounded. Postural stability is an absolute requisite to good health. All parts of the body tend to suffer to some degree if the structural foundation is unstable.

After the postural examination, the patient is checked for bone-muscle-nerve involvements. The two great American sciences of Osteopathy and Chiropractic provide the source material for the great bulk of this examination. In recent years, however, we have increasingly begun to investigate the various nerve reflex centers away from the spine itself, and we have also investigated many of the Oriental methods such as Acupressure and Acupuncture.

From our correlation of these therapies, we find that there is a common pattern behind much of the mechanical distress each of these methods purports to treat. We find that they are all effective, even though, in theory at least, they work on somewhat different principles. The Chiropractor works on bones in order.to remove pressure on nerves; the Osteopath works on bones and muscles to free blood supply. Oriental physicians work on both muscle and nerves but do not attempt to move bony structures. In the end, however, all the results seem similar if the practitioner is knowledgeable and skillful.

From our extensive work and experimentation, we have hypothesized that most of these mechanical defects occur in the following manner:

First, the patient undergoes some sort of assault on his system. It could be nervous tension, physical exhaustion or strain or even some type of trauma (accident) that affects his structural integrity. This assault may in turn cause a nervous tension that is transmitted to the muscles, producing a muscle spasm. This muscle spasm exerts more pressure on the nerves, thereby increasing the spasm through the effect of the reflex arc created. This spastic muscle in time can pull on some of the bony structures of the body, causing what the Chiropractor calls a subluxation. When the bone, if it happens to be a vertebra, slips out of alignment, it in turn may further increase pressure on the nerve, the whole cycle being aggravated further. In certain traumatic cases, it may be that the injury will first of all cause the bony displacement, in which case the same bone-muscle-nerve disorder is caused except that it begins with a different component.

With this type of disorder, a so-called vicious cycle is produced that therapeutically can be broken by working with any of its separate components. Thus, if the vertebra or other bony parts are replaced and kept from exerting their abnormal pressures, it is wholly possible that the nerve and muscle components will, in time, relax, resulting in a cure. If one works on the muscles with deep massage and other therapeutic methods to reduce their inflammation and spasticity, it is theoretically possible that the resulting muscular relaxation would remove the pressure on the nerve, enabling the bony component to return to its normal position.

Finally, if we were therapeutically able to reduce the nerve irritability, the muscle would relax and with luck the bony displacements would also be corrected.

It therefore is possible to cure a single entity by a variety of means; simply because a specific therapeutic method is effective in these cases does not mean that this method is the only useful therapy or that its explanation of the disorder is thereby verified and substantiated.

At our Healing Centers we attempt to understand bone-muscle-nerve disorders as single entities and we attempt to treat them on all levels of involvement—that is, we correct bony displacement, we work to relax the muscle and we make every effort to reduce the nerve inflammation.

In our structural examination of patients, we attempt to find whatever bone-muscle-nerve disorders may be present. Although such problems are definitely far less romantic than the complicated chemical ones we may discover by other means, they nevertheless can cause much more patient distress and discomfort than some of the more exotic chemical imbalances.

Some of the most important of these structural problems are fully discussed in Chapters 3, 4 and 11.

Further Diagnostic Measures

Besides the *adaptometer* mentioned above, many medical diagnostic instruments have been designed that are particularly useful in detecting chronic disorders and in ascertaining optimum body functioning. Many of these are used routinely in most medical Centers and will not be discussed here. A number, however, are rarely used by orthodox physicians but we have found them to have great diagnostic value. Among these are the oscillometer, the doppler vascular units, the phonocardiograph, the plethysmograph and the Telefunken Clinical pH meter.

The Oscillometer, Doppler Units and Plethysmograph

Although designed to work on different principles, the oscillometer, doppler units and the plethysmograph are all capable of giving us a direct measurement of the circulation capabilities in the body extremities.

Restricted blood flow is a part of many chronic ailments, such as diabetes, Raynaud's disease, scleroderma, arteritis obliterans, varicose veins and thrombophlebitis. Besides these severe conditions, we find this difficulty in a great variety of lesser conditions in which the patient complains of cold hands and feet or of burning and tingling in the extremities.

The only truly scientific way we have found of ascertaining the degree of circulatory activity, or of evaluating the extent of improvement of such conditions without invasive procedures, is by the use of these instruments.

The oscillometer has been with us for some time and is produced by several manufacturers. The one we use is produced in Germany and has proven particularly efficient because it is able to measure both legs or both arms at the same time, thereby making an immediate and direct comparison of the bilateral circulation.

The oscillometer, in itself relatively simple, is composed of a blood pressure cuff-like mechanism wrapped around the extremity and containing two rubber bladders. One bladder functions as in the blood pressure cuff to constrict the vessel; the other is a sensing unit that sends the pulse wave beat back to the meter in the instrument. Such pulse waves are then recorded for each extremity and comparisons are made with those considered normal. From these readings a most accurate measurement of the arterial circulation in the extremities is made.

Their circulation must be reduced to at least half of normal before the average patient shows any particular symptoms. If the arterial circulation is less than normal, but above half normal, and we detect no serious organic diseases, we usually place the patient on a special diet and supplementation to improve the arterial circulation. If the patient's circulation is less than half normal, we usually suggest a course of chelation treatments, for this patient is on the brink of trouble, and chelation alone usually produces the improvement needed at this stage. Chelation as a method of treatment will be thoroughly discussed in Chapter 22.

While the oscillometer is extremely valuable diagnostically, it has proven even more beneficial as a therapeutic guide. Once the circulatory disorder is discovered and the patient placed under treatment, the oscillometric evaluation of such treatment is imperative. It is most difficult for the average patient to honestly know in the early stages of such treatment if they are improving or not. Conditions of weather, emotions and diet can all affect their subjective responses to such a degree that they may unwittingly mislead the physician about the efficacy of the treatment being used. The oscillometer is unaffected by such influences. It accurately informs the physician if his therapy has been effective. In these vascular problems, it is often necessary for many treatment methods to be tested before the most useful and effective for each patient is discovered. In this search, the oscillometer has proven invaluable.

The doppler vascular analyzer and plethysmograph are much more complicated instruments than the oscillometer. They are also considerably more expensive. However, they can detect many conditions that elude the oscillometer and are thus essential to a complete evaluation of any vascular disorder.

The plethysmograph records the degree of capillary circulation in a finger or toe. Such a measurement is made by a small sensing unit attached to the finger or toe by a Velcro strap. By the action of a minute photoelectric cell, the pulse wave in the capillaries is read and graphed by this instrument through complicated electronic means. From this we obtain a measurement of circulation at the point where arterial blood flow ends and venous blood flow begins—the point where circulatory trouble usually begins. The plethysmograph therefore enables us to discover difficulties in blood flow at the earliest possible time.

This instrument also has one other advantage over the oscillometer. Because oscillometer readings are made in the forearm of the upper extremities and in the calf of the leg for the lower extremities, if a vascular lesion should occur in the wrist or hand, or in the ankle or foot, the oscillometer reading would not show abnormalities. Plethysmograph readings are made at the tips of the fingers and/or toes, and such lesions would thus immediately be discovered.

An important recent development is the doppler effect vascular analyzer. With this expensive but fascinating instrument, the accurate flow of blood in the vessels can be measured and graphed, thereby facilitating the discovery of all sorts of circular difficulties. This vascular analyzer permits the doctor to readily evaluate the most important treatment procedures and to choose rapidly the most effective method.

This instrument is applied similarly to the oscillometer but is considered to be far more accurate in its readings than this much less costly tool.

The Phonocardiograph

The phonocardiograph is an instrument for analyzing heart problems and it differs in certain fundamentals from the more common electrocardiograph (EKG). This latter instrument reads the electrical impulse potentials as they traverse the heart, while the former uses a microphone to graph the sound of the muscular contractions of the heart.

The electrocardiograph's measurement is a very important indicator of heart activity and it is used in all general examinations at our Centers. However, certain heart malfunctionings do not substantially affect the cardiac electrical impulses, and these disorders usually are not easily detected by the electrocardiograph. For analysis of these conditions, we turn to the phonocardiograph. The phonocardiograph consists of a sensitive microphone that feeds a wide-band amplifier, which in turn drives a stylus to produce a graph on a motor-driven piece of waxed tape. If the phonocardiograph microphone is placed over the areas on the chest where a physician would normally listen for heart sounds with a stethoscope, it will produce a graph of these sounds. This graph gives us a permanent objective record of the heart sounds instead of the fleeting subjective impressions obtained by using a stethoscope.

The phonocardiograph, although capable of detecting tachycardia, bradycardia, and other heart irregularities as readily as the electrocardiograph, is most specific and useful in analyzing muscular disorders of the heart. One of the most common heart problems is that in which the heart muscle itself becomes somewhat weakened and unable to respond to the electrical impulse to its fullest capability. If this muscle weakness becomes severe enough, it can readily be detected by orthodox diagnostic means. In the early stages of muscle weakness, however, most orthodox tests, including electrocardiography, will be normal. Such early muscle weakness, however, is rapidly and easily detected in properly run phonocardiography. It is in the detection of these early muscular defects that phonocardiography has proven invaluable to us. We find such muscular weakness much more common than generally realized and a not uncommon cause of unexplained tiredness that does not respond to general therapeutic measures. This subject is discussed in detail in Chapter 19.

Along with its use in detecting cardiac muscular weakness, the phonocardiograph has proven successful in diagnosing many forms of nutritional deficiencies. It would·appear that various forms of nutritional deficiencies cause rather sudden but subtle effects on heart function. Many of these deficiencies can be detected at very early stages with the phonocardiograph and proper corrections made before any permanent damage has occurred.

Some phonocardiograph operators are so proficient that they perform the following test to display their skill. The phonocardiogram of ten persons are taken. They all leave the room and rest for ten minutes, except for one who is asked to smoke a cigarette. They all return and phonocardiograms are run again. When this is done, the operator is able to pick out the person who smoked the cigarette because of the adverse changes in his heart's phonocardiogram.

The Telefunken Clinical pH meter

The wonders of electronics and miniaturization have recently provided us with a new, exciting tool in the diagnosis of digestive problems. The Telefunken Clinical pH meter allows us to follow the digestive enzyme production of the body without the usual distasteful and unreliable methods of the past. The patient swallows a small non-toxic radio transmitter no larger than an ordinary capsule and a receiver outside the body records the pH (acidity or alkalinity) of the entire digestive tract. This information allows the doctor to pinpoint exactly which part of the digestive system may be malfunctioning and is thus able to prescribe the needed healing therapies.

Therapeutic Diagnosis

Therapeutic diagnosis is a technique used by most physicians in one form or another. It is mentioned here, not because it is unique with us, but because it is generally misunderstood and maligned without good reason.

In discovering an unknown factor—and this is the basis of all diagnosis—we must travel from the known to the unknown. If we have a patient with an unknown condition who is taking unknown supplementation or medication, following an unknown diet and living in an unknown and uncontrolled environment, our chances of making a diagnosis of a complicated metabolic problem are almost nil. This patient's problem is compounded with so many variables that the physician doesn't know where to begin to make a proper diagnosis.

To bring some reason out of this diagnostic chaos, the physician must reduce the number of variables to a minimum. To accomplish this end, in our Centers, the patient is first placed on one of our Basic Health Maintenance Diets, which is a balanced, nutritionally oriented diet, the results of which we know well. Next, the patient is placed on certain specific nutrient remedies whose nature is also well known to us, and that seem indicated by his symptom grouping. We then await results.

In this way we have removed as many unknown variables as possible and have substituted in their place a diet and nutritional substances with which we are very familiar. The way in which these substances act on the patient's constitution tells us much about his body functions. For our diagnostic purposes, it matters little whether he feels better or worse, or shows no improvement. Each of these responses tells us a story that is important in ascertaining his basic difficulty. This is the nature of the procedures involved in therapeutic diagnosis.

If the patient is not well-informed about the nature and purpose of such testing, he may feel that the physician is "experimenting" on him. Nothing could be further from the truth. Properly used therapeutic diagnosis is just as valuable and useful as any laboratory or X-ray examination. It has the particular advantage of examining the body in action and as a functioning entity, rather than measuring only one small part of the body chemistry.

Unfortunately, patients may compare our therapeutic diagnosis to the testing of their responses to various drugs by medical practitioners. Because most drugs have more or less serious side effects, no one likes to take them unless absolutely necessary. Any physician, therefore, should be loath to use such remedies in therapeutic diagnosis; such methods are not generally used by reputable physicians.

The natural remedies at our disposal are all inherently nontoxic and they can therefore be used in such diagnosis techniques with complete safety. At times, some momentary physiologic upsets may result, but because this is an integral part of the therapeutic diagnosis, such upsets are very helpful to the final diagnosis and only rarely do these reactions become greater than slightly annoying.

Esoteric Diagnostic Methods

There are a group of diagnostic measures that have been advanced by various groups at one time or another, but that have never been fully accepted by the general medical body. Some of these have been developed by medical doctors, some by drugless practitioners and some are of unknown parentage. The real value of most of them has never adequately been ascertained, though in general they are condemned as quackery by the political active portion of the orthodox medical profession.

The Beverly Hall Corporation Healing Research Center has been established as a research center for all forms of natural therapy and diagnosis. We are always in the process of investigating various methods of diagnosis (as well as treatment), some of which may prove useful in our future examinations. Below we describe a few of the methods now under investigation. I do not, however, want such a description to be confused with an endorsement, for such is not the fact. I make no claims of value, nor assume any responsibility for the accuracy of these unaccepted methods.

Albert Abrams and Radionics Diagnosis

The radionic diagnosis technique was developed by Albert Abrams, M.D. in the early 1930s. This man, a true genius, was so far ahead of his time that even today his ideas are considered fantastic (read quackery) by most physicians. Abrams, a scientist and medical practitioner, developed many revolutionary concepts during his lifetime. Surprising as it may seem, he was originally an avid medical conservative who embarked on a program to disprove the medical heresies of the day. His work brought him into pointblank confrontation with Chiropractic, Osteopathy and Homeopathy. Not too surprisingly, his investigations did not succeed in disproving the theories of these irregular sciences, but, on the contrary, offered considerable scientific justification for their precepts. Because Abrams was more of a scientist than a politician, he accepted his discoveries even though they were not what he had expected and in true scientific fervor continued to investigate until he was able to establish to his satisfaction methods and techniques in diagnosis and treatment that went not only well beyond anything within the medical profession of his day, but also well beyond anything the other irregular schools had to offer as well.

In his later research, Abrams began to develop a strong belief in the vibratory nature of disease and health. This work resolved itself into his acceptance of the theory that the cellular structures of all healthy tissues have specific normal vibratory rates. According to Abrams, when these tissues become diseased, this normal cellular vibratory rate changes, each disease producing its own specific change in the affected cells vibratory rate. He also found that the various toxic elements in the body cause a specific change in the vibratory rates as well. He then postulated two concepts. First, if he could develop a machine that measures these vibratory rates, it would be possible to determine if any specific organ system was in good health or was diseased and by measuring the vibratory change, he could ascertain exactly the type of disease that was afflicting the organ. Second, because he knew that the various toxic substances, bacteria and viral agents each had individual vibratory rates, if he could detect these specific vibratory rates within the body, he would know that the body was contaminated by these elements and could proceed accordingly.

This was the foundation of his theory of radionic diagnosis. While I cannot discount the validity of Abrams' theory, I am, however, somewhat skeptical of the value of the instruments he and later practitioners of this method have constructed to carry out, in practice, the tenets of this method.

The instruments that Abrams and his disciples have constructed are purported to measure individual vibratory rates, either from the patient directly, or from a drop of the patient's blood on a specially prepared piece of filter paper. In a good radionic analysis, well over one hundred various disease entities and body organs are tested. Unfortunately, although the construction of the machines is impressive, the final detecting mechanism has always been the human nerve arc. That is, the detection method depended on the ability of the operator for its sensitivity. This factor alone has kept Abrams' wonderfully conceived method from being accepted by the most of the scientific community.

In operating the radionic diagnostic device, the patient, who is connected into the circuit of the machine, rubs his fingertips over a piece of Bakelite or rosewood until, through changes of the dials, a certain resistance is felt at his fingertips—the readout signal. The setting of the dials at the times of the read-out signal indicates the disease involved or the specific state of organ activity.

In practice, some people seem much more capable of making the radionics instrument work than do others. In operation, the whole procedure reminds one of a Ouija board. I say that, not disparagingly, but only as an observable fact. I personally know of many fine physicians who used this method almost exclusively in their diagnosis and who were noted far and wide for their diagnostic ability and cures.

It has also been my pleasure to meet a younger generation of physicians who are interested in radionics and who hope to be able to substitute a sensitive electronic sensing unit for the human nerve reflex, so that this method could be placed on a firm, scientific foundation. I don't know whether they will be successful, but, if they are, the advantages of radionic diagnosis could then be made available to many of our sick and ailing.

Iridiagnosis

Iridology (iridiagnosis, as it is referred to by some practitioners) is the science of diagnosing diseases by examining various markings in the iris of the eye. According to early naturopathic practitioners, each organ or section of the body is represented by a specific area in the iris. Furthermore, they thought that if the organ were diseased or abnormal, certain distinct changes would occur in the corresponding area of the iris.

If this theory were correct, it would be possible by a careful examination of the iris to detect the various sites of disease or abnormality that may exist in the examined patient. Owing to the nature of the alterations in the iris, some authors also claim that they can ascertain the exact state of the disease process—if it is acute, chronic, or at an in-between stage.

The problem of verification in iridiagnosis is somewhat different than that in radionics. The technical problems of iridiagnosis have been solved. It is possible to take a sharp color photo of the iris and of the lesions that are supposed to exist. The basic contention is whether the theory itself is valid.

Our own research has not yet given us a definitive answer to this question, though we plan to continue our investigation until we think all avenues have been exhausted, or until we are convinced of its value.

Though we make no claims, we include an iridiagnosis chart, on the next page, which you may use for your own amusement and/or investigation. This chart comes from Henry Lindlahr's great landmark of natural healing *Nature Cure* originally published in 1914. The chart, though not as complete as those of later years, will nevertheless give you adequate information for experimentation.

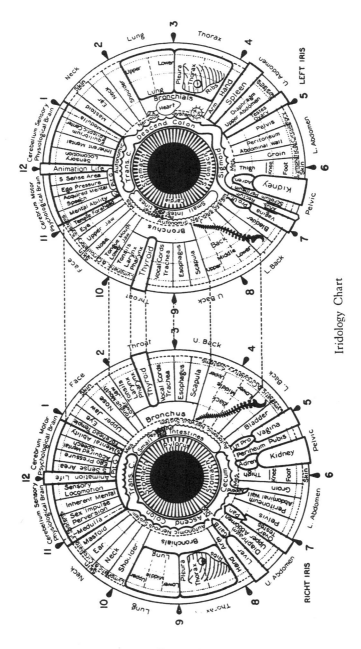

Iridology Chart

Figure 1

27

Reflex Diagnosis

The theory behind all forms of reflex diagnosis goes like this: An internal organ is in trouble. Nerves from that organ grow to some specific area of the skin. If one touches or presses on this specific area, it will produce pain. This indicates that the organ whose reflex center is at this point is in trouble and therefore a diagnosis can be made of organ disease from the mere finding of a specific sensitive area of skin.

The foregoing has been somewhat intentionally vague because there are many theories about where these various reflex areas are. Certain acupuncturists tell us that there are places on the ear that correspond to most of the disease entities of mankind. The so-called reflexologists, or zone therapists, tell us that these reflex centers also occur on the feet and that if we know exactly where to touch or press on the feet, each of the various organs and portions of the body can be tested. Others say that the reflex areas occur all over the body and testing thus must be made in a very widespread and intensive manner.

Probably the most common use of this method in recent years has been the use of the foot reflexes. Eunice D. Ingham, in her book *Stories That The Feet Can Tell*,* has had a very profound effect on this type of diagnosis and treatment.

In the hands of a knowledgeable practitioner, the various reflex methods of diagnosis can prove most effective and in some instances they are not to be despised over any other known form of diagnosis.

In our own humble way we have developed a group of reflex diagnostic areas known affectionately as "Poesy's Points." These points are most commonly found in the neck area on either side of the cervical spinous processes. They are present in many conditions but demonstrate their most painful presence in our Chronic Fatigue patients.

Intuitive Diagnosis

When all the other diagnostic measures have been exhausted, one final factor often may be the most important of all in diagnosis and helping a patient to an optimum health status. This factor is the intuitive feeling of the physician about the nature of his patient's difficulty.

After interviewing a patient, an experienced physician often is aware of a sense of calmness or peace and an inner knowledge that his patient is going to be all right. In another case, even though diagnostic signs may indicate otherwise, the physician is not able to shake a sense of

---

*Eunice D. Ingham: Stories That the Feet Can Tell. Eunice D. Ingham P.O. Box 948, Rochester. N.E .

uneasiness or impending difficulty. Such feelings are definitive signs of diagnostic intuition. The more materialistically inclined physicians have recognized such signs but usually dismiss them as merely the subconscious reactions of a highly developed state of mental perception. Those of us who are more liberal in our feelings on this matter consider these feelings to be intuitively perceived help from unknown forces that help man in times of trial and tribulation.

Dr. R. Swinburne Clymer, to whom our Centers are memorials, told me one time that all true physicians had such intuition, and it would grow in strength and vitality if they would but listen to it. Unfortunately, most physicians disregard such hunches and tend to stick to the so-called strict scientific examination procedures.

I mean in no way to discredit any of the scientific methods of diagnosis; at our Centers we make full use of them all. But I do believe that subconscious attention to this intuitive nature was probably the secret that made the family physician of a hundred years ago the equal, or sometimes even the superior in the long run, of some of our modern practitioners. Today, we often find an attempt to depersonalize medical care. This is especially true as more and more medical care is dictated by insurance companies instead of physicians.

There is, in medicine, an increasing desire to computerize medical investigations so that errors are minimized. As far as this goes, it could be used for good. Unfortunately, a computer has no intuition; I think that if this trend goes far enough to further injure the already weakening rapport between doctor and patient, much of great value will be lost from the practice of medicine.

At our Healing Centers, we encourage the use of this intuitive diagnosis and treatment. We try to establish a close understanding and rapport with our patients. We take time to get to know our patients as individuals. We believe this is far more important in the long run than any so-called professionalism we may lose by such a close association. We try to make our patients feel at home and to make them feel a part of one big happy family in the truest and most useful sense of that word. This is our final diagnostic *tour de force*. It is something that can't be put down into figures, nor can we show it to you in a picture. Yet, it is there and can be felt by almost everyone. In the last analysis, we believe that it is an absolute essential to the functioning of a true Healing Center.

Chapter II
Stress And You: Hypoadrenalism, Chronic Fatigue Syndrome, Environmental Disease

When we first published *It's Only Natural* , more than twenty years ago, Chronic Fatigue Syndrome, Fibromyalgia, Candida infections, Epstein Barr infections and the various Environmental Diseases were all unheard of. Patients with these conditions were considered to be malingerers or neurotics by the vast majority of physicians. We were considered a "quack" to even intimate that there might really be something wrong with these patients. All this has now changed. Not that we have been given any credit or respect for our pioneering work (that would be asking too much), but that at least these patients are no longer considered to be only hypochondriacs.

In the original edition of this work I used the name functional hypoadrenia to describe these patients. Since there is no evidence that this is not the underlying cause of these various conditions I will retain this nomenclature in this chapter.

To further the cause of individuals with these conditions I later wrote two separate books entirely devoted to this subject. They were *Adrenal Syndrome* and *Chronic Fatigue Unmasked*. The latter of these works is still available and is recommended for all those who see themselves or someone they love in the type of patient presented here.)

Many years ago, Dr. Hans Selye presented papers on the adverse effects of stress and what he called the general adaptation syndrome (GAS). This research showed that when the human body is placed in a situation that produces a degree of pressure greater than can be handled by its normal homeostatic organ functioning, a series of chemical and glandular changes are produced that he called the General Adaptation Syndrome.*

One of the most important factors in the GAS was found to be a previously often neglected gland, the adrenal. This small gland, which weighs about as much as a nickel and sits like a Bishop's cap on top of each kidney, is now recognized as one of our most important endocrine glands (glands that produce hormone-like substances discharged directly into the bloodstream).

---

*See figure 2.

31

The adrenal glands are composed of two parts—the medulla (inner portion) and the cortex (outer surrounding portion). The adrenal glands produce many substances, the most noteworthy of which are epinephrine, (previously known as adrenalin), which is produced by the medulla; and the various sterols such as cortisone and aldosterone, produced by the cortex.

Many observers believe that in hormonal responses to stress the adrenal medulla is the primary agent. According to this view, stress on the body stimulates (probably by way of the sympathetic nervous system) the adrenal medulla to increased epinephrine production. This hormone increases the secretion of adrenocorticotrophin (ACTH) by the pituitary, which in turn activates the adrenal cortex to a greater production of corticoids such as cortisone.

Cortisone and its related sterols have been used for years in treating all forms of inflammatory reactions, from extremely severe diseases to mild skin conditions. Inflammatory conditions usually respond quite rapidly to cortisone therapy. Unfortunately, in chronic disorders cortisone usually doesn't bring about a cure but only temporary relief. The reason for this is simple. The production of cortisone and allied sterols represents only one step in the general adaptation syndrome (GAS). These sterols rid the condition of inflammation but they don't resolve other problematic aspects of the condition. This must be done by other agents of the GAS activity. If the endocrine gland system is weak and not able to carry on these activities, the condition will revert to its inflammatory stage as soon as cortisone is withdrawn. Because cortisone is notorious for its side effects when given for any length of time, every physician tries to withdraw it as soon as possible, if at all feasible. Although sterols are useful in serious cases and undoubtedly have relieved much suffering, they are definitely not the answer to a balanced glandular system. It is in the search for this balance that this chapter is devoted.

About this time, you may be asking yourself, "Very interesting, but what does all this have to do with me?" It concerns you in this way. The General Adaptation Syndrome is reacting in your body every moment of the day. As long as it functions well, you should be healthy and contented. If it functions poorly, you undoubtedly will be vexed with problems that often tend to cause consternation among orthodox physicians. In fact, at the Beverly Hall Corporation Healing Research Center our experience shows that most of the misdiagnosed, neglected, and rejected patients who come to our doors are victims of a malfunctioning General Adaptation Syndrome. Most of these exhibit hypoadrenalism (also called hypoadrenia)—functional (nondisease-caused) adrenal insufficiency. The

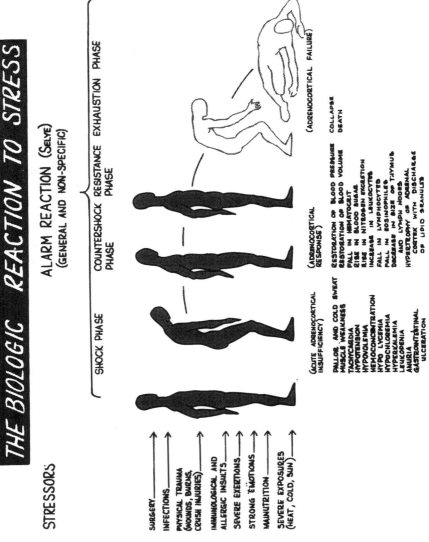

Figure 2

adrenal glands of these patients, through exhaustion, have ceased to function as well as they should, and· they aren't capable of putting out the normal complement of the substances required for proper body function. Interesting in many of these patients they are over excited when they should rest and sleep and tired and weak when they need to function. This seeming paradox is the "signature" of this condition.

There has been much research, particularly by Dr. John W. Tintera, relating this condition to another common metabolic defect—hyperinsulinism (low blood sugar). A great deal has been written of recent years about this connection. The nutritionist authors—Carlton Fredericks, E. M. Abrahamson, and Allan Nittler—have all presented in great detail the symptoms, the methodology, and the basic nutritional and supplemental care for these patients. Although I agree with Tintera and others that many cases of hypoglycemia are caused by malfunctioning adrenal glands, it's been my experience that patients can have functional hypoadrenalism and all its symptoms without necessarily having the hyperinsulinism of the low blood sugar syndrome. And hypoglycemic patients do not always have lowered adrenal functioning, but many do.

Many patients come to our Center with typical symptoms of low blood sugar who have had one, two, or even more normal glucose tolerance tests. Often, as an empirical treatment, these patients had been placed on the low-blood-sugar diet by their previous physician, but to little avail. Upon examination, we usually find these patients suffering from adrenal exhaustion, which has not yet manifested as hypoglycemia. Under treatment, these patients usually respond well; almost without exception, they have been able to return to a normal, productive life.

Functional adrenal exhaustion is poorly understood by most physicians, and very little has been written for the general public on this condition. Surprisingly, the earlier investigators in hormones and hormone therapy knew it well. The reason it has been so ignored is difficult to explain. I personally think this apathy has been produced by the general vagueness of its character, the seeming neurotic symptoms of its victims, and the slowness of its correction, even with the most advanced therapy. In our Center, I always meet the newly diagnosed hypoadrenal patient with mixed feelings. I am, on the one hand, very pleased to know that we have a patient who will once again become useful and productive instead of being only half-functioning. On the other hand, I always groan a little bit inside when I think of all the care, time, and constant loving support necessary to carry this patient through the seemingly nonproductive early stages of treatment. With perseverance, however, they all respond. In the end, they prove to be among our most appreciative patients, which gives the physician a great sense of accomplishment. (While this paragraph was written over twenty years ago it is still as true today as it was then.)

I mentioned earlier that the hypoadrenal syndrome has been known for some time. To verify this statement I want to quote from one of the great early investigators in glandular therapy, Dr. Henry R. Harrower, M.D., F.R.S.M. (London). In his book *Practical Organic Therapy, the Internal Secretions in general Practice*, Harrower had this to say:

"Since the adrenals are so extremely susceptible to so many outside influences, it is likely that they would be easily worn out, and as a matter of fact, *functional hypoadrenia* is as common a condition as any endocrine manifestation. From a practical standpoint, this is an extremely important symptom complex." Remember this was written just a short time after World War I. Harrower goes on: "It is quite some years since Sajous began to emphasize the importance of this condition, and while his opinions were scouted, and some of his ideas declared visionary, it must be admitted that our present knowledge of this subject is very much in harmony with the following quotation from Sajous' monumental work: 'Functional hypoadrenia is the symptom complex of deficient activity of the adrenals due to inadequate development, exhaustion by fatigue, senile degeneration, or any other factor which without provoking of organic lesions in the organs of their nerve paths, is capable of reducing their secretory activity. Asthenia, sensitiveness to cold and cold extremities, hypotension, weak cardiac action and pulse and anorexia, anemia, slow metabolism, constipation, psychoasthenia are the main symptoms of this condition.' "

Therefore we see that this condition was not only known in the early 1920s, when Harrower wrote, but Harrower himself quotes Dr. Charles Sajous an even more famous endocrinologist, who discussed it at a still earlier time.

Harrower goes on to say that "Hypoadrenia is a complication of all the serious acute infectious fevers, since the adrenals are so intimately connected with the driving of the body and are so susceptible to toxemia, that the ultimate reduction of the accustomed adrenal stimuli is responsible for a slowing down of many of the sympathetic controlled functions of the organism. Too often this sympathetic asthenia is the actual cause of death from disease of this character."

In such cases Harrower stated that, "Asthenia is the rule and muscular tone (both striped and unstriped muscle) is poor. Exertion is difficult, if not impossible, and the fatigue syndrome is prominent. The intestinal musculature is inactive. Stasis, a common cause of hypoadrenalism, is also a usual result of it. Mental exertion, even the simplest exertion, often causes so much weariness and exhaustion as to be prohibitive. Mental elasticity is lost, and there is both mental and physical depression with the fear that the individual now can not accomplish his accustomed good mental work; and the story that he 'has lost his nerve.' With this, one frequently notes a fearfulness of making wrong decisions and vacillating and indecisive frame of mind. This is the most usual form of adrenal insufficiency. It is chronic both in origin and in its course."

Another section in Harrower's book is entitled "Neurasthenia as an adrenal syndrome." The word neurasthenia isn't used as much as it once was, nor is it well-understood by the general public as it was at one time. Neurasthenia means weak nerves. Although they may not have heard of neurasthenia, we frequently hear people speak of their weak or sensitive nerves and upset nervous system. I personally still find neurasthenia an acceptable term and an exact description of many patients we see daily.

Again, Harrower's report is so lucid that I am presenting the entire section on neurasthenia:

Neurasthenia as an Adrenal Syndrome.

"The minor form of functional hypoadrenia is more common than some have appreciated, and the fact that there is a psychic origin as well as the other physiologic causes already considered, allies it to the fashionable neurasthenia of today. In fact, some have stated that what is improperly called 'neurasthenia' is not a disease per se, but really a symptom complex of ductless glandular origin and that the adrenals are probably the most important factors in its causation. Campbell Smith, Osborne, Williams and others, including the writer, have directed attention to the importance of the adrenal origin of neurasthenia (though a pluriglandular dyscrasia is practically always discoverable), but so far this is not understood as well as its frequency and importance warrant.

"A few quotations from the literature will firmly establish the importance of this angle from which to study this common and annoying symptom complex. Quoting from the Journal A.M.A. (Dec. 18, 1915): 'The typical neurotic generally has, if not always, disturbance of the thyroid gland. The typical neurasthenic probably generally has disturbance of the suprarenal glands on the side of insufficiency. The blood pressure in these neurasthenic patients is almost always low for the individuals and their circulation is poor. A vasomotor paralysis, often present, allows chilling, flushing, cold or burning hands and feet, drowsiness when the patient is up, wakefulness on lying down and hence insomnia. There may be more or less tingling or numbness of the extremities.'

"Again, Kinnier Wilson in his monographs on The Central Importance of the Sympathetic Nervous System, makes the following pertinent remarks: 'Many of the common symptoms of neurasthenia and hysteria are patently of sympathetic origin. Who of us has not seen the typical irregular blotches appear on the skin of the neck and face as the neurasthenic patient 'works himself up into a state'? The clammy hand, flushed or pallid features, dilated pupils, the innumerable paresthesias (tinglings), the unwanted sensations in head or body, are surely of sympathetic parentage. In not a few cases of neurasthenia, symptoms of this class are the chief or only manifestations of the disease. Here then, is a condition of defective sympatheticotonus; may it not have been caused by impairment of function of the chromophil system? [Adrenal System] .... There does not appear to me any tenable distinction between the asthenia of Addison's Disease and the asthenia of neurasthenia. Cases of the former are not infrequently diagnosed as ordinary neurasthenia at first. It is difficult to avoid the conclusion that defect of glandular function is responsible for much of the Central picture of neurasthenia.'

"Later this same author makes the following apothegm: 'Sympathetic tone is dependent on adrenal support, and until the glandular equilibrium is once more attained, sympathetic symptoms are likely to occur.'"

Interestingly, this quotation from the Journal of the American Medical Association of 1915 postulates a relationship between neurasthenia and low adrenal function. Yet to this day, such a relationship is rarely considered in medical treatment. At the Beverly Hall Corporation Healing Research Center, we consider such a cause and effect very common, and we treat accordingly. We have become internationally known for our treatment of the weakened nervous system.

Our treatment methods aren't so original or revolutionary; it's just that we are willing to get down to causes and accept as facts the postulates of Harrower, Sajous, and the many other brilliant investigators of those earlier days. Their work showed that many emotional states have glandular causes. We believe our duty as physicians is to find these causes and correct them whenever possible. The path to follow has been shown. Harrower established the basic treatment more than fifty years ago; yet today, not one physician in a thousand is familiar with this malady even though his office may be jammed with patients suffering from it. (This was true twenty years ago but not now. These patients are now beginning to be recognized. The only problem is that most physicians still have no idea of how to treat them or of the underlying glandular weaknesses. Maybe in another twenty years?)

How can one tell if they have adrenal insufficiency (Hypoadrenalism-Chronic Fatigue Syndrome-Environmental Disease)? Usually the first and most obvious symptom is tiredness, apparent laziness, or lack of ambition. A young person often feels as if he has some serious wasting disease. The young hypoadrenal patient usually is by nature a go-getter, smart in school, and extremely conscientious. With hypoadrenalism, he finds it more and more difficult to concentrate. The harder he tries to work, the more tired he becomes. Parents and friends become alarmed, and the patient is usually taken to a variety of physicians to correct the enigmatic condition.

In middle age, the hypoadrenal person usually feels he is just slowing down, or that he is beginning to grow old prematurely. Again, he tends to push himself to added effort. Sometimes he takes special exercises or courses to stimulate mental activity. As in the younger person, the harder he tries, the less he is able to accomplish. The situation can become so bad that the hypoadrenal person may even become dizzy or have fainting spells, which usually brings him to a physician.

In the elderly, this condition is blamed on old age. It is believed that Mom or Dad is finally wearing out. But the symptoms of senility and of hypoadrenalism are not the same; usually the difference can be discovered by a physician reasonably versed in the latter disorder.

If hypoadrenalism is not diagnosed and treated in the early stages, the patient will start to manifest symptoms that he takes as signs of mental deterioration. He becomes more and more forgetful; he begins to have small blacking-out incidents, and dizziness is particularly prevalent, especially that which occurs on arising from a seated or reclining position. He begins to fear that he has a brain tumor or perhaps cancer of some vital organ. The most common fear however is fear of a mental disorder. This is the point at which he is driven to seek medical attention.

Let's take a look at this picture. We have a person who is tired, much more than he should be, has occasional dizzy spells, and has disturbing mental aberrations—all contrary to his usual physical and emotional status. This person had always been bright, overconscientious, a perfectionist by nature, had an overabundance of energy, and had been able to drive himself constantly to accomplish what he would with his life. Now this whole pattern is reversed—not that his desires are gone, but the physical and mental entities are no longer able to carry out the dictates of his will. This is most frightening to any intelligent person, and is the sad story he pours out to his physician.

Now let's put ourselves in the position of his physician and listen to his story. You find before you a patient who is obviously intelligent, able to present his symptoms with great lucidity, and yet whose symptoms don't seem to fit any disease that you're familiar with. You find the patient excitable, agitated, and apparently overly concerned. Although you aren't one to pass snap judgments, your first thought is that he is becoming neurotic because of the pressures in his life. You are, however, very thorough so you give him a complete physical examination, a reasonably complete blood chemistry examination, a urinalysis, and all the other things any physician should do to discover a known pathologic condition that may cause such symptoms.

The tests all are within the normal range. The physical examination is unremarkable. The patient's blood pressure might be slightly lower than normal, but not seriously so, and of course it's only high blood pressure to be worried about anyway. Slightly lower pressure just means that the man will live longer.

Your examination confirms that you have before you a strong, healthy person with symptoms that obviously are of a neurotic nature. He is probably just overworked. So you talk to him. You recommend that he slow down, that he find himself a hobby, or that he take a vacation.

You give him a mild tranquilizer, and if he feels depressed, you give him a gentle antidepressant. (Today Prosac is the fashion) Because he doesn't sleep too well at night (insomnia being one of the symptoms of the second stage of hypoadrenalism), you give him a mild sedative. You send him home with a comforting pat on the back, reassuring him that there's nothing really wrong with him, he's just been working too hard, and he's to settle down a bit, keep on his medication, and try to get some enjoyment out of life.

This, in a nutshell, is the therapy most patients with hypoadrenalism received twenty years ago. It was very professional and was usually given with the best of intentions. Unfortunately, not only was it insufficient, but it also was usually detrimental, because the various drugs put a greater strain on an already overloaded glandular system. And so more problems are heaped on those that already exist.

Today a few knowledgeable physicians will prescribe a more rational treatment program, but even today, if our patients are any indication, the majority of physicians are still treating this condition as they did in 1975.

Many patients, not realizing they have organic problems, continue with this archaic treatment. Unless certain changes occur in their life that remove much of the stress originally causing the condition, they will continue to go downhill as they become more and more dependent on their drug therapy. The drugs don't help the basic condition at all; the imbalances are all still there. The drugs simply mask the patient's ability to be affected by the symptoms.

39

If this condition goes unabated in some persons, it can in time lead to mental institutionalization. Knowledgeable investigators frequently have found both hypoadrenal patients and hypoglycemic patients in mental institutions. Many of these patients are willing to admit themselves to mental institutions because they have been told very clearly that they have no physical condition that could cause their symptoms; yet these symptoms are so severe the patient no longer feels capable of coping with society. This is a sad commentary on a condition whose cause and treatment have been known for more than seventy-five years.

When we first wrote about these patients we were seeing most of them in the early stages of this condition. That is not true today. The majority of our new adrenal patients today are in the second or third stage of the GAS as outlined in the diagram of Dr. Selye (Fig. ***). Rather than exhaustion being their major complaint, nervousness, panic attacks and insomnia take first place with fatigue being there but it is these other symptoms that bother them the most. What is happening, as outlined in Dr. Selye's chart, is that their body is over-stressing the gland and nervous system to keep them going despite the serious glandular weakness. They are running on vital reserve energy and when this runs out total collapse may well ensue. (Again see Dr. Selye's chart)

We now run a test called the ASI test on all suspected adrenal patients. This test can pinpoint exactly where the individual patients is in the Selye sequence. Once this is known, then the correct treatment plan can be implemented. Without this knowledge it is entirely possible to worsen the condition if the first stage treatment is given to a second stage patient and vice versa.

Nature of Hypoadrenal Patient*

Before discussing the treatment of hypoadrenalism used at our Center, let's consider the nature of the person who is most likely to develop this disorder and the manner in which it is produced. If I could describe the hypoadrenal patient in one single word, that word would be sensitive. He is cognizant of all that is going on around him, and he perhaps feels an overconscientious sense of responsibility about those near and dear to him and even about the whole world. This person's nervous and glandular systems are delicately balanced; yet he is willing to take the cares of the world on his own shoulders.

However, such a nature, by itself, is not sufficient to cause adrenal insufficiency. In my own estimation, a hereditary weakness of adrenal

---

*This entire subject is discussed in great detail in the *Chronic Fatigue Unmasked* from the Beverly Hall Corporation, P.O. Box 220, Quakertown, PA 19851.

structure must be present for this condition to manifest. There are many sensitive persons who, though they fit this description, nevertheless have sufficient glandular vitality to avoid adrenal hypofunction. On the other hand, we do find persons who are by nature not perfectionists or are not inclined to drive themselves, yet suffer from this ailment. In these persons, it would appear that the hereditary weakness is so strong that even a relatively normal amount of stress is sufficient to trigger adrenal hypofunction.

To understand the hypoadrenal patient further, it is necessary to understand exactly what stresses cause this condition in susceptible persons. When I was in medical school, I was taught that the adrenal gland helps us with our "flight or fight" demands. You probably have heard of cases in which persons under excitement or stress have been able to accomplish feats of tremendous strength and endurance well beyond their normal physical abilities. These are all moderated by the effect of the adrenal gland, which is a storehouse of hormones that can be dumped into the circulating blood to stimulate body function if needed. If the need is great enough, large amounts can be dumped, which can produce for short periods a prodigious degree of physical strength and endurance. Afterwards, however, a period of rest is needed to replenish the depleted hormones from these glands so they will be prepared to produce this dumping action when needed again.

The classical example of this acute stress is the cave man who encounters a sabertoothed tiger. When he sees this dangerous animal, his adrenal glands pour forth a great abundance of the required hormones into his bloodstream. He could use this sudden strength either for fight or for flight. He could either turn on the tiger with superhuman strength and attempt to subdue it, or he could take flight and through the use of adrenal support run faster and further than he had ever run before. Finally, after he reaches safety or subdues the beast (assuming the tiger was not victorious), he rests or recuperates, gasping to draw in large amounts of oxygen in an attempt to replenish his supply of this vital gas. He is now exhausted and his body requires rest for a few hours or even a day or two if the drain on his adrenal glands is to be rectified.

It is postulated by most authorities on this subject that this, in general, was the specific function for which this gland was used. However, many other stresses are applied to the body for which its secretions are useful and even vital. Some of these stresses, however, are of such a nature that they do not provide the proper periods of rest for the recovery of the gland; this type of unremitting stress tends to cause hypoadrenalism .

The various forms of stress to which man is susceptible can be broken down into those of a physical, a chemical, or an emotional nature.

Among the physical stresses; we include extreme cold or heat, overly dry or humid air, trauma of various kinds—for example, a broken leg, broken ribs, crushed hand or surgery—and almost any form of physical entity that causes the basic body function to make adaptations beyond the rather narrow limit of homeostasis (physiologic equilibrium due to a balance of functions and chemical composition).

Chemical stresses include the various types of toxins due to infections, and toxic substances that may come in any chemical form—carbon tetrachloride, lead, mercury, gasoline fumes, cigarette smoke, or even alcohol in abundance. Any chemical substance that the body must detoxify is a stress on the adrenal gland. These can also include allergies in those susceptible to them and things not often considered as stresses such as immunizations and prescription drugs.

Emotional stresses are so multitudinous that I can name only a few examples. Parents that don't understand you, children that don't mind you, a husband that drinks, a lazy wife, a boss who is hard to get along with, employees that don't do their jobs properly—all can cause adrenal stress. But situations don't cause strain on the adrenal system; our internal reactions to these situations do. In other words, people around us don't cause our adrenal insufficiency; our reactions to these people and stressful situations are the culprit.

All these stresses may lay the foundation for hypoadrenalism. However, at least three factors must be present to produce hypoadrenalism in the average person.

The first of the three factors is the nature of the stress. The adrenal gland, designed to help us during stressful periods, tends to atrophy with nonuse, and it grows stronger with proper use. Thus, the adrenal gland doesn't exhaust itself by reacting to stress; it actually becomes stronger if the stress is applied in a reasonable fashion and needed periods of rest allowed for regeneration. What does exhaust the gland is if the stress is so applied that its effect is unremitting and no proper time is provided for the adrenal gland to accomplish its normal regeneration.

The second factor is our response to stress, and the third is the degree of hereditary influence. Let me give an example to show these three points. Hypoadrenalism (Chronic Fatigue Syndrome, Fibromyalgia, SBS, etc.) frequently occurs in a person who has cared for a loved one through a long, extended illness. Let's take, for instance, a woman whose husband has developed cancer and has been operated on unsuccessfully. The physicians have given up all hope, but the man has a sturdy constitution and he lives on for maybe a year or two before he finally succumbs. The family is not wealthy and can not hire nurses or other help to care for him, so his wife must care for him. She is often up day and night, watching out for his needs. The man she has loved for many years is now gradually changing. He is little by little withering and dying before her eyes. His emotional nature often changes and he becomes a very difficult person to live with. There are times she would like to scream at him; yet she knows that this is not socially acceptable, so she holds it in. She can't get her proper rest. She doesn't eat properly because the whole situation has made her lose her appetite. So she snacks on foods that don't supply her body with the vital elements she especially needs at this time. Her adrenal glands, the willing servants that they are, keep pouring out hormones to sustain her during this time. Unfortunately, they, like she, get little respite.

As time goes on the stress is now unremitting and constant. Although the glands can recuperate during sleep to some degree, her rest is less than normal and her glands have little time for their own regeneration. But they are valiant friends; they don't give in. They keep functioning and working well beyond their normal requirements.

Finally, death comes to her husband, but stress is not over for her. She must deal with the undertaker and then the lawyers. Then come the government, inconsiderate relatives and the other people who disturb or even prey on a recent widow.

During all this additional stress, her steadfast adrenal glands keep working their best to produce the substances she needs to keep going. Finally, she is able to rest. The undertaker, the relatives, the lawyers and even the government are satisfied. At last she can relax. What about her adrenal glands? They are exhausted. They too now demand a well-earned rest. As soon as the stresses are removed and the adrenal glands aren't needed to the extent they once were during heavy stress, their function slows to enable regeneration for the preservation of the whole physical system. Our widow suddenly feels tired and exhausted. At this point, she may or may not develop hypoadrenalism. Much depends on the basic hereditary integrity of the adrenal glands. She may well go into a period of depression and of exhaustion. If the glands are basically strong and healthy, she will recuperate and be able to go on with her life in a reasonable time. If the glands are inherently weak, she may develop chronic hypoadrenalism. The glands become so exhausted, so weakened that even with the rest they now receive they aren't capable of regenerating to their normal state. They still function, or the woman would die, but they function at a far lower level than they did before the prolonged period of stress; much lower than the level needed for a contented normal daily existence.

We have just reproduced a classic case of functional hypoadrenalism. Although there are many other ways of producing this syndrome, certain specifics can be derived from this case history about the nature of the stress most likely to produce this condition.

First, although the stress itself isn't necessarily great, it is generally unremitting. Also, we sensitive humans aren't able to overcome it, either because of a sense of responsibility or because of our own emotional dependency. For example, even though it was exhausting her adrenal glands, there was really nothing else for this wife to do but to take care of her husband. For her own physical well-being, she could have abandoned him, turned him over to relatives if such existed, or tried to get the State to take care of him. These actions may have prevented her developing hypoadrenalism, but her own sense of responsibility would not have allowed it. In my experience, most stresses that produce hypoadrenalism come from doing what we believe to be our duty. If we are to prevent hypoadrenalism in those who are susceptible, we must teach them to learn to control their response to this and other forms of stress.

Besides unremitting stress, the second factor necessary for adrenal insufficiency is our own emotional response to this stress. In this day and age, we can't escape stress; not even unremitting stress. From the radio, television set, and newspapers, we are constantly bombarded by stress-producing news. The events in the world today occur too rapidly for our adaptive systems to absorb and adjust. These stresses alone can produce hypoadrenalism in a susceptible person. A stress—especially one due to emotional factors—isn't a stress because it is applied to us. It is a stress because of our reaction to it. The real stress is our reaction to the stimulation.

This of course is not true of most chemical and physical stresses, only those of an emotional or psychologic nature. Even with chemical or physical stresses, however, there can be an emotional component that can greatly increase damage. For example, if the fear of a disease and what it might entail is superimposed on the disease itself, an additional stress is produced that may affect the body more than just the disease. This is often true of physical stresses. A knee injury to an athlete that prevents him from playing in an important game, or causes him to lose income, may readily produce far more stress than the actual injury on his glandular system.

Our attitude—what I call acceptance of the stress—is often equally or even more important in producing reaction than is the stress itself. In

44

the example of the woman with the dying husband, if she could have rearranged her life, much of her later trouble could have been prevented. She could have called in relatives to help care for her husband on various nights, enabling her to get her sleep. She could have arranged her own life so that her diet was more adequate for her needs, thereby reducing the nutritional stress on her body. She could have eaten the foods and nutrients that are best able to build up and support the adrenal glands during her difficult period. With more knowledge she could have changed her basic attitude toward her husband at this time, to a complete acceptance of his condition and of his unavoidable death.

The third and perhaps most important factor in hypoadrenalism, but unfortunately the one we are least able to change, is heredity. After nearly forty years of treating these patients, it is my belief that some adrenal glands are almost incapable of becoming exhausted, no matter what the stress or in what manner it is formed or accepted. On the other hand, I know that there are people who, no matter how well protected, are fated to have some degree of hypoadrenalism at some time in their lives. Most of our cases fall somewhere between these two extremes.

I believe that, even though there is an adverse hereditary factor, the average susceptible person, if he takes care to follow the regimen we recommend, can avoid functional hypoadrenalism. Also, the average hypoadrenal patient is capable of responding readily to proper treatment, thus returning to normal function.

Diagnosis of Functional Hypoadrenalism at the Beverly Hall Corporation Healing Research Center

When a patient first presents himself at our Center, we take an extensive history. Nine times out of ten, a tentative diagnosis of hypoadrenalism can be made from this alone. The patient usually tells us about symptoms similar to those already described. We hear tales of the various physicians they have been to, and of the multitudes of medications that have been prescribed. I will never forget one patient who told me she had fifteen different types of tranquilizers in her purse. I asked her how she knew which one to take. She replied that she really didn't know. She would just keep taking first one and then the other until she felt better.

After the history of a suspected hypoadrenal patient is taken, we begin the physical examination and laboratory work. Although it is possible to measure such adrenal secretions as the 17ketosteroids, we rarely find this test sensitive enough to detect functional hypoadrenalism. This test is used to detect the organic adrenal diseases such as Addison's disease, but these factors are usually within normal levels in functional hypoadrenalism .

One laboratory test we do suggest in suspected hypoadrenalism is the 5 to 6 hour glucose tolerance test. Because there is a frequent relationship between hyperinsulinism (low blood sugar) and functional hypoadrenalism, we always check to make sure that both conditions do not exist in the patient. It has been my experience that where a physician knowledgeable in these metabolic disorders has discovered one and treated it unsuccessfully, it usually was because the other had also been present but not treated.

We do extensive blood and urinary testing of these patients. Usually, however, except for the glucose tolerance test, we generally don't discover abnormal findings, unless the patient also has a concomitant disorder. It is possible of course that a chronic systemic ailment may be aggravating the functional hypoadrenalism. If this is true, this condition must be treated concurrently with the adrenal problem.

In recent years a new test (ASI test) has evolved that allows us not only to determine whether or not functional hypoadrenalism exists but, more importantly, exactly where the patient is in the Selye progression of stress adaptation.*

This test is essential for all our patients suspected of any of the many conditions related to functional hypoadrenalism. It is fully explained in the book *Chronic Fatigue Unmasked*. If you need more information on this essential test, please ask your Center physician.

One of the most important diagnostic features of the physical examination is what is known as the postural (orthostatic) blood pressure test. In this test, which is routine in our office, the patient is placed in a reclining position 4 or 5 minutes; the blood pressure is then taken and recorded. The patient is brought to a standing position with the blood pressure cuff still in place on his arm. The blood pressure is immediately taken and recorded. The pressure is again taken in a minute with the patient still standing.

In the patient with full adrenal integrity, the blood pressure will be five to ten points higher in the standing position than in the reclining position when they first rise because of the increased tone of the abdominal blood vessels, which are under control of the adrenal glands. When you lie down, the heart relaxes, and all the large vessels tend to relax, because every vessel is at approximately the same height as the heart, and gravity has little effect on the blood flow. When you suddenly

---

*See Selye stress chart Fig. 2

46

stand up, however, there is a tremendous downward pull of gravity on all the blood in the upper body, the tendency being for the blood to flow down into the large abdominal vessels and pool there. If there was not some compensatory mechanism to correct this, most of us would go into a state of oxygen deprivation (anoxia) whenever we stood up, immediately becoming dizzy or faint. However, there is a mechanism, mainly under the control of the adrenal glands, that increases tonicity (constriction) in the large abdominal vessels whenever we stand up. This abdominal constriction produces a slight rise in blood pressure that occurs normally upon standing. In adrenal insufficiency, however, this mechanism functions weakly. In fact, it reacts in inverse ratio to the integrity of the adrenal glands. Thus, the more the adrenal glands are depressed or unable to function, the less this mechanism is able to work. When a patient with hypofunctioning adrenal glands stands up from a reclining position, the blood pressure tends either to stay the same or drop slightly in mild cases. In the more severe cases, the drop may be considerable. I have seen patients in whom the blood pressure dropped forty points upon standing. These patients usually become quite dizzy upon standing—of all the symptoms of hypoadrenalism, this dizziness upon arising from a reclining state is one of the most consistent.

Because the degree of blood pressure drop is usually a dependable indication of the adrenal state, it is used at our Center to measure patient improvement. As a patient is treated and makes subjective improvement, we also find objective improvement in the orthostatic blood pressure readings. Although not the most important adrenal function, it is the easiest to measure, and such improvement generally parallels improvement in the other particulars of adrenal function.

The difference in nature between the first and the second standing reading is also important. In my experience I find the first standing reading indicative of the short term stress on the adrenal gland while the second reading is more inclined to give us information on the nature of the regeneration of the adrenal gland itself. For instance if a patient would read 110-70 lying down, 100-65 when first standing but 120-75 on the second standing reading, I would surmise that they have had some recent short term stress but that the adrenal gland on a long term basis is regenerating. On the other hand if the respective readings were: 110-70, 100-65 and 95-60, I would deduce that this patient is not regeneration and needs more stress reduction and increased treatment. If the first standing reading is lower than the reclining reading it means that the patient has been under some recent stress and would do well to back off their lifestyle until the adrenal gland is able to catch up to their needs. If the third reading is lower than the reclining reading it shows that the stress on the adrenal gland is such that it is deteriorating, not regenerating, and measures must be instituted immediately to correct this situation or it could become difficult to correct.

Although this test was developed many years ago, we find it used little by most physicians. However, I find it an unerring indication of this rather enigmatic condition. One can even predict a patient's feelings for several days following the test once one becomes in tune with the patient and the test. The postural blood pressure varies from day to day and even from hour to hour in some cases, as does adrenal function. If I have a patient who has been doing well under treatment, whose orthostatic pressure suddenly drops considerably more than usual, I know that he is under some new or sustained type of stress that even he may not be aware of. We can then search for the new problem and correct it, even before it can produce viable symptoms. Physicians who do not regularly use this test deprive themselves not only of an effective diagnostic tool but also of a therapeutic guide par excellence.

To us, a combination of the history, the lab tests, and a positive postural blood pressure test is considered sufficient to make a diagnosis of functional hypoadrenalism; however, it is only with the ASI test that we are able to determine exactly the state of the patient in this condition. Of course, the programmed intuitive nature of the physician also enters into the diagnosis. When one has handled many hypoadrenal cases, they tend to stick out like sore thumbs. Their whole nature and being help make the diagnosis. The physician must only look and listen. The only real way to miss functional hypoadrenalism is to not be aware of its existence, or as the Bible says: "There are none so blind as those who will not see."

Treatment

Treatment of this condition is both very simple and extremely complicated. It is simple in that the instructions, diet, and remedies used aren't particularly difficult to use or extensive in nature. On the other hand, complex emotional factors are always present and involved and these must be dealt with or the treatment will fail. The physician who is not in emotional harmony with his patients, or who does not have unending patience, should not take on himself the treating of this condition.

The diet used for this malady is of great importance though no single diet will help all patients. We usually suggest a low-stress diet—one that provides in as readily assimilable form as possible and as pleasantly as

48

possible all the nutritive materials needed for satisfactory body function with especial emphasis placed on those compounds that are needed to regenerate the adrenal glands. The diet should be arranged so these foods are most easily digested, absorbed, and metabolized. It should exclude all foods that contain toxic substances, that place an added stress on the system, and that require more energy in their digestion and assimilation than they actually return to the body in nutritive value (refined foods, heavy fatty meats, etc.) .

We have found that a modification of our hypoglycemia diet and our basic maintenance diet best fulfill these requirements. (See the diets in the appendix of this book). The frequent meals, the high protein, and the increased fruits and vegetables of the hypoglycemic diet also seem to fit the needs of the hypoadrenal patient. However, the hypoadrenal patient is usually not as sensitive to a small amount of starch as is the hypoglycemic patient.

All foods chosen should be as free of pesticides and additives as possible. Although organically grown foods are not an absolute prerequisite, we find that where they or their home-grown counterparts can be obtained, recovery is more rapid. An attempt should also be made to obtain chicken, fish, lean meat, and other proteins from as reliable a source as possible, so that they are fresh and free from the chemical additives that are still being used in many of these products today.

The hypoadrenal patient frequently has a poor appetite (anorexia), and it is often difficult to get him to eat any but minuscule amounts. In these patients, it is all the more important that every mouthful of food be as nutritious and as non-stressful as possible—that is, free as possible from chemical contamination. All chemical compounds not normal to the body place stresses on its adaptive apparatus, of which the adrenal is a prime factor. It is usually important to have these patients eat small amounts frequently. Gradually as the treatment progresses, the anorexia will abate. In time, they may develop such ravenous appetites that you end up having to control what you took great pains to stimulate in the early stages of care.

Experience has demonstrated that one of the first functions to weaken in functional hypoadrenalism is the digestion. Therefore it may be necessary to offer digestive aids to these patients to help them utilize the foods they ingest. In may be well to use some of the more advanced diagnostic procedures such as Complete Stool Analysis, Heidelberg pH digestive test and other hi-tech procedures to determine exactly what the individual patient requires in the way of help with their digestion and assimilation.

With poor digestion and assimilation these patients often exhibit multiple allergies due to incompletely digested proteins entering the blood stream. In many of our patients this has advanced to the degree that they are known as Universal Reactors, that is someone who reacts to everything. In these patients the physician must not only test for the digestive weaknesses but also for incomplete assimilation (Leaky Gut Syndrome.)

Once our patient has been tested for digestive and assimilation imbalances and placed on a proper diet, specific supplementation for supporting the adrenal gland can be begun. Now that we have the ASI test we are able to individualize all such remedies. What each individual requires depends to great degree where they are in the progression of this malady according to the chart of Dr. Selye. Those remedies that would be indicated in the exhaustive stage would not be best in the resistive stage and vise versa.

In the exhaustive stage we usually suggest a supplement containing vitamin C, calcium pantothenate, vitamin B6, and raw adrenal and spleen substances. These last compounds—which we believe to be absolutely vital to proper adrenal regeneration in the exhaustive stage—are made by desiccating bovine adrenal gland at below body temperature, so as not to destroy any of the delicate RNA and DNA factors necessary to promote a rapid recovery.

Occasionally, we find a patient sensitive to some of the auxiliary substances in this product and in this instance we substitute an item that contains mainly the desiccated adrenal gland substance without added amounts of specific vitamins or other glandulars.

As this condition is beginning to be recognized by more and more physicians there are ever increasing efforts to produce natural products that will help these patients. Therefore, we are always on the lookout for better remedies. Several new ones have shown promise. You can be certain that as the premiere Center in the nation (world?) that treats this condition that we will always have the most advanced remedies available to help you.

Besides those agents mentioned above, we see to it that our patients have adequate amounts of the other supplemental elements needed to insure rapid recovery. Unfortunately, as also mentioned above many of our patients have difficulty with their digestion and so we must choose such remedies carefully so that they do not cause reactions due to poor assimilation of their various components.

In years past we often supplemented our basic therapy for the more serious patients with certain injectable compounds. These were not drugs in the usual sense, but were nutritional compounds that could only be satisfactorily absorbed when placed directly into the muscle or blood-stream.

The three we used most commonly were a calcium preparation called Calphosan, adrenocortical extract (ACE, an aqueous solution produced by several companies) and injectable vitamin B12.

A few years back the FDA decided that the ACE was an "obsolete" drug. This was a true stroke of genius on their part. Since ACE had been used for decades without adverse side effects there was no way the FDA could outlaw it. However, by declaring it "obsolete" they effectively re-moved its "grandfathering" and so before a drug company could again produce it they would have to go through the multimillion dollar process of resubmitting this compound for FDA approval. Since there simply was not enough demand for this remedy to offset the tremendous ex-pense of gaining FDA approval, all manufacture of ACE was discontin-ued in this country. Thus forcing any physician who desired to support the adrenal gland to use the expensive preparations of the established drug houses. Substances that, unlike the ACE, only weaken the adrenal gland in the long run.

Now that our government, through its FDA, has done all it can to prevent functional hypoadrenal patients from obtaining the substances they require to get well we have had to seek such healing in another direction. We have found the use of certain physical therapeutic modali-ties can be used to take the place of the "obsolete" items. We use a treat-ing unit called the Magnatherm,* which produces a pulsed, electromag-netic wave that can be directed to pass through the adrenal glands, liver, and spleen. In our experience—perhaps through increased blood supply to these organs— the Magnatherm acts as a regenerating agent to aid in adrenal regeneration. Through the use of these treatments, we have been able to replace the ACE to great extent. The Magnatherm and other modalities that we use to help our functional hypoadrenal patients are discussed in greater detail in later chapters.

It's been my observation that most hypoadrenal cases also have nerve-muscle-bone displacements and tensions in the area of the shoulder blade and along the upper thoracic and lower neck areas. These we treat with mild ultrasound therapy and with finger pressure, working the sensitive areas to gradually eliminate the muscle-nerve spasms and in turn any bone displacements. In some of the more sensitive patients, this work must at first be handled with great delicacy; but as improvement occurs, the pressure may be increased. In fact, we find that as the adrenal condi-

---

*Manufactured by the United Medical Equipment Co., Kansas City, Mo.

tion of our patient improves, he becomes less and less sensitive to this treatment, and he finds it increasingly more pleasant. This phenomenon is discussed at greater length in our chapter on Tissue Sludge. We find his Tissue Sludge is present in many conditions besides adrenal insufficiency.

This gives you some idea of the basic therapy we use to help functional hypoadrenalism. The big secret with such therapy is knowing just when to use each of the items and just how much of each modality to use. This cannot be taught; it must come from long experience. However, as difficult as it is to select each day the best treatment schedule for each patient, this is still the easiest part of the treatment. The most difficult part is that which must take place *within* the patient by his own efforts. From the beginning, he must realize that his present way of life has caused his problem and this lifestyle must be changed if improvement is to be expected. We usually ask the patient to analyze his entire lifestyle and to make every effort to reduce or eliminate all the habits that may cause stress on his adrenal glands. In addition, we try to make the patient realize that he has a physical condition. Most patients are convinced they have some kind of emotional or psychologic disorder.

Because the condition is physical, there are certain physical requirements for its correction. The first and most important of these requisites is rest. If the adrenals are to recover, even under the treatment I have described, the patient must have a great amount of rest. Only in these rest periods can the adrenal glands regenerate. This, of course, is true of any organ but is particularly vital for the adrenal.

Normally the adrenal glands regenerate during a night's sleep the vitality they expended during the previous day. They are then ready the following morning to go through another day of equal rigor. In hypoadrenalism, the glands are exhausted. They have expended more vitality than they can make up for in a single night's sleep. Thus, if they are going to return to normal, they must regenerate more than the body expends. If the glands can't do this, they won't recover. They may not get worse, but they won't get better. For this extra regeneration, rest is required—much more than the usual eight hours a night.

The example I usually give my patients compares them to their bank accounts. The reserve of the adrenal glands is like money in a bank account held for emergencies. Let's say you have a thousand dollars in the bank, and every night you deposit a hundred dollars. If during that day, you spend a hundred dollars, the reserve fund is still intact.

In the same way, the adrenal glands have a considerable reserve held for emergencies, and they are able to regenerate (deposit money) at night while they rest. During the day, if we expend no more energy (money) than the adrenals are able to build up at night, we still have our adrenal reserve (the thousand dollars). If an emergency arises and we must use some of the thousand dollars, we must do one of two things. We must either make more money or spend less so we can deposit more into the bank account to build it up to its reserve level. This same philosophy works with the adrenal glands.

When the adrenals are exhausted, to produce regeneration it is necessary to expend less energy during the day than the adrenals build up during rest. In this way, some of the energy the adrenals build during this rest can go toward building their reserve.

No matter what therapeutic means are used, there is one vital fact all hypoadrenal patients must remember. The only way that the adrenal glands can regenerate is for the patient to expend less energy than the adrenal glands can regenerate during that same day. Every part of our treatment helps the patient toward this objective, but if he doesn't get sufficient rest or he places himself in stressful situations that use more energy than the adrenals can regenerate during that day, he will never recover from hypoadrenalism.

When our patients come to me and tell me they are not improving under our treatment and their postural blood pressure and other indicators of their condition verify this fact, I must lay the fault directly at their own feet. In no instance has this blame yet been unjustified. If they expend more energy during a day than they are able to rebuild at night, they will surely retrogress. When this situation is explained to the patient and they start living within their glandular means, they invariably improve.

The patient will often ask, "How much rest must I have?" The answer is simple—whatever is necessary to produce proper adrenal regeneration. Some people have to make only a very small change in their daily routine. While other patients with severe hypoadrenalism must have near total rest for long periods. The average is somewhere in between.

The rest needed is indicated by the patient's response pattern. It is necessary to reduce his activities until improvement falls within expected limits. The patient must reduce his activity and obtain enough rest to produce a steady but consistent improvement. If they are not improving, they are doing too much and allowing too much stress in their lives. There are no exceptions to this.

Even though the hypoadrenal patient often believes he has a mental or psychologic problem, it is not the neurosis that causes the symptoms but the symptoms that cause the neurosis. The feelings he fears are the symptoms of the adrenal condition which are physically caused. I find it good therapy to constantly confirm this fact to the patient. In the early phase of treatment I find myself constantly restating "Now remember you are as sane as anyone. This is a physical condition you have and it will be corrected in due time. All you have to do is listen to me, follow my instructions, keep up with your medications and treatments, and you'll be just fine." This by the way is not just positive thinking; it is a fact.

The psychologic problems in hypoadrenalism are usually intensified by past therapies. Before we see these patients, they usually have been to physicians who have either assured them that there is nothing physically wrong with them, or have suggested that they see a psychiatrist.

Now, we at our Center come along and tell them just the opposite— that there is something physically wrong with them and that they don't need a psychiatrist. Whom should they believe? Their other physicians are usually well thought of in the profession, and after all, the Beverly Hall Corporation Healing Research Center is not the *Mayo Clinic*, so just why should they listen to us? The only way I can prove that we are correct is by getting the patient well. Unfortunately, this takes time in hypoadrenalism. And so the period from the first interview and diagnosis until the real improvement begins can be a time of frustration and doubt for the average patient. What we say sounds practical, and they certainly hope we are right because no one else has given them any real help but they cannot forget the fears that have been such an integral part of their lives for so long.

At this time, all the psychologic skill and diplomacy a physician possesses must be called into play. I mentioned earlier that I groan a little whenever I discover another hypoadrenal patient. This is the main reason—I know that this period must come and that during this time I and my staff will be called on to use all the tender loving care we can muster. To shorten this period, we have tried to incorporate into our therapy every legitimate, harmless, nontoxic method known to hasten improvement. It is a happy day when the patient finally says, "Doctor, I'm getting better. I feel like a new person." They will often say, "You know, Doctor, yesterday I felt better than I have in five years." When this happens, the physician breathes a sigh of relief, for he knows that the first critical period is over.

Another incident in the early stages of hypoadrenalism should be mentioned. A type of negative feed-back occurs in the hypoadrenal syndrome; it works in the following manner. The symptoms of hypoadrenalism produce worry and concern in the patient, which in turn produces stress tending to worsen the condition. However, these emotions also stimulate the adrenals forcing them to keep going even though near exhaustion. This stimulation keeps the patient going at the expense of the adrenals, which go into debt in regard to their own reserve of energy. Much like our own country's huge national debt.

After the patient comes under our care and accepts his problem as a physical condition that is going to be overcome, he stops worrying about it to a certain degree, and the stimulation due to worry and anxiety is removed from the adrenals. The glands will now begin to rest and regenerate by reducing their hormonal output. The patient consequently feels more tired and exhausted than he did when he first came to us. At this time, we intensify our treatment and usually our efforts more than offset this hormonal withdrawal period. If the adrenals have been badly abused, however, there is usually a lag period between the time the glands begin to rest (because of the removal of anxiety) and the time before therapy has an opportunity to build new strength into the glands. Because of this, for a week or two after we first see the patient, he may seem to worsen.

In the early days of my practice, I lost some patients because they thought that the advice of other doctors was correct, for our treatment at first made them feel worse, not better. I wasn't certain at that time what was happening physiologically. I did know, however, that those who persevered soon improved and all got better in time.

Now that this lag period is understood, I can forewarn patients. In some patients, the lag period is very short; in others it isn't noticed at all. Surprisingly, if the patient is very bad and the glands are near complete exhaustion, anxiety has little stimulating effect because the glands are incapable of responding. Thus, we have a mechanism that spares the most severe and the mild cases from this exhaustive stage, but is most likely to be noticed in those of medium severity (the average patient). At least the patient who experiences this lag time can be reassured that his condition is not severe or the glands would not react in this fashion.

If we again examine the chart of Dr. Selye, we can see what is happening to these various patients. Note that there are two exhaustive stages and two stages in which the patients may seem somewhat normal. Also remember that in order to regenerate a patient we must move him from the right to the left of the chart. The first exhaustive stage is the mild case of functional hypoadrenalism. We have only to move him one place to the left for a cure. Usually this patient responds well to our therapy and has no or only a slight "lag" period. Basically he has nowhere to go but up.

The second exhaustive stage is a much different is a much different matter than the first. The patient, at this stage, is near complete adrenal collapse. When he is properly treated, he will pass through all the various stages to his left on the Selye chart. The physician must take this into account so as to know exactly what is required by this patient in each of the stages he must go through to complete recovery.

In the center, or resistive stage of this condition (where most of our patients now fall), we find a patient who experiences the strange combination of anxiety and exhaustion at the same time. They are exhausted but they often have difficulty sleeping because their adrenal gland is being over stimulated in an effort by the body to "keep up." This combination of anxiety and exhaustion is unique to functional hypoadrenalism and can truly be understood only by those who experience it. It is these patients who, as they are moved back to the left on the chart, go through the first stage of exhaustion again. Actually, what really happens is that the artificial support from their body that created the anxiety is corrected and they are then able to feel the exhaustion that has been a part of their nature since they first began their travel to the right on the Selye chart.

With these resistive patients the physician must use his diplomatic skills to explain the situation thoroughly to the patient and his family. Unless the family understands what the doctor is attempting, they will often do much to offset his therapy. The family can make or break the best of treatments. Unless they understand the phases and purposes of the treatment, they can cause anxieties that thoroughly debilitate the hypoadrenal patient.

It is advisable to call family members in for another reason. Hypoadrenal weakness is often hereditary. If one member of the family has this tendency, others may also, though perhaps not as severely. I always suggest to the family members that we take the postural blood pressure, an ASI saliva test and perhaps a glucose tolerance test if their histories are suspicious. It is rare not to find one or two in the family who show signs of early adrenal weakness. Suggestions on diet and instructions on controlling stresses around them do much to prevent full-blown hypoadrenalism from developing.

When the patient reaches the stage where he finally starts feeling some of his old strength, energy, and ambition returning, the second traumatic period in his control is at hand. Now he becomes cocky and feels his condition is nearly cured. He over-expends his new-found energy. He may get away with it for two or three days, and then boom! He is practically flat on his back. He feels almost as if he had had no therapy at all. He can't understand what's happened.

Using our bank account analogy, we can explain this circumstance. Because of his treatment, the patient has gradually built some adrenal reserve and the glands finally have started to secrete more hormone into the bloodstream. He begins to feel normal. What does he do then? He goes on a spending spree. Instead of making $100 a day, he now makes $125. Unfortunately, he feels so affluent, he spends $200. But he can overspend for just so long; then the reserve is gone. Like the spendthrift, the hypoadrenal will rapidly overspend what little reserve he had built up.

This frequently happens two or three times to patients in the second stage. I warn my patients what will happen, but they all do it anyway. It seems that one experience is worth a thousand warnings. So when the patient tells me of his troubles, I very carefully (as I have done before) explain exactly what has happened and that he must be careful to accept the improvement without over-expending. If he doesn't listen and continues to repeat these episodes, his recovery is retarded and much valuable time is lost.

Another interesting effect of the adrenals is the lag period between actions done and reactions upon the person—making it difficult for the patient to relate cause and effect. Let me explain. When activity expends adrenal secretions, the glands valiantly keep trying to pour them out. Even after this activity, the adrenals keep going for a short time before they rest. Then, sometimes hours, sometimes a day or two after we have stopped our activity, the adrenals relax. It is then that the reaction becomes apparent.

Patients constantly say to me, "I am so tired today, Doctor, and I can't understand it. I've been resting the last couple of days." I always say, "Yes but what did you do over the weekend?" "Oh, that was fun, Doctor." The patient went bowling or skied, but really he felt good. The little old glands were just working their heads off, and it wasn't until two or three days later that they finally relaxed to regenerate. This is a typical adrenal pattern. Once explained to the patient, he can learn to judge his own activities and govern himself accordingly. We always attempt to teach patients responsibility for their condition. We tell them what will happen if they overdo but allow them to make the decision if they desire to overdo or not. As they do so they learn to control their destiny.

A few more comments on small things that can affect hypoadrenal patients are appropriate here. Crowds of people seem to have a strong enervating drain on all hypoadrenal patients. The worst seem to be meetings in which banality and bickering are rife.

If we subject the patient to treatment or remedy costs he is not readily able to pay, an unrequited stress is placed on him that worsens his condition. Thus, it is easy to aggravate the very condition that we are trying to correct. This is another factor not taken into account by many Centers, and yet it does have an undeniable effect on the patient's improvement.

Long telephone calls also exert some strange weakening effect on those people who are sensitive. I usually ask my patients to limit all calls to five minutes. I personally feel that the restricted frequency range of the telephone somehow adversely affects the adrenal gland.

The most difficult part of the therapy is to teach the patient how to prevent stresses from affecting him. We can't avoid stresses, so we must learn to deal with them. In truth, the stresses that seem to cause the most common forms of hypoadrenalism really don't exist in the first place. Worry over things that might happen often causes more anxiety than the consequences that do occur.

Often patients are concerned or anxious about problems that are none of their business. Events that befall us generally fit into two categories. First are those for which we must take some action because they are directly related to our own existence and responsibility. The only way of overcoming them—which must be done if we are to remove the anxiety and stress involved—is to take some kind of action to correct the situation. Our responsibility here is to take action as rapidly and as thoroughly as possible. The more we procrastinate, the greater the anxiety and adrenal tension we build.

On the other hand, some problems beset us that no possible action on our part can correct. Most of these are none of our business in the first place. I find one of the most common problems of this nature is that of parents worrying about their grown children, a sister worrying about a brother, or a daughter worrying about her mother. Except for minor children under our own personal care, we have no control of other persons. If we have no control, we have no direct responsibility. I know it is useless to tell a mother not to fret about a grown child or a wife not to be upset about a husband's bad habits. Yet in all my years as a counselor, I have never seen such anxiety produce any beneficial results. Can it do anything but injure us? Admittedly the whole world is imperfect. We are imperfect creatures, each trying to do his best to seek salvation in some shape, form or manner. There is yet no unanimity of opinion about what is the best way. Yet some of us are filled with concern as we judge the actions of others. Jesus would not judge, how then should we? It has been my experience that such anxieties cause more hypoadrenal disorders than all the other causes put together.

We, at the Beverly Hall Corporation Healing Research Center, are now in the planning stage of a new Center we consider to be a Healing Sanctuary. In this Healing Sanctuary we will be able to take patients and remove them from as much stress as possible thereby allowing their body to begin the regeneration of the adrenal gland in a controlled environment. This will allow us to minimize the early lag period that so frequently accompanies the patient with functional hypoadrenalism. This same Healing Sanctuary will be available for all patients who feel the need to reduce stress in their lives so that their bodies can begin the healing process. The body is a marvelous healing entity but it requires the proper atmosphere and environment to do so. That we intend to provide in our new Healing Sanctuary. This Center will be the culmination of my own long experience with stress related conditions. No detail from the paint and wall covering to the music available is too small not to have my personal attention.

Although long, this is one of the most important chapters in this book. Almost all known diseases are affected by the stability of the adrenal glands. Many authorities now believe that hypoadrenal function may cause symptoms of allergy, asthma, chronic inflammatory states, and a great variety of other conditions affected by the many secretions produced by these glands. The therapy applied in hypoadrenalism is also helpful in many of these conditions. In almost every chronic ailment treated in our Center, some form of adrenal support is used, and I believe that further research in the medical field will continue to substantiate our work in this field.

Chapter III
The Low-Back Syndrome

When I first graduated from The Western States College of Natural Medicine some forty years ago, I had planned to devote most of my practice to nutrition, the use of herbs, homeopathic specifics, and the counseling of marriage and sexual difficulties. Owing to its proximity to my home, I established my first office in one of the suburbs of Seattle, Washington. Most of my patients were teamsters or aircraft workers, or were employed in local shipyards.

Many problems brought to me by this hard-working group of people centered on the low back. These low-back problems, and other difficulties related to it, composed well over half my early practice. Because a fledgling physician can't pick and choose his patients, to subsist it was necessary for me to develop methods to correct this distressing orthopedic difficulty rapidly.

Although I was a trained and licensed Chiropractor as well as a Naturopath, I soon discovered there was much more to these low-back problems than mere adjustment. Not only was it imperative for me to correct these difficulties in order to build a successful practice, but it was also necessary to do so as rapidly as possible and with an absolute minimum of time loss for the patient. Most of my patients lived from pay check to pay check, and even a few days off work could materially upset their budgets. Therefore out of pure necessity for my own survival, I was forced to develop methods of treating this common and agonizing problem with speed, yet at the same time keeping the patient ambulatory and productive.

The low-back syndrome, and in particular sacroiliac slippage (subluxation, dislocation), is not only common in those doing heavy labor, but is also one of the most common and often ignored conditions that can beset all of us. It wasn't surprising therefore to find when we started the Beverly Hall Corporation Healing Research Center that while our patients now came from all walks of life, a very high percentage of them, at one time or another, were afflicted with this rather troublesome disorder.

The ramifications of this difficulty extend well beyond a simple backache. I find that the sacroiliac slip is capable of initiating many other reflex symptoms apparently unrelated to the low back. In fact, a good third of all these patients have symptoms that occur in some apparently unrelated portion of the body. Even a casual listing of these must include such conditions as enigmatic headaches and neck difficulties, tension in the upper shoulders, stomach upsets, hernia-like pains in the groin, shooting pains down the leg, knee difficulties, and pains in the feet and ankles.

Menstrual difficulties in puberty and in the immediate postpubertal period frequently are complicated by this condition, and the menstrual problems almost invariably improve once the sacroiliac distortion is corrected. In many of these patients with discomfort in a part of the body other than the low back, previous practitioners have rarely corrected the sacroiliac subluxation. Usually only the symptom area was treated, and thus only partial success was achieved.

In the earlier days of medicine, syphilis was known as the great masquerader—it could cause a great variety of symptoms and physical abnormalities, and it took an astute physician to find the true cause. Today, the sacroiliac distortion can act in the same manner. This slippage is so common that one of the first physical checks we make on any patient, no matter what his difficulty, is to ascertain the integrity and mechanical functioning of these joints. If this area is in subluxation, all other work the doctor may do for his patient will fall short of his desired expectations until this infirmity is properly corrected and joint stabilized.

The pelvis is made up of three bones—two large ilia (singular, ilium) and the sacrum (Fig. 3). The following relationships are important to our subject: The spine, and therefore the whole of the trunk of the body, sits on the sacrum. Each ilium articulates with the sacrum, one on either side, in a joint that is more dependent on the integrity of the ligaments than on any bony apposition. The femur (upper bone of the leg) articulates on each side with the corresponding ilium in a socket called the acetabulum. The two ilia meet in front at an articulation (joint) called the symphysis pubis, which is a simple butting style articulation and is also supported mainly by ligament structures. The interrelation of these various structures and its importance to anyone with a low-back problem will be made apparent shortly.

The classic subluxation of this area is a slipping or sliding of the ilium on the sacrum, upward or downward, and either one side or both (Fig. 4). There are theoretically eight possibilities for movement in this area, although, in practice, two of these account for most of the difficulties. Either ilium may move upward or downward on the sacrum. The left ilium may move upward while the right ilium moves downward, and vice versa.

The most common subluxation occurs when one ilium moves upward or downward. If the situation remains for more than a few days, the ilium on the other side will usually move in the opposite direction because of the instability produced by the first subluxation. The situation

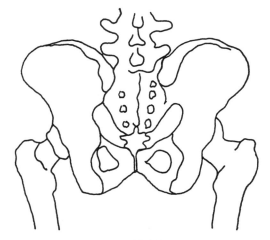

Normal Pelvis

Figure 3

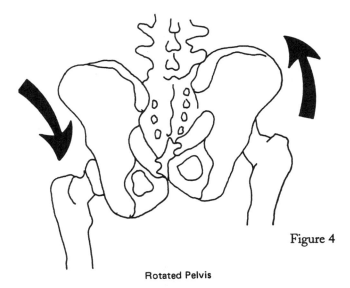

Figure 4

Rotated Pelvis

in which both ilia move either upward or downward is uncommon, although it does occur and can often make diagnosis very difficult unless the physician is aware of its possibility.

Now let us examine why such displacements occur and what consequences may attend their occurrence. Many investigators of the body's mechanical integrity believe that the sacroiliac articulation was formed when man began to walk upright; the horizontal position of this joint in lower animals rarely causes difficulty. Although I don't entirely accept this evolutionary explanation, I agree that the sacroiliac is more susceptible to strain and subluxation than any other joint in the body.

We have here two bones that are seemingly slapped together and then surrounded by strong fibrous bands (ligaments) to keep them in proper alignment. On top of this, the joint is located in an area where it is subjected to almost constant strain, even in an only moderately active person. As long as the ligaments remain firm and taut, however, the joint is still serviceable; but if these fibers lose some of their integral strength, the joint becomes most susceptible to slippage and subluxation. Luckily within the past few years, we have discovered certain nutritive elements that can help sustain and rebuild this ligamentous integrity. Thus, it is now possible to stabilize sacroiliac joints that were once overly susceptible to subluxation.

The sacroiliac problem usually doesn't arise from heavy lifting, but rather from twisting or turning motions. When the body is in this position, the sacroiliac joint is opened slightly, one set of muscles pulling on the ilium, while another pulls on the sacrum. If at this time movement is made in just the right manner, the sacroiliac joint will slide. If the slide causes impingement on a nerve, pain can be almost instantaneous. Such pain usually occurs as a dull aching sensation in the low back, on the side of the slippage. It may occur as a pain radiating down the back of the leg (sciatic nerve) or around the side and to the front of the leg (anterior cural nerve). The patient may actually hear a click when the joint slides, or there may be no noise sensation.

Although pain may occur with the movement of this joint, it is possible for the joint to move in such a manner that no nerve is impinged on. In this situation, the person does not usually know when the slippage takes place. Later in the day, he may begin to notice some sensation in the back or in the leg on the affected side. This sensation usually manifests itself as a vague uneasiness ·in the hip and low back. Numbness or mild tingling down the leg may occur along the nerve pathways already described. At times the condition may not be noticed until the patient attempts to rise from a sitting position, only to find that his back is stiff and must be "loosened" before he can move properly.

The extent and intensity of the symptoms can vary widely from one patient to another, even though the basic subluxation is the same. Some patients are in such severe pain that they can't move from a reclining position without great difficulty. At the other extreme, some experience only a slight discomfort that seems to leave after a few days, only to bother them occasionally if they place a mild strain on this part of the back.

Those with more severe pain are the luckier of the two; they are forced to seek professional help and seek it rapidly. If they are attended by one trained in manipulative therapy, their condition should respond to his help, and they'll be back in shape shortly.

On the other hand, if they seek help from one not so oriented, rest and muscle relaxants usually are prescribed. This in time will relieve the acute inflammation and enable them, after a somewhat longer period, to return to their regular activities. They'll find, however, that they're constantly having some low back difficulty on the side of the slip that will continue until they consult someone versed in correcting the mechanical slippage.

Of patients who have moderate difficulties from this subluxation, some will seek professional manipulative help and overcome their difficulty, but many will undergo no treatment or ineffective treatment, remaining mildly aware of a "weakness" in the low back. We often discover this type of patient during an ordinary physical examination. Frequently they have completely forgotten when or how the original injury occurred. Many have come to accept the residual pain and stiffness as a sign of aging. Strange to say, I hear this same remark even from some patients in their 20s and 30s. Most of these patients respond rapidly to manipulative therapy and are very pleased to find that their so called aging aches and pains are nothing more than a simple misaligned sacroiliac.

At this point, I'd like to explain just exactly why I called this condition "the great masquerader." When a sacroiliac articulation becomes subluxated, there is a tilting of the base of the sacrum. This in turn causes a lateral bending (scoliosis) of the spine (Figure 5). If the sacroiliac subluxation is corrected within a few days of its original occurrence, or at the most a few weeks, the spine will return rapidly to its normal position and there will be little difficulty beyond that manifested in the low back itself.

On the other hand, if the subluxation persists, as it so often does, the spine in time must compensate to correct for this tilt because the balancing action of the semi-circular canals in the inner ear requires that the head be carried vertically or the person feels unstable. If the base of the spine is tilted, the only way the head can be carried vertically is for other portions of the spine, particularly the lower cervical (neck) and upper thoracic area, to tilt in the opposite direction. First the body produces what is called a "C" curve (figure 5) and then, if the pelvic torsion is not corrected for years, an "S" curve (figure 6). When this occurs, it is very easy for abnormal nerve pressures, muscle spasms, and tensions on affected ligaments to produce symptomatic problems in the shoulder, upper back area, and neck. Frequently these will reflex to cause headaches that don't respond readily to ordinary forms of therapy.

It is often their neck difficulties and/or headaches that finally bring the patient to our office. Upon examination we find our old friend, the sacroiliac subluxation. Natural treatment of the upper back, along with correction of the original sacroiliac subluxation, soon gives us a patient who is symptom-free in both areas.

If this upper-back scoliosis is allowed to persist, a variety of structures are eventually affected that may involve, through irritated nerve pathways, the various internal organs. When a patient has had sacroiliac subluxation for many years, it becomes almost completely impossible to track down the full ramifications of the malalignment. In our own treatment, we correct the pelvic distortions and then make every effort to relieve the various nerve irritations and organ disorders that remain. We usually have excellent success with this type of person, although it does take time for him to gain complete recovery. Of course, it would have been easier for both patient and physician had this relatively simple problem been taken care of years earlier.

When pelvic rotation occurs, not only does the difficulty reflex upward, but there are also manifestations from the pelvis downward. Through a group of nerves called the pelvic plexus, it is possible for the bowels and the urogenital organs to be affected. Unexplained constipation may suddenly occur in these patients. Bladder irritation and urinary incontinence (the inability to retain urine) aren't unheard of. I've even had an occasional case of impotency that seemed to be aggravated by this subluxation. Pains similar to so-called ovarian pains can be mimicked by this slippage, and, in my experience, it is also possible for these nerve irritations to cause true congestion of the female organs.

The most frequent problems in the lower portion of the body stemming from this subluxation occur in the legs, knees, and feet. In some manner not yet fully understood, this condition may cause blockage or sluggishness of venous return, usually on the affected side. If the patient tends to have varicose veins, the condition can be intensified by this subluxation. I have had patients in whom this restriction of fluid return

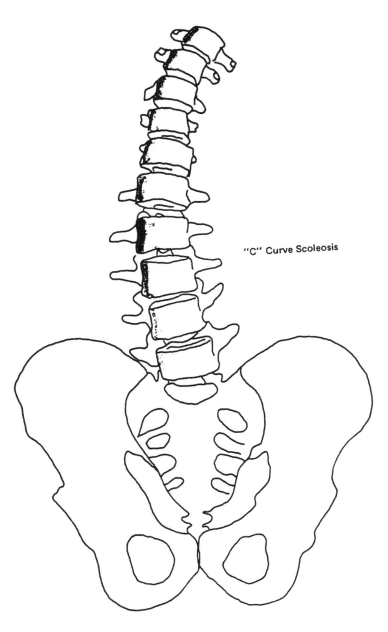

"C" Curve Scoleosis

Figure 5

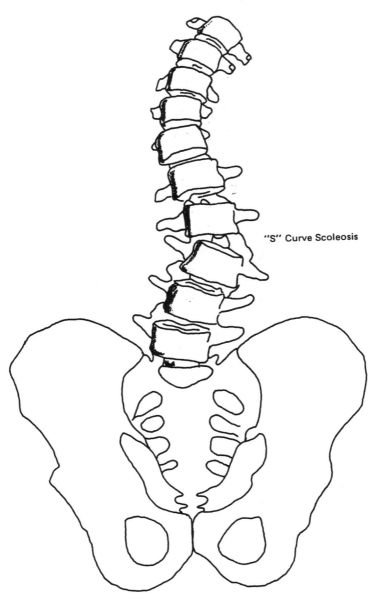

"S" Curve Scoleosis

Figure 6

was so severe that the leg swelled to half again its normal size and looked very much like thrombophlebitis. When the pelvic malalignment is corrected, however, the leg rapidly returns to its normal size within a few days, and all signs of fluid congestion disappear. It is possible that this condition is due to lymphatic congestion rather than venous congestion. Whatever its cause, it is rapidly corrected by the simple pelvic manipulation.

The knee is often involved when the pelvis slips. At least 50 per cent of all so-called knee problems I have seen in the last 40 years have been due to sacroiliac problems. These affected the knee, either through the postural changes due to this condition, or by direct impingement on the nerves supplying the knee.

Because sacroiliac shifts change the center of body weight, the greater proportion of this weight usually falls on the leg of the affected side, which in turn places abnormal stress on this knee with each step. The longer the sacroiliac is out of alignment, the longer stress is placed on the knee and the greater the possibility of trouble. If the pelvic subluxation is allowed to persist for months or years, permanent knee damage can be caused demanding treatment of both the pelvis and knee. Even with the best treatment, returning such a patient to a completely symptom-free status is difficult, though persistence usually will be rewarded.

When the knee problem is caused by nerve impingements, complete recovery, usually rapid, attends the pelvic correction. Even here, however, the speed of recovery depends on how soon the pelvic slip is corrected after the injury.

Foot and ankle problems due to the sacroiliac condition sometimes occur. Nerve-pressure symptoms are the most evident, usually occurring as numbness, tingling, or even as burning sensations felt throughout the foot. Occasionally, ankle weakness or pain occurs owing to the change in body weight distribution. These problems usually respond more rapidly than knee conditions, and they don't generally cause the knowledgeable practitioner much difficulty.

It isn't practical here to describe all the conditions that may stem from this subluxation. The ones I've described are the most common.

In addition to difficulties that may occur in an otherwise normal patient, many patients already have pre-existing ailments that may become aggravated or intensified when this condition is superimposed. One of the most common of these diseases is arthritis.

If part of the body is affected by both the slippage and arthritis, all the previously mentioned conditions can be intensified. For example, cervical (neck) arthritis may be intensified by a superimposed scoliosis.

Such an aggravation can occur at any point of stress in the body. The knee is a very common area for arthritis to be intensified by a sacroiliac problem. In all these cases, it is first necessary to correct the pelvic problem, and then specific therapy can be used to overcome the aggravation of the arthritis. When such arthritic areas become aggravated, they don't necessarily subside of their own accord after the cause of the aggravation is removed. Frequently additional therapy is required.

Statistically the most common condition "stirred up" by the sacroiliac slip is a compression of the disc between the last lumbar segment and the sacrum, or between the last two lumbar segments The discs in this area of the spine are subjected to the greatest wear and tear of any in the body, and it is here that the thinning process so frequently associated with age is first observed. Because this disc thinning develops slowly, the body has time to adapt, and many times the patient is only vaguely aware of difficulty in this area. If a sudden sacroiliac subluxation occurs, such acute stress will often precipitate a reaction in the disc area, and the patient will suffer acute pain, which is only slightly relieved by correction of the sacroiliac subluxation. Whenever we have a patient whose back corrects very well posturally but whose painful symptoms don't improve considerably after the fourth treatment, we routinely request an X-ray of the lower back. In 75 to 80 per cent of these patients, we find some degree of disc degeneration. With proper natural therapy, most of these patients can be made symptom-free without surgery. This subject is described in more detail in the next chapter on traction therapy.

Sacroiliac Treatment

The basic treatment for this condition is very simple for any manipulator (chiropractor naturopath, or adjusting osteopath) worth his salt. Mere replacement of the joint, however, is not sufficient therapy in most cases, for almost invariably the joint soon slips out again. Only when the joint is *stabilized* can we consider the condition truly corrected.

A stabilized joint is one that has been replaced in correct alignment, had its inflammation reduced to a normal status, and its spastic muscles returned to normal muscle tone, enabling the ligamentous structures to regain their full integrity. Sometimes such a state is easily and rapidly attainable. In other instances, only through long and arduous work on the part of both physician and patient can such true stabilization be achieved.

The sacroiliac subluxation may be replaced in a variety of ways. The well-known lumbar roll with its Gonstead variations is perhaps as useful as any, although I have seen patients in whom only a direct thrust over

70

the sacroiliac joint itself was effective. In some, a rotary leg movement is useful, and in certain cases only the very mild Gilete move proves to be possible. By the use of a proprietary rotation move perfected at our Center we are able to painlessly correct many sacroiliac subluxations that defy all other methods.

Because the actual correction should be left strictly to the professional, I won't dwell on the details here. Some bits of information, however, a patient should know in order to help the physician stabilize his condition. In my long experience with this subluxation, I find that after the first replacement the joint usually slips again within twenty-four hours. I have found nothing effective to prevent this re-slippage. In our own Center, we insist the patient return a day or two after the original correction for his second treatment. In 75 to 80 per cent of all patients, the joint will begin holding after the second treatment. What causes this I don't exactly know but it is my belief that the body isn't able to create the necessary healing rapidly enough to hold the joint with the first treatment. However, most systems seem capable after second correction to reduce inflammation sufficiently to hold the correction .

I stress this point of the need for a second and even a third treatment for this condition because many practitioners are aware of the simple nature of the sacroiliac subluxation and will make the proper adjustment, but fail to follow the patient's progress until the joint is stable. They frequently say, "That's back in place now. If it causes you any further trouble, get in touch with me." Unfortunately, the joint will probably slip within a day or two, and the patient, still suffering pain, often will assume this pain is just muscle or nerve irritation. After a week or two, when the pain doesn't disappear, the patient will return to his physician (or seek another one because he thinks the first physician didn't correct his problem). All too often this scenario will be repeated again and again. New patients often come in and tell us, "Oh my hip is always out of place." All this means is that the previous physician knew how to replace the joint but not how to stabilize it.

If this joint is corrected a second time within two or three days, it will usually hold. However, if the interval between the first treatment and the second is a week or longer, inflammation in the area may well return to the same degree as before the first replacement. If this occurs, this late second replacement must actually begin all over again. This situation is often repeated again and again, the patient returning to the physician once a week or so for months, resulting in only partial improvement in the condition. In our offices, we watch the sacroiliac patient closely until we know the joint is back in place and the attendant inflam-

71

mation is reduced sufficiently so that there is only minimal chance of further slippage.

After the sacroiliac articulation remains in position, we request the patient to return at least once more to assure us that the joint is stabilizing and to enable replacement of the lower lumbar vertebrae, which are almost always put into a minor twist or rotation by the sacroiliac subluxation. While the sacroiliac is misplaced, the muscle tension on these vertebrae prevents correction. Only after the sacroiliac joint has been in place a day or two is it possible to replace these rotated lumbar vertebrae.

After this last correction, if the patient is relatively pain-free and the muscle tension seems minimal, he is discharged. However, he should be told that the sacroiliac joint will be sensitive and weak for a week to ten days, even after a proper correction, and he must take care in its use during this period or he risks another subluxation. In can take this time for the supporting ligaments to return to normal tone and until this happens the joint is weaker than normal and more susceptible to slippage.

At the time of the first replacement, each of our patients is warned to refrain from certain types of movement that may cause the joint to slip again. We usually suggest that he refrain from any form of twisting to the side, particularly to reach or to pick up anything. If he wants to pick something up, we suggest that he face the object, bend down directly in front of it (bending the knees at the same time), grasp it, and then rise the same way.

The patient is also requested to make all efforts to keep his knees together, or one in front of the other, as much as possible. The patient should refrain from any form of movement that moves one knee laterally (out to the side) from the other. One of the most common movements to be avoided is the usual method of getting into a car. The sacroiliac patient should not get into a car one leg at a time. Rather, he should open the car door, turn around, sit down on the seat, and then bring in both legs together keeping the knees close together. He should get out of the automobile in the reverse order, keeping both knees together and moving both legs at the same time. This last admonition is difficult for the patient to remember. He will carefully get into the car and drive to where he's going, only to forget entirely our instructions when he gets out. However, it is just as important to exit a car properly as it is enter it correctly.

If you ever have a sacroiliac problem remember these precautions and observe them; they have proven invaluable for all our patients.

Although manipulation of the low back is the basic and essential therapy for sacroiliac subluxation, other modalities are of great help in most patients. We often begin therapy with short-wave diathermy, which is a specific deep-penetrating form of heat used to relax the muscles and ligaments in the affected area. This makes our correction easier and more thorough. After correction, we use ultra-sound to help reduce inflammation in the affected area, and then sine wave to help control pain and aid in achieving greater mobility. Recently we have added the new Low Level Laser Therapy to our more traditional modalities. This new marvel has allowed us to heal some difficult sacraliliacs in days that used to take weeks. All these modalities are discussed at length in Chapters 7, 9 and 25. I mention their use here only to describe our full therapy program.

The therapy just described is usually adequate for sacroiliac disorders that are seen within a few days of the original accident and that are only moderately severe and don't cause many complications. At least half our cases, however, don't fall into this category; with these, greater skill, care, and experience are needed to produce sacroiliac stabilization.

Where the condition has existed for a week or more, we often find a fairly high degree of muscle irritation and spasm present. In these instances, the modalities mentioned previously prove extremely helpful. We also utilize a method of muscle goading and relaxation. In this treatment, a lubricant, usually olive oil, is rubbed into the patient's lower spine, and the large muscle groups contiguous with the pelvis are then deeply massaged by the practitioner. Sometimes these areas are exquisitely tender, and great care must be exercised at first. But as therapy progresses, the muscles lose much of this sensitivity and the patient's pain greatly diminishes. In these spastic patients, more treatments than the basic three are usually needed for proper stabilization. Generally, the program should not run much beyond six treatments, however. If six treatments have been given with the sacroiliac in place and the patient is still having difficulty, there is probably something else involved, perhaps a mild disc problem (see Chapter 4).

In some patients, the sacroiliac joint won't stay in place by the third treatment, or it may stay in for a few days and then slip out. Where the joint has been out of place for some time, it is common for it to react normally for the first three treatments, only to slip out again within a week or so as the patient resumes his usual activities. It usually requires an extra replacement, or at the most two, to finish stabilization in this patient, and he usually makes rapid recovery after this second set of corrections.

Some sacroiliac joints continue to slip out of alignment, even with the most careful replacements and diligent use of the other modalities.

In this type of patient, the ligaments that hold the articulation in place have been so overstretched that they won't return to normal by our usual therapeutic methods. The joint thus remains loose and doesn't hold an adjustment. This type of patient at one time was the bane of all manipulators. Nothing seemed to correct their problem completely. Luckily, within recent years, it has been discovered that the mineral manganese, (along with other synergistic nutrients) if used in fairly large but nontoxic doses, helps to normalize their ligamentous function and, used along with the basic sacroiliac therapies, enables joint stabilization.

To help these patients further, we may need to fit a man's six inch elastic rib belt around the pelvic area. This is fit outside the underclothes, to add support to the weakened ligaments. These patients are instructed to wear this belt day and night, until we think satisfactory ligament tone has been established.

This treatment usually produces satisfactory joint stabilization within a few days. The belt usually can be discontinued in four or five days, though some patients must wear it a week or two. Usually, the manganese dosage is reduced after a few weeks, but we suggest that these patients continue a low dosage of this supplement for at least a year, because ligament problems, perhaps owing to their poor blood supply, repair very slowly. If the tablets are discontinued before complete stabilization is achieved, the joint may once again become loose, making another sacroiliac subluxation a distinct possibility.

Even with the foregoing therapy, some patients don't improve completely. These are of two general types. First is the patient whose sacroiliac isn't capable of staying in place, even with support and the use of the manganese supplementation. The second type is one whose articulation defect is corrected but whose symptoms remain or even become worse.

In the first instance, we usually have a patient whose body tone is so poor that it can't hold these structures in proper position, or we have a patient who has a sacroiliac inflammation that produces a constant swelling that interferes with proper setting of the joint. We occasionally have someone with a congenital anomaly, someone like my wife, who was born with a very small amount of the surface between the sacrum and ilium actually articulating. In her case, the bony articulating surfaces are seemingly insufficient to produce the proper surface for a normal joint.

Each of these cases requires individual professional care. They all can be helped by natural methods and although the treatment may be more involved than what I have described, it is usually very successful.

The second type of case is more common than the first and luckily is easier to correct. When a sacroiliac has been adequately corrected and the patient given sufficient time for the inflammation to subside—usually ten days to two weeks— he should be pain-free with normal movement fully restored. If free movement is still restricted and the pain, though improved, still considerable, we insist on an X-ray of the lumbosacral area.

We have certain X-ray views taken in a postural or standing position. The bottom of our film is parallel with a platform at the base of the X-ray machine, on which the patient stands. Four views are taken, an AP (front to back), a lateral (through the side), and two obliques (at an angle through each side of the back) .

The standing AP tells us whether there is any anatomic difference in leg length, any spinal curvature, arthritis, ankylosis, or spurring of the spine. It also shows us the integrity of the hip socket, and from it we can visualize the sacroiliac joint to determine if any pathologic or congenital problems are there. This view also shows us if any pelvic rotation still remains.

The lateral film provides us with the most information about the disc integrity. Disc thinning or narrowing is best demonstrated in this view. Spinal lordosis (swayback), straight military spine, tipping, and arthritis may also be seen in the lateral view.

The oblique view is used to determine the integrity of the articulating surfaces—the points at which the lumbar vertebrae are joined together. Arthritis in these areas is common and will cause difficulty. Owing to deviations in the spine itself, sometimes caused by sacroiliac subluxation, these articular surfaces (called facets) may jam, a situation caused by an irregularity of pressure where these two vertebrae meet. This situation can cause a variety of problems in the low back and can be greatly aggravated by a sacroiliac slip.

The most common X-ray finding is a disc thinning between the last lumbar and the first sacral segment; next most frequent is a short leg. This short leg (anatomic short leg), must be differentiated from the apparent short leg found in sacroiliac subluxation. If the sacroiliac joint slips upward and backward, it tends to draw the leg on that side upward (Fig. 4). Conversely, if it slips downward and forward, it tends to draw the leg downward (fig. 4). In this manner, an upward sacroiliac on the right gives the appearance of a short leg on the right, and a downward sacroiliac on the left gives the appearance of a long leg on the left. When the proper sacroiliac correction is made, these apparent short or long legs correct themselves automatically. An anatomic short leg is actually shorter than the other leg and can only be detected accurately by a postural X-ray. It is possible for an anatomic short leg to produce many of the symptoms that we have heretofore attributed to sacroiliac slippage. This is especially true of the knee symptoms and of problems related to upper trunk scoliosis.

For a true anatomic short leg, the best therapy is the judicious use of heel lifts. We usually begin with a very small lift and gradually, week by week, increase its size until we have brought the patient to a point where he can accept a lift approximately half the size of the leg shortage. Any attempt to build the lift higher usually upsets the physiology of the spine to such a degree that its use is not justified.

Because of its frequency, I have taken the time to discuss lift therapy. However, I don't recommend that you experiment with this treatment. A lift should be used only after its need is fully demonstrated by postural X-ray. There is no other way to my knowledge of accurately ascertaining whether a lift is needed. If a lift is used where the real problem is a pelvic distortion and not an anatomic short leg, the basic condition is intensified and the reflex symptoms may worsen.

Of all the conditions we find on the postural X-ray examination, the compressed disc is the most common. Two basic types of disc problems afflict the lower back. One is the slowly developing chronic form known as a degenerated (narrowed) disc. The other is the herniated or slipped disc. In this latter form, the jelly-like substance in the center of the spinal disc forces its way through the tougher surrounding material and protrudes into the spinal canal. This pressure may even irritate the spinal cord itself. This condition may come on very suddenly; in 80 per cent of cases it corrects itself after a period of complete bed rest. In severe cases, the orthopedist may need to perform an operation. In this operation (laminectomy), the surgeon cuts through the back of the vertebra and removes this offending gelatinous disc center. The main hard fibrous section of the disc is left intact, and often the patient experiences a very dramatic and much appreciated sense of relief after surgery.

Most disc cases we encounter aren't of the herniated variety but rather are the degenerating or thinning variety. In this case, the whole disc—particularly the outer tough circular layers—is compressed or thins from wear and tear. Bed rest is not particularly helpful for these patients, except for an occasional acute manifestation. Once the disc thins to a certain point, there develops a steady nerve impingement due to a telescoping of the normal nerve opening, because as the disc thins the vertebra above settles down on the vertebra below. When this occurs, the normal opening formed by these two vertebrae for the spinal nerve is narrowed, and the bones may put sufficient pressure on the nerve to cause pain along the nerve pathway.

Because this situation occurs slowly over the years, this area of the body makes every attempt to adapt to keep the nerve and its allied elements from injury. However, if a patient with such a disc problem suddenly suffers sacroiliac subluxation, a sudden shift in the pressures on the disc area is produced, usually aggravating the area to such a degree that severe muscle spasm and nerve inflammation ensue. Even though this patient seeks professional care soon and the sacroiliac subluxation is corrected, he is usually left with an irritation of the pre-existing degenerated disc.

Because the Beverly Hall Corporation Healing Research Center is noted for its success with difficult low-back cases, we see a good percentage of these patients. Often the patient has had a history of back trouble for years, though until recently it was readily corrected with a few treatments by his local chiropractor or osteopath. Now he has what seems to be the same old sacroiliac slip, but his physician is not able to help. He is at a loss to explain his physician's sudden incompetence. The truth is that not his doctor but his back has changed. His slowly degenerating disc has finally reached a point where the body can no longer adapt to its pressure.

An operative procedure can be used on these patients; however, it isn't as universally successful as the laminectomy, nor anywhere nearly as simple. In this procedure (called a fusion), the surgeon cuts into the back, removes what he can of the degenerated disc, spreads the opening, and puts a section removed from the patient's own bones or bone dust into the area between the vertebrae to ankylose (fuse) the two vertebrae together, producing an artificial disc between the two.

In the state of Washington, a very thorough survey a few years ago taken of all industrial lowback cases showed that the operation was successful in only 50 per cent of cases—at least half the workers undergoing this operation were never able to return to work. Knowing the odds against such an operation being successful, we very rarely recommend it.

In a recent survey of all acute back treatments by the U.S. government the same results were found and they recommended that fusion operations be used seldom.

Physiotherapeutic methods can be used to keep most of these patients productive and relatively comfortable. We are able to return most of them to full activity completely pain free.

Chapter four is devoted to this and similar disc problems, but because many of these patients are found during the treatment of a superimposed sacroiliac disorder, I thought it best to begin the discussion here.

Here too the new Low Level Laser Therapy has proven to be of great help. As one eighty year old patient, who was treated with this Laser for an old chronic disk compression, said, "For the first time in many years the Laser made my back feel normal again."

I have written much about such an apparently simple problem because of its high incidence and because many otherwise highly competent physicians almost totally disregard it. If you have any unresolved vague problems in the neck, shoulders, back, knees, legs, or feet, I suggest you find someone versed in manipulative therapy to check the integrity of the sacroiliac articulation. Don't be surprised if he confirms that you too are one of the multitude having this simple but rather aggravating condition.

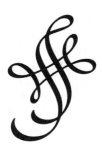

Chapter IV
Intermittent Motorized Traction and Allied Therapies

As we look at a picture of a spine, we see a group of thirty-three irregularly shaped bones sitting one on top of the other, the smallest at the top, largest at the bottom, and between each a cushion or disc shaped like a doughnut with a nice wad of jelly in the middle. The main part of this doughnut consists of tough cartilaginous material that is hard and unyielding. The center part of the doughnut (the jelly) consists of a substance called the nucleus pulposus, a gelatinous material surrounded by a membrane sheath, which acts as a shock absorber to give resiliency to an otherwise inflexible spinal component.

The spine is not straight front to back, but is shaped like a letter S. This adds to the shockabsorbing effect of the spine by providing a spring-like action that absorbs much of the pressure and stress on the lowest spinal segments.

Despite this wonderfully designed structure, the spinal discs, like all other parts of the body, are susceptible to wear and tear. This degeneration would cause few problems were it not for the serious consequences that can arise when the degeneration narrows the intravertebral foramen (the opening through which the spinal nerves pass from the spinal cord to the periphery).

The upper portion of this foramen (opening) is formed from a surface of the vertebra above and the lower portion from the adjacent segment below. The spinal disc separates the two vertebrae in such a manner that the opening is adequate for the nerve and allied tissue to function freely (Fig. 7). The size of this opening is thereby controlled by the integrity of the spinal disc. If the spinal disc between these two vertebrae deteriorates, the vertebrae are jammed together and the opening for the spinal nerve becomes smaller. This causes pressure on the nerve and allied parts, producing a *pinched nerve*. Although, theoretically, this may occur at any level of the spine, it most commonly takes place in the lower lumbar (low back) and/or cervical (neck) regions.

The Low-Back Disc Syndrome

The lowest part of the spine must carry the weight of the entire upper trunk of the body. It is this area—the 4th and 5th lumbar vertebrae and the first sacral segment—that receives the greatest stress. And it is here that spinal disc degeneration occurs most commonly .

Injuries to this portion of the spine are relatively common. Almost any form of heavy lifting produces its greatest strain at this level. Many types of falls cause injury destructive to this area. It isn't surprising, therefore, that treatment of disc compressions in this area comprises a considerable part of our low-back work.

The neck vertebrae are only slightly less frequently affected than those of the low back. There are three common causes of disc degeneration in the cervical spine.

The first is arthritis, which apparently affects neck discs more readily than those of the other spinal levels. This may be because the neck discs are much smaller than the others and therefore more easily damaged by arthritic calcium deposits. The second most common cause of cervical disk narrowing is the later consequences of whiplash injuries. With the increase in the number of automobiles, rear end collisions have been growing by leaps and bounds; the injuries to the spine caused by this accident tend to produce cervical disc problems some time after the accident. Such narrowing may not show up for several years after the original accident and, therefore, all physicians should be very careful in discharging such accident patients too soon after the injury.

The last cause of cervical disc problems is the general neck trauma (injury) caused by a variety of falls or accidents. When we discover a neck disc lesion through X-ray where there has been no whiplash injury and the patient is free of arthritis, we can usually trace the patient's trouble to some neck injury that occurred previously, often during childhood. This early injury may have been quite minor, but the neck is delicate and such minor assaults often show up later as cervical disc compressions.

Disc Treatment

Most disc problems can be treated satisfactorily by the use of traction and various other modalities designed to help the traction perform its needed task. Most of you are probably familiar with the regular hospital traction generally used for these patients. In this type of therapy for the low back, weights are attached to the patient's ankles by a system of ropes and pulleys. Up to fifteen pounds is placed on each leg, and it is necessary for the patient to remain in bed for a considerable period while under this therapy. Recent studies on this type of traction found that patients given it did *not* recover any faster than those who were treated without it. These results confirm our own experience with this type of steady traction for the low back.

A similar form of traction is used for the neck, except that a halter is attached to the chin and head, a rope that goes over pulleys is connected

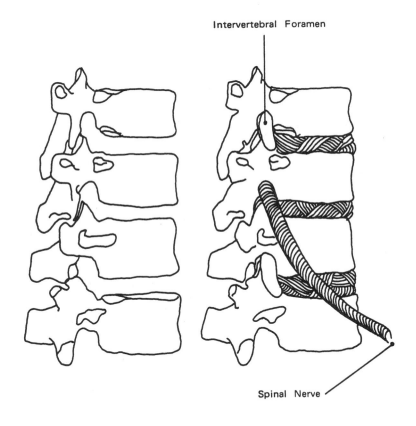

Intervertebral Foramen

Spinal Nerve

Figure 7

to this and a weight is attached to the end of the rope. We have found this type of traction *to be useful* as a home treatment in some varieties of cervical disk compression but only in conjunction with other therapies that we use at the Beverly Hall Corporation Healing Research Center.

In all low back patients and in many cervical (neck) patients we find that this type of steady traction has several disadvantages. Most of these disadvantages are overcome by the use of intermittent motorized traction (IMT), the method used in our Center.

One of the most obvious disadvantages of orthodox steady traction is the inconvenience to the patient. Not everyone has the time to spend two or three weeks flat on his back in bed, not to mention the cost involved. Because hospital traction is applied to the ankles in low-back syndromes, the knee and hip are both placed under tension before the force reaches the lumbar area. Stretching in these joints dissipates much of the applied force and thus as little as one or two pounds of traction force is actually delivered to the injured disc.

Also, when a steady traction is applied to an area, the musculature goes into spasm to protect the part from this abnormal pressure. Often this muscular spasm not only increases the patient's pain, but also acts as an effective counteracting force to diminish still further the traction's usefulness.

Because the need for effective traction therapy was so great and the accepted methods so inadequate, many fertile minds went to work in search of a better way. From this work evolved the theory and mechanism of intermittent motorized traction. In IMT, a belt is applied immediately around the hip area, and a nylon rope is attached to this belt by a special "tail," which is secured to either side of the affected disc area. This rope is attached to a computercontrolled motor unit that can be adjusted to intermittently pull and release the rope at any chosen poundage. The holding time of the traction and the resting time between tractions are also variable so that they may be set for the best possible patient response.

A special table for this unit enables the upper part of the patient to remain fixed while the lower portion of the table (on rollers) is free to move, thereby assuring an absolute minimum amount of friction during the treatment. The feet and knees are elevated by a special stool that provides the most restful posture as traction is applied.

Treatments are usually given for twenty minutes at a time, two to three times a week, depending on the severity of the case. Pressure may vary between fifty and eighty pounds.

Because of the ingenious use of the belts described above, which enable the major part of the traction to be applied directly to the area of involvement, twenty to fifty times more pressure can be applied to the vertebral area than by regular steady hospital traction. Also the alternate pull and release of this form of traction doesn't allow sufficient time during the pull cycle for a buildup of the muscle spasm that is a frequent component of the more static forms of traction, thus effectively preventing counteracting muscular forces. With the use of IMT, the patient is kept ambulatory and only the most severe cases must refrain from their regular employment.

Cervical Traction

This type of traction can be used just as readily for the neck as for the low back. In cervical traction, the patient is reversed on the table, the sliding component of the table secured, the position of the motor head raised to produce the proper angle for the neck and then an appropriate neck halter and spreader bar are used to secure the patient. The hold period of traction pressure is usually reduced because the neck muscles are more sensitive than those of the low back and greater care must be taken to prevent a spastic reaction. The poundage ranges anywhere from twenty to forty-five, thirty-five for women and forty-five for men.

The average low-back disc patient will notice improvement after the third or fourth treatment, though in some resistant patients, it may take six to eight treatments before observable improvement becomes evident. Cervical patients are more variable in their response. Some show improvement with the first traction, while some old whiplash patients may require up to ten treatments before real help is felt.

Other Modalities

The usual form of therapy we use for low-back disc patients consists of diathermy to relax the musculature, intermittent traction to open the disc area and take pressure off the spinal nerves, and finally ultrasound treatments directly over the affected discs to stimulate their regeneration and reduce the inflammation always found in these areas. Recently, we have added the phenomenal MicroLight 830 to this program. This Low Reactive Light Laser Therapy has revolutionized the pain control of these patients in our Center. While at the time of this writing, this hand held wonder is still in the investigational stage, we have found it to be without peer in bringing long desired relief to many cervical and low back patients. See the section later in this book for a complete run down on this "magic" little unit.

Because we at the Healing Research Center believe that all chronic conditions are aggravated by improper nutrition, we recommend that our low-back patients follow our basic maintenance diet. In addition we supplement this diet with vitamin C, vitamin E, manganese phytate, and any other special nutrients that we have found are important to the patient's recovery from such maladies.

In the last forty years, I have handled thousands of these low back cases, yet I can count on the fingers of one hand those that required surgery when the treatment outlined above was used. Of course, the earlier in the condition we are able to treat the patient, the quicker and more complete will be the results but even in most advanced cases, the intermittent traction therapy and the other modalities are not without considerable success.

Whiplash Injuries

Intermittent cervical traction is particularly beneficial in all types of old whiplash injuries. These patients usually begin to exhibit symptoms many years after the original accident, and often they have nearly forgotten the causal incident. Problems usually begin as numbness or tingling in one hand, particularly at night. It may even awaken the patient with an arm that has "gone to sleep." When the patient is up and around, his head and neck are in motion and there is no constant pressure on the affected nerve in the neck. But when he goes to sleep or perhaps sits down to read a book, the lack of motion of the head and neck may put sufficient pressure on the spinal nerve to produce the sensations down the arm. These symptoms are caused by vertebral pressure due to thinning discs or calcium deposits. Both problems are usually rapidly improved by IMT, the MicroLight laser and the other modalities we us.

Arthritis

Intermittent cervical traction is also useful in certain arthritic problems of the neck and upper back. The procedure must be done carefully, but it seems that gentle pressure to counteract the daily effects of gravity will alleviate these troublesome symptoms, even in some of the older and more chronic cases.

We have even used cervical traction to good advantage in many cases of cerebral arteriosclerosis (hardening of the arteries of the brain). While certainly not specific, it seems the mild rhythmic stretching of the neck structures increases the circulation to the brain and helps relieve many of the distressing symptoms of cerebral anoxia.

Cautions to be Observed

IMT is an active form of therapy in which care must be taken not to begin treatments with too much pressure. We always start with mild pressures and gradually build up the tension along with the patient's ability to accept it. Some patients can take two hundred pounds of pressure in the low back; others feel that fifty to sixty-five is too much.

After every IMT treatment on the low back, it is very important that the patient remain on the table for at least five minutes before going on to the next therapy. The patient usually doesn't feel the full effect of the traction until he tries to arise after the treatment. Very often while under treatment, the patient says that he hardly feels any pulling at all. Yet when he tries to move after traction, he soon finds that his muscles and ligaments have been stretched and they need a little time to adjust before he can walk easily. This is also true in neck patients, so all our intermittent traction patients are asked to rest five minutes after their IMT treatment.

Except for a little muscle stiffness after the first or second treatment, the patient will usually feel no discomfort from this type of traction. If the patient does experience discomfort after a few treatments, the therapy should be discontinued. Even though IMT is the therapy of choice in most low-back disc cases and in many neck problems, not every patient can accept it readily. For these patients, other forms of therapy must be instituted. It's been our experience that patients who can't take IMT readily, do respond satisfactorily to some of the less energetic forms of physical therapy. This is especially true now that we have the Low Level Laser to offer them.

Although IMT is relatively simple, it is most effective and nothing else quite takes its place. It is not commonly available, however, in most hospitals or doctors offices and very few of our patients had heard of it before their treatments at our Center. Few doctors in the manipulative field use this therapy. It is even rarer in the offices of the orthodox medical profession.

Cost may be a factor as to why this method is so little used; the equipment is quite expensive and many physicians may believe that they wouldn't treat enough patients to justify the expense. At the Beverly Hall Corporation Healing Research Center we do not place cost first when it comes to the welfare of our patients and so we are often the first to offer such advanced therapies.

For low-back disc problems or for neck troubles that don't respond to manipulation, don't be talked into surgery until you have investigated the possibility of our intermittent motorized traction and the modalities that go along with its use.

Chapter V
Whiplash

There is probably no other condition in the annals of medicine about which so much purposeful confusion has been created as the post accident condition known as "whiplash."

(These words were originally written over twenty years ago and I had trusted that by now this situation would have changed and the true nature of this injury would have been accepted by all interested parties. I was naive. It seems to me that the purposeful misinformation on this condition and its sequelae is as blatant today as in the past, if not more so.)

This injury, classically caused by a rear-end automobile collision, produces a whipping trauma to the neck that can cause dire future consequences. The immediate injury done to the patient's neck, however, is of such a nature that X-rays and other examinations made shortly after the accident usually show nothing worse than minor muscle spasm. The real damage only shows up much later.

Because much of the early and continuing pain and discomfort from this type of injury can't be substantiated by ordinary medical investigation, insurance companies attempting to minimize their liability, have attempted to convince the medical profession that whiplash injury is a figment of the patient's imagination or merely a guise to bilk the insurance companies. When I first entered the healing profession, forty years ago, I too was much influenced by this insurance company propaganda. I too treated most of these patients only for minor cervical strain and suggested that they settle their claim with the insurance company as soon as their neck felt comfortable.

My rather smug attitude toward this condition was suddenly altered when within a week's time two patients whom I had discharged months earlier returned with their neck condition greatly aggravated. Because I had suggested that both of these patients settle with the insurance company, I felt a certain responsibility to take care of this later aggravation Pro Bona and so treated both of these patients for almost two years without charge. As you can imagine, such an incident is likely to leave a permanent impression on a young struggling physician. After this, I began a thorough investigation of whiplash on my own. From the information I gathered, I became certain that the condition is not a figment of the patient's imagination, but is a very real, physical entity not particularly well understood by any of the healing professions, orthodox or alternative.

The Three Stages of Whiplash Injury

This investigational work and subsequent clinical experience have led me to determine that whiplash may well present three different stages (phases). The first occurs immediately after the accident, the second begins thirty to ninety days afterward, and the last stage, which may or may not occur, becomes manifest only five to twenty years after the original injury.

Surprisingly, the degree of pain and discomfort present in the first stage doesn't necessarily accurately indicate the degree of trouble in later stages. In our experience, those who may exhibit little discomfort in the first stage frequently have severe problems in the second and third stages. Because of this possibility, I consider every whiplash injury potentially serious and capable of permanent disability. I believe it is the physician's duty to inform the patient of this possibility and, whenever possible, to aid the patient in receiving proper compensation for the full extent of this injury from the insurance company involved. As you may surmise, I am not on the insurance companies Christmas list.

The First Stage

Most patients with whiplash suffer some degree of discomfort within a day or two of the original accident. Such disability may be mild or severe, depending on the actual structures affected by the whipping action. This primary discomfort usually abates within a week or two. I reiterate that one can not tell the true significance of the injury by the degree of discomfort and pain experienced in the first stage. Some patients have almost no discomfort at this time, yet years later they develop severe calcium deposits and disc degeneration. On the other hand, some have severe discomfort during the first stage, yet never go into the second or third stages. It is imperative that both physician and patient remember this so they don't gauge insurance liability by the severity of the discomfort experienced during the first stage.

First-stage discomfort is usually treated best by mild physical methods, such as ultrasound, diathermy, and sine wave therapy. Now-a-days we also use the **MicroLight 830** low level laser. As mentioned in the last chapter it has revolutionized the treatment of such pain and spasm. An occasional manipulative treatment to the neck may be beneficial, although we strongly recommend against too many or too energetic cervical adjustments at this time. The neck has been injured, the muscles and nerves need time to heal, and they must have rest and relaxation to do this, not constant manipulative aggravation. There are exceptions, but the physician in charge must be aware that treatment should be tailored to the patient's needs and desires at this time.

Many patients benefit from a neck collar during this phase. I usually provide one for each patient, but I don't insist that they wear it unless the neck feels better while the collar is on. Many times the patient experiences less discomfort if his neck is allowed a certain amount of movement, unfettered by such a collar. To many patients, however, the neck feels weak and uncontrollable unless a collar is worn. If used in such a manner, the collar is of great benefit and without adverse effects. Although I've used all types, I now prefer the soft foam collar for most patients.

Low-Back—Neck Syndrome

A reflex injury to the sacral-iliac joint frequently follows the first stage of whiplash; it is too consistent to be coincidental and yet it can't be explained from our knowledge of normal nerve relationships. In approximately 90 percent of my whiplash patients, the sacroiliac joint slips out of alignment a few days after the original accident, whether or not there was any injury to the lower back during the accident. It seems that this is produced by a reflex-caused weakness due to injury of the cervical vertebrae. Although the occurrence of this sacroiliac subluxation is enigmatic, its cure is conventional. It usually is corrected quite rapidly by normal therapy for the low back (see Chapters 3 and 4). The only difference between an ordinary sacroiliac problem and this is that it is often necessary to replace these joints several times before an adequate stable joint is obtained. The joint probably won't stay in place permanently until the neck irritation is reduced to a point where it no longer initiates the causative reflex.

The Second Stage

If the second stage is to occur, it will usually begin to show up a few weeks after the first-stage symptoms have abated. The second stage begins with symptoms such as unexplained headaches, tingling down the arms into the hand, pressure on the chest, dizziness, vertigo, recurring lowback pain and other reflex symptoms related to nerve pathways of the neck. These second-stage symptoms are usually due to nerve and soft tissue damage that occurred at the time of the accident but that is just now beginning to cause actual reflex disorders. These symptoms can be so bizarre and severe that many patients think they are losing their minds. Physicians may be mystified—although the symptoms are positive and concrete to the patient—because a cursory physical examination usually doesn't disclose any physiologic or anatomic reason for these symptoms. They are real, however, and usually respond well to the physical therapy methods used at our Center

In this second stage, great help can be obtained from the careful use of cervical traction. We use intermittent motorized traction; this, combined with gentle manipulation and other relaxing physical therapeutic methods, can usually relieve second-stage symptoms within a reasonably short time. In selected patients benefits may be obtained by the use of home cervical traction but if used the patient must be very carefully trained in its use.

These second stage patients often require a considerable amount of emotional support from the attending physician, particularly in reassuring them that their condition is physical, not psychologic or emotional. If this is not given, the doctor will usually be disappointed in the patient's progress.

The Third Stage

It is a very fortunate whiplash patient who does not progress beyond the first stage, and one should be pleased if the disorder stops at the second stage. Unfortunately, many patients suffer the consequences of third-stage developments. The third stage may occur as late as ten to fifteen years (or longer) after the original accident. It is even possible that some patients who had minor first-stage discomfort and no second-stage discomfort may later develop third-stage problems. Unfortunately, in these cases, even when attended by the most conscientious physician, all insurance liability will probably have been discharged years earlier. It is therefore usually necessary for the patient with third-stage trouble to foot the bill himself. It is routine in our Center to suggest to patients that they do not settle a whiplash claim for at least eighteen months to two years after the original accident. Obviously, however, even this rather conservative approach won't cover many of the really delayed third-stage problems.

Third-stage difficulties arise from the fact that when this type of injury occurs, small areas of necrosis (dead tissue) are produced in various sections of the cervical spine. As the years pass, the body lays down calcium deposits in these necrotic areas in an attempt to support the injured tissue. The calcium deposits may, in the ensuing years, cause pressure on nerves and muscles, preventing proper bony articulations. Such pressures and impingements cause many of the thirdstage symptoms. It is also possible that some of the nerves and small blood vessels that feed the cervical spinal discs are also destroyed or injured in the original accident. In time, the nutrition to these discs is diminished and they

90

gradually atrophy, causing the vertebrae they separate to move closer together. This produces nerve root pressure which in turn may cause added symptoms to this stage of whiplash.

Third-stage problems are not likely to go away as rapidly or as completely as those of the first or second stage. Once the calcium has accumulated and the discs have thinned, the patient is confronted with a permanent chronic malformation of the cervical spine.

Symptoms sometimes begin as pain in the neck or shoulders, but more commonly as pain or tingling in the arm or hand, particularly when the patient tries to sleep at night. These latter symptoms are caused by direct root pressure on the cervical nerves.

The most useful therapy for third-stage afflictions is intermittent motorized traction to the cervical spine, diathermy to the neck, and ultrasound to the whole of the upper back. To these old standbys may now be added home traction in selected patients and the use of the **Low Light Laser** in all patients.

Because the injury is permanent, it is necessary to have the patient return occasionally for maintenance traction therapy after his acute problem has abated. Most patients faithful to this maintenance schedule remain nearly symptom-free.

Parting Words

This discussion of whiplash is based entirely on my personal experience of the last forty years and that of the other physicians at our Healing Research Center. To my knowledge, there has been little research into the pathologic aspects of these three stages. These last forty years, however, have assured me that these stages exist and that they can be treated successfully as I have described. I would like to include, however, a few closing admonitions for those so injured.

If you are ever "rear ended" while riding in an automobile or have any other reason to think you have a whiplash type injury, look for a physician familiar with the methods described here. Don't let anyone convince you that it isn't a serious injury or that your symptoms are imaginary.

If you have been injured, be sure that the accident is properly recorded and that you contact any insurance carriers involved in the case so they can be prepared to cover you properly as early as possible. See to it that a full set of X-Rays of the neck are made shortly following the accident. These will usually not reveal damage at this time but they will allow you to prove that you were normal prior to the accident if later X-Rays show third-stage damage as described above.

Don't settle any whiplash case as long as you have any degree of pain. In our own Center, we don't settle for at least eighteen months to two years after the original accident.

After the whiplash injury, be very careful about who you let adjust your neck. Frequent chiropractic or osteopathic adjustments at this time can be injurious.

If you have a physician who understands the whiplash injury as I have outlined it here, please follow his instructions. Don't think he is being overly cautious if he doesn't want to release you when you think you feel well. Very few patients understand the possible consequences of a whiplash accident.

If your physician doesn't seem to understand or accept the consequences of your accident, give him this chapter to read. If he still isn't interested or doesn't think our presentation valid, find another physician. Your future health and welfare depend on it. Many physicians have been, and still are, so influenced by the literature published by insurance companies that they still can not accept that whiplash is the potentially serious injury it is.

Chapter VI
You and Your Sinuses

The most common ailment seen by physicians is what is generally referred to as an upper respiratory infection. In this category are such things as colds, blocked stuffy noses, congestive deafness, sinus problems, and what in the old days used to be called "catarrh of the head."

I have a personal affinity for this problem, because as a child, I was personally plagued by sinusitis (inflammation of the sinuses). My doting grandmother was greatly pained at seeing her favorite grandson thus afflicted, so beginning at a tender age I was toted from one physician to another. I was washed, drained, injected and baked; and this vaccine and that serum was used on my poor unsuspecting body—all, I might add, to no lasting benefit except to the soothing of my grandmother's conscience.

I remember one physician in particular who was a great favorite of my grandmother. She kept insisting he must know all there was to know about sinus trouble because "he had it all his life." I must have been only ten or so at the time, but I remember thinking even then that if she wanted to take me to a doctor, I'd rather she found one who had cured himself of sinus trouble rather than one who had suffered from it all his life.

My grandmother never gave up; but unfortunately, neither did my sinus trouble. In my late teens, I met my future wife, and she introduced me to a new idea of treatment for my ailment. It was through her and her family that I first became acquainted with natural healing. She suggested that I see a naturopath. Although I wasn't exactly eager at first, I finally consented, assuring myself that he couldn't do much more damage than had already been done by the legion of previous medical practitioners.

His approach was refreshingly new. He spoke of congestion and non-congestive food elements. He talked of constipation problems causing mucosity. We discussed certain treatments designed to build up the integrity of the inflamed and swollen tissues themselves. Through his treatments and the diet he suggested, (Which I have followed with certain modifications ever since) my sinus problems soon vanished and they haven't returned in more than fifty years.

Having suffered from this agonizing condition, it has been easy for me to empathize with my sinus patients, and much of our work at our Healing Research Center is devoted to correcting these cantankerous respiratory difficulties. More patients come to us from great distances for this type of work than for any other we do at our Center with the possible exception of the Chronic Fatigue Syndrome.

I personally was very fortunate in my medical training to have studied under Dr. Frank Finell of Portland, Oregon, who was the only practitioner in the natural healing field to devote his entire practice to eye, ear, nose and throat work. Dr. Finell treated the whole gamut of these cases using only natural methods of therapy. Some of the methods he used were classic in our field; some were developed by colleagues of Dr. Finell, but many were personal discoveries and developments of this devoted man himself. Few of the students he taught really appreciated the uniqueness of his work and, only later, after extensive discussions with our contemporaries, did we, who were his disciples, discover that the methods taught so freely by Dr. Finell were almost unheard of elsewhere. To my knowledge, this is the first time that this important subject has been presented in a publication for the laity. Although it isn't my purpose to present an exhaustive treatise on all the natural treatments for the eye, ear, nose and throat, I will attempt to describe the methods that are most often used at our Center.

Chronic Congestion of the Head

Most chronic catarrh (inflammation of mucous membranes) is manifested as congestion and infection of the sinuses, Eustachian tubes, and nasal and throat membranes. This condition may go under many names: sinusitis, pharyngitis, laryngitis otitis media, and blocked Eustachian tubes, to name a few. The symptoms presented by these difficulties can also be numerous, such as headaches, breathing difficulties, irritations in the nose, sore throats of all sorts, pressure on the ears, tinnitus (ringing in the ears), and pains in the ears.

This problem can occur at any age. We have treated patients two months old, and we've also done endonasal work on some in their late nineties. The condition can be acute, such as a cold with its attendant after effects; or chronic, in which the symptoms, though perhaps not as extreme as in the acute form, do not abate but persist for weeks, months and even years.

The various anti-allergy agents and decongestants may prove useful to patients in the early stages of the acute form, but once the condition has become chronic, which it does all too often, medical science has little to offer in the way of a true cure. This last statement is not mere opinion but is admitted by many physicians in this field. Sam E. Roberts, M.D., associate professor of otolaryngology at the University of Kansas School of Medicine, says this:*

---

*Roberts. S. E.: *Ear. Nose and Throat Dysfunctions due to Deficiencies and Imbalances.*

"I have practiced medicine for almost half a century. For twenty-five years my methods were strictly orthodox, just as I was taught. During that quarter of a century, I viewed each patient as a candidate for surgery of some sort; my thinking stopped just there." (There are many well-meaning, sincere surgeons whose thinking still stops just there! It means one thing—faulty teaching.)

"At the end of this twenty-five year period, I weighed my accomplishments and found them wanting. For months I kept a daily tabulation of my patients' progress. The observations were recorded under four headings: (1) those really helped, (2) those for whom I did little to relieve their troubles, (3) those for whom nothing could be done with our present store of knowledge and (4) those who were made worse by surgery.

"There were far too many patients in the last three classifications. The foregoing critical self-analysis is suggested for all branches of medicine and surgery.

"If it were positively known how many surgical procedures could have been avoided had all physiologic dysfunctions been carefully investigated and given adequate therapy, the revelation would be shocking. Equally shocking would be the facts as to how many patients are now in hospitals and mental institutions who in the beginning had only physiologic and easily correctable dysfunctions."

Dr. Roberts, although not the first, was probably one of the most thorough men of the orthodox medical profession to study the nonsurgical methods of correcting ear, nose, and throat difficulties. He goes on to say:

"Many patients with acoustic, ocular, cardia, and scores of other dysfunctions—including nervous and even mental disorders—with negative laboratory findings, are too frequently categorically classified as 'Irreversible.' Little thought is given to the possibility of arresting or reversing these dysfunctions, thereby preventing further degenerative tissue changes.

"Since I have frequently been profoundly astonished by finding dysfunctions somewhat reversible which I had previously considered irreversible, I now hesitate to give a dour prognosis without a vigorous therapeutic effort to help the patient."

Chronic Upper Respiratory Difficulties

In treating both acute and chronic ear, nose, and throat (ENT) cases, we usually divide treatment into two basic areas— first, treatment the patient must do himself, and second, treatment that can be given only by a knowledgeable natural healer with the proper equipment. In the long run, the first type of treatment is just as important or even more important than the treatment he receives from the physician. No matter how skillfully the physician does his work, unless the patient does his part, the condition will return. After healing the sick, Jesus would leave them with this admonition: "Go thy way and sin no more lest a worse thing come upon thee." It is possible for us at the Healing Research Center to correct almost any form of ENT difficulty; however, if the patient doesn't stick to the maintenance program we outline (to go his way and sin no more), the same or a similar problem will usually appear in the future.

What the Patient Must Do

The most important factor the patient can use to correct or control these problems is diet. Most ENT problems stem from a diet consisting of too many sugars and carbohydrates and an insufficient amount of fruits, vegetables and protein of high biologic quality. In the beginning of our treatment, we also restrict dairy products because these tend to produce mucous and congestion. Cottage cheese, yogurt and to some extent, buttermilk seem to have less of a tendency than the other dairy products and, therefore, are allowed to patients in limited quantities after the more congestive stages of the disability are corrected. Egg yolks also have a low congestive tendency in comparison with the white and they are allowed at this later stage as well. Dairy products that combine milk and sugar, such as ice cream, are particularly bad for these conditions, as are most hard cheeses, because of their concentrated food elements. The food allotment, in the acute stage, should consist mainly of fruits, vegetables (both raw and cooked) lean meat, fish, seafood, and herb teas. As the condition improves, the patient may add small amounts of yogurt, cottage cheese (as natural as possible) and good whole grain products.

Other dairy products are allowed in small amounts after the severe symptoms are controlled in patients who aren't sensitive to them; even here it is important that the patient attempt to obtain milk that is raw, preferably certified, and also to use other dairy products that are as natural as possible. Even though I can't give specific scientific evidence to prove that pasteurized or processed dairy products are more congesting, forty years of private practice has satisfied me on this subject.

As the patient improves with treatment, some of the more healthful starches can be brought back into his diet. Products such as natural brown rice, baked potato, small amounts of whole-grain breads, whole-grain cereals, honey and natural raw sugar may be added. These must, however, be regulated in amounts and, even with the most successful case, should not be allowed to exceed the recommendations in our Basic Health Maintenance Diet. It is nearly impossible to correct these ailments without attention to a corrective diet, though only rarely is diet sufficient to elicit a cure by itself.

Almost all such problems require a specific amount of local treatment and nutritional supplementation to bring about their proper resolution. The main function of the diet is to prevent a recurrence of the inflammatory congestive process once it has been removed by specific natural therapeutic treatments.

What the Physician Must Do

The most useful single form of local treatment for these catarrh problems is *endonasal therapy*. This is the basic treatment used to initiate the draining and cleansing processes necessary to remove the congestion common to all these difficulties. With a twinkle in his eye Dr. Finell used to refer to this procedure as "finger technique." In a moment you will see why this truly heroic therapy goes by such a rather plain and ignoble title.

Behind the nose and up above the tonsils is a small indentation called the "fossa of Rosenmuller" (Fig. 8). In this area the proximal end of the Eustachian tube opens into the throat. The Eustachian tube begins in the middle ear, passing downward, to come to an end in this fossa (Fig. 9). Owing to the nature of the surface anatomy and of the draining pathways of the mucus, the fossa of Rosenmuller invariably becomes clogged with this draining fluid in catarrhal conditions.

With the passage of time, the material that accumulates in this small cavity solidifies and becomes jelly-like. In this stage, it may clog the opening of the Eustachian tube and even some of the sinus drain tubes. In time the accumulated material becomes harder; both small capillaries and adhesions may form in this mass as time goes on. I find the accumulation of this material in this vital area of the nasal pharynx is one of the most consistent causes of ENT difficulties. Until this deposit is removed, no case of sinus or related disease will be corrected permanently. Such disorders may be alleviated by other therapies, but they will return again and again until this accumulation is eliminated.

Because of this material's placement at the end of the Eustachian tube, its persistent pressure can cause catarrhal afflictions of the ear. Many cases of partial deafness and tinnitus can be corrected only by the removal of this material. Many cases of recurring earaches in children and others are immediately alleviated by attention to this deposit. The procedure for its removal takes less than three minutes. Often the improvement is immediate and if a patient follows the proper dietary instructions, the procedure almost never needs to be repeated. If sinus sufferers knew what help is available to them through this method, I would never have time for any other therapy. I know of no other therapy that is so quickly done and yet so thorough and long-lasting.

This therapy has been around for some time, but unfortunately it is little used, even by those trained in its techniques. Perhaps, like some other good therapies (colonic irrigations, for example), it is considered messy and troublesome in execution and for this reason many physicians have avoided it. A second reason for its rare use may be that a certain amount of skill and dexterity is needed in its proper execution, but not more than that required by many other medical procedures

The mechanics of the treatment consist of passing into the open mouth a rubber-cotted forefinger, which is carefully advanced between the uvula and the tonsil, passing up behind the soft palate. By turning the hand to the side, the fossa of Rosenmuller is found. A careful but rapid examination of the area is made with the finger. If deposits of mucoid material are found, they are removed with an agile sweep of the finger-tip. As the hand is removed, the adjoining areas are gently massaged and the soft palate is pulled, or "sprung" as Dr. Finell like to refer to it. The hand is then removed, and the procedure for that side is complete. The patient is given some time to enable the freed material to drain from this side and then the other side is done. The entire procedure is finished in just under three minutes. The actual time the finger is within the nasal pharynx is about six seconds. In addition to this basic technique, we use many modifications at our Healing Research Center that make the procedure more effective and comfortable. To best show these nuances, let me describe the procedure exactly as we give it in our Center.

The patient is first given **chlorophyll nebulization**—a therapy in which water-soluble chlorophyll is placed in a standard glass nebulizer, which in turn is activated by a tank of oxygen. For about ten minutes the patient breathes in this aerosol through the nose. This chlorophyll-oxygen compound is very healing and helps decongest the tissues without using the usual decongesting drugs, which tend to have a rebound congesting effect after their primary use is finished.

After chlorophyll-oxygen nebulization, the patient is prepared for surgery. He is given a plastic pan to hold containing a small amount of water and beside him two glasses of hot water are placed—one salted and one plain. If the patient wears artificial dentures or elaborate removable bridgework, these are removed before the operative procedure begins. The physician then wets his cotted finger in the glass of plain

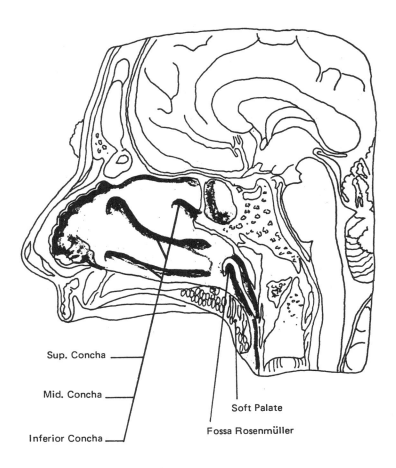

Sup. Concha

Mid. Concha

Inferior Concha

Soft Palate

Fossa Rosenmüller

Figure 8

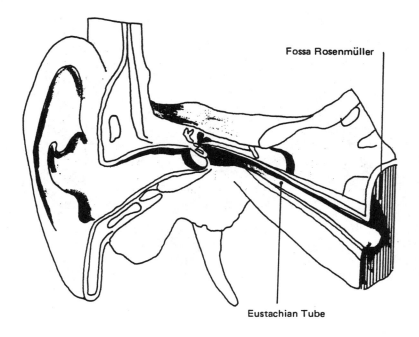

Fossa Rosenmüller

Eustachian Tube

Figure 9

100

water, gently enfolds the patient's head with his free arm and proceeds with removal of the congested material as previously described. As soon as he is finished, the patient is given the glass of hot salt water to gargle. In some patients, large amounts of accumulated mucoid material will come out almost immediately; in others, who will benefit just as much by the treatment, almost no discharge is immediately evident. Some of these eliminate the material later and in a few it passes out the nasal passages.

After a short wait, the other side is also corrected, with the foregoing procedure repeated. After this therapy, the patient is again given the chlorophyll-oxygen nebulization, which now helps allay any minor irritation caused by the procedure. After nebulization, the patient is given a cleansing diet and specific nutritional products to help return his chronic inflamed mucous membrane to normal. He is then discharged with the admonition to gargle with hot salted water if there is any soreness in the throat following the procedure.

Although not exactly pleasant, the procedure is not particularly painful. It is over in a few seconds and there is little discomfort afterwards. There is less distress to endonasal work than there is to filling a tooth. A few moments of discomfort in a properly executed endonasal procedure can mean months and years of freedom from severe pain and suffering. All too often we are offered situations that subject us to years of regret and suffering for a few moments of pleasure. It is refreshing to find something that gives us a reverse choice.

The Character of the Endonasal Procedure

When Dr. Finell discoursed enthusiastically on this procedure in class, most of us considered it the ravings of a near-senile old man. Only years of experience and my own medical maturity have proven to me that, if anything, Finell was conservative in his praise. It is difficult to estimate the full beneficial ramifications of this therapeutic measure. Besides cleaning out the congestion in the fossa of Rosenmuller, this treatment revitalizes all the tissues of the nasal pharynx. Many congestions and inflammations of the upper respiratory tract not directly connected with the Eustachian tube or the fossa often respond to this therapy. Even eye problems are often improved when congestive orbital pressure is removed by its use.

I originally used endonasal therapy only on a select group of sinus problems. Other upper respiratory conditions were treated by more traditional natural means. A reappraisal of my work showed, however, that disorders for which the "finger technique" was not used very commonly recurred and an honest cure could not be claimed. In recent years, endonasal therapy has become almost routine for ENT cases in our Center, and the rate of satisfactory recovery has been higher than at any previous time.

Follow-Up Treatment

The endonasal procedure is only the beginning of the curative process in chronic ENT problems. Once these vital passages are cleared, they must be drained and kept open, and the tissues returned to their normal tone and vitality. This work should begin a day or two after the original surgery. At this time, the patient is once again given chlorophyll nebulization, after which a special form of oxygen called Octozone is instilled via the nostrils up into the nasal pharynx and sinus areas. After Octozone instillation into the nasal pharynx, there is a mild burning sensation from the membranes, similar to that caused by placing a weak antiseptic on a wound. The action is very similar, for in this type of a concentration, the oxygen released from the Octozone acts as an effective stimulant and antiseptic. The main purpose of the Octozone, however, is to liquify old accumulated mucus so that the body can more easily eliminate it. Sometimes the patient may appear to be catching a cold. He is not, the Octozone has merely produced a healing crisis in his nasal passages. A healing crisis is an acute reaction created in a chronic condition to stimulate the body's inflammatory mechanism to heal the old ailment.

The common cold is an example of a disease crisis. We have here a virus infection in which the body reacts to an inflammatory state to such an extent that the inflamed tissues involved are rapidly and completely regenerated. Therefore, at the end of a properly handled cold, one is just as healthy or perhaps even healthier (if naturopathic theory is correct) than he was at the beginning of the acute episode. In a chronic ailment, however, a low-grade inflammatory or degenerative state is present that the body is not able to correct unaided. And therefore a sort of cold war is established between the body and this offending pathologic condition. The condition is not strong enough to destroy the body, but the body is not strong enough to cast off the offending ailment.

We in natural healing believe it possible to stimulate the body to produce a healing inflammatory reaction in chronic ailments that enables the inflamed tissues to return to a normal state. It is difficult to do this with all conditions, but it is accomplished in many and in ENT congestion our batting average is near a thousand.

After the Octozone has worked a few minutes, the patient is again given chlorophyll nebulization to act as a soothing agent. At this time in our treatment, we often use a special diathermy (Magnatherm) treatment to stimulate tissue regeneration.

Now that we have the *MicroLight 830* low level laser this treatment is also used to help reduce the inflammation of these conditions. As in all the other things treated by this modality the results have been very rewarding.

Manipulative therapy (chiropractic and osteopathic) is also helpful, as is selective massage therapy over the affected sinuses. This last therapy is not well known but has proven most effective at our Center. In performing this treatment, a thin layer of olive oil is first put over the cheeks and forehead. The physician then uses the tips of his thumbs to gently but thoroughly massage these surfaces. Of particular interest is the area just below the eyes, for nerve centers there help drain the maxillary sinuses (in the cheek bones). Many sinus difficulties are centered in this area, and drainage and resolution can be greatly encouraged by correct massage treatments.

Endonasal therapy is usually performed only once but the other treatments are continued until the membranes are no longer sensitive to the Octozone and the patient is basically symptom-free. When he is finally discharged, he is encouraged to follow a rational low-stress, low-congestion diet to avoid recurrence. Where patients have been even moderately faithful in this admonition, most have remained symptom-free for many years.

Some patients may require variations of this fundamental endonasal therapy because of the specific manifestation of their problems or coexisting problems unrelated to the ENT condition.

Hearing Problems

The endonasal procedure may be used successfully for hearingdifficulties and ear noises. In these cases, the basic therapy is accompanied by regular Magnatherm treatments to the ears and tissues of the repair system. Also we now are using the Low Level Laser on these conditions as well. Specific herbal and homeopathic remedies designed to help the regeneration of the Eustachian tube, middle ear and tympanic membrane (eardrum) are also prescribed. Both deafness and ear noises may come from a variety of causes; however, we have a sufficiently high percentage of response to the endonasal therapy to make its use worthwhile in most cases. Even though we can't guarantee success in these conditions by the use of this therapy, I can not remember one case in which the patient was not helped to some degree. This is also true in cases diagnosed specifically as nerve deafness. I don't want to imply that the diagnosing physician has been incorrect, but we find in most cases of nerve deafness that some congestive deafness aggravates the condition. By the use of our basic treatment, this congestive component can be diminished and the patient thereby improved.

This same multiple cause may also exist in tinnitus. Almost any injury to the eardrum or auditory nerve can cause forms of tinnitus. However, many of these are complicated by congestive pathologic conditions; when these are corrected, the tinnitus improves, even though its primary cause may not have been overcome.

Our success in such cases, however, suggests another possible reason for the improvements. The effects of endonasal treatment are far more widespread than can be accounted for by the simple mechanical congestion removal. It is my personal feeling, after many years of using this therapy, that there may ensue a revitalization of the auditory nerve itself, plus other nerves in this area, which may account for the success we find in many of our patients. I know that it is a medical axiom that nerves, once damaged, do not readily regenerate, but I remember what Dr. Roberts said in his book on ear, nose and throat work. He found, as have others, that many things that supposedly can't be regenerated do regenerate. Dr. Clymer said to me many years ago, "There is only one sure road to failure, only one sure way to not help a patient and that is to never try." So I sincerely suggest that those readers who may be troubled with hearing and tinnitus problems look into constructive endonasal treatment. I have never yet known a case made worse by this therapy and I have known thousands made better.

Polyps and Allergies

Allergies of all forms are common in our practice, and many allergies produce symptoms of the ear, nose and throat (ENT) system. Although many allergies respond well to endonasal therapy, most of these patients also have the hypoadrenal syndrome or hypoglycemia. Unless this systemic defect is treated (see Chapter II), no permanent improvement of the allergy can be expected.

At Woodlands Medical Center we have developed procedures for ascertaining and correcting specific allergies and this work is often essential to help some of these patients.(See Chapter XXIII)

Nasal polyps is a rather common and resistant condition. The polyps usually result from an allergy that weakens the wall of the nasal mucous membrane causing ballooning of this wall followed by a filling of the sack with a clear liquid. These polyps sometimes become large enough to completely occlude the nasal passages, making nose breathing almost impossible.

Although polyps are generally easily removed surgically, they have a nasty habit of returning rapidly because the cause hasn't been found and removed. We have had patients whose polyps have been removed twelve or more times with no real curative results.

Polyps usually should be treated somewhat similarly to regular allergies, with a careful check of the adrenal and sugar levels. We have found, however, that even when all known methods of therapy are utilized, the polyps are often resistant to treatment. We have had extremely good results with the use of certain specific homeopathic remedies in these cases. Thuja, in the proper dosage, has proven invaluable in preventing polyp recurrence after surgery and even in causing polyps to regress in many patients who haven't required surgery.

We are now beginning to see what the **MicroLight 830** will do for polyps. As this is written we have not enough experience to say whether this therapy will help or not. If you have polyps ask your physician at our Centers, by the time you read this we should have more information on the Laser treatment of this condition.

Lymphatic Swelling

A rather enigmatic problem often encountered is that of the patient who complains of chronic sensitive, swollen glands. We have found many diverse reasons for this condition, from the patient who had cat-scratch fever and nearly died, to one with a salivary stone caught in one of the ducts. Most cases, however, are due to a toxic condition of the general system, which responds to an eliminative diet such as suggested for endonasal conditions. Herbal therapy using our special herbal remedy known as EMP-Plus and specific nutritional support, particularly that with elements of the RNA and DNA factors from the various lymphatic substances, is usually very helpful in these patients.

These swollen glands are inflamed lymph glands. The lymphatic system is one of the most outrageously disregarded functioning systems in our body. The lymph is a very important substance that helps keep our body in a healthy, normal state, yet it has been almost entirely ignored by the medical orthodoxy. I believe that some day a bright-eyed medical researcher will suddenly discover the lymphatic system and through his discoveries a whole new form of therapy will be instituted. But even then, this man—so far ahead of his time—will still be about seventy-five years behind the natural therapist.

Other specific therapies are used in our Clinic for treating ailments of the ear, nose and throat, but because each is specific for the patient involved, it is not practical to discuss them here. I can say, however, that natural therapy has great hope to offer sufferers of ENT difficulties, so don't let a discouraging medical prognosis keep you from investigating the possibility of natural therapy. In the whole field of medicine, no other group of disorders seems to respond so poorly to orthodox treatment and yet so well to natural therapeutics as does this group.

The Eye

Dr. Finell devoted many years of his life to the treatment of eye conditions. He would travel across the country to see a man purported to have a new treatment for glaucoma or cataract. He also did much work using the Bates method of eye care, in which use of eyeglasses was replaced with eye exercises and visual training. We have attempted to carry on his work in this field at the Beverly Hall Corporation Healing Research Center. We don't say that we have a specific cure for cataracts, although we have many patients with this condition who seem most satisfied with our care. Many local eye specialists can't understand why some of their patients are doing as well as they are. They can't explain why some patients' cataracts that are supposed to get progressively worse are getting better. These patients, of course, don't tell their physicians they are also visiting us at the same time they are under their care.

Sight Without Glasses

The Bates method of sight without glasses has been utilized by our Center since its inception. We use it not so much to encourage people to get rid of eyeglasses but rather to correct the basic eye strain that often precipitates need for them. We endeavor to remove the strain, not the glasses. We teach various exercises to relax the whole ocular mechanism, and the results have been most encouraging. Such treatment has proven useful, not only for eye difficulties, but also for many other apparently unrelated nervous problems. The eye, because of its natural sensitivity, is one of the first organs to show signs of bodily strain and stress. If we take this as a warning signal and begin to treat the nervous condition at the first sign of these early warnings, it is possible to prevent many far more dangerous problems. Chapter 18 is entirely devoted to the Bates method of eye care, and the system is explained in detail there.

In summary, I wish to reiterate the success of natural therapies in eye, ear, nose and throat problems. The orthodox treatment for most chronic ailments in this area has been surgery, but it has only rarely produced satisfactory longterm results. Patients willing to give natural therapy a fair trial very rarely must go for surgery. So I leave you with this optimistic note. Nearly 95 per cent of eye, ear, nose and throat patients respond successfully to natural therapy. The odds are in your favor. Why not try it?

Chapter VII
Miracle Healing With Photons

One of the latest healing advances at our Centers is a miniature marvel known as the **MicroLight 830** low level laser. This unit is at the time this is being written still in the efficacy investigation stage, though I expect that by the time you read this it will be fully approved by the FDA. At this time we are a part of the investigational team assessing the therapeutic advantages of this treatment. Before we give you some of our own experience with this unit, which I affectionately call "the world's most expensive flashlight," we want you to hear from Dr. David G. Williams who had an opportunity to evaluate the **MicroLight 830** before us.

The nature of this therapy and the various conditions that it is designed to treat are discussed in the following articles that first appeared in the newsletter, *ALTERNATIVES*, by Dr. David G. Williams.

"If you've ever watched an episode of the old science fiction television show *Star Trek*, or its newer spin-off, *Star Trek, The Next Generation*, you'll undoubtedly remember how simple and quickly health problems were eliminated.

"Regardless of the problem, the futuristic doctors treated each patient by simply holding a small device directly over the afflicted area. I'm not sure if the little playing-card sized device emitted some kind of gas, electromagnetic waves, or what. I just know the patient quickly got well and there was never any cutting, bleeding or removal of organs or tissue. Hey, it was just a television program. Nobody could actually develop such a device. That's what I thought, anyway, until a couple of months ago.

"For the last several months, I've been investigating a small flashlight-looking device that will probably revolutionize certain segments of health care as we know them today. A small company near Houston, Texas has developed a portable, infrared, low energy cold laser device that has demonstrated remarkable healing powers. The unit was created by Lasermedics, 13600 Murphy Road, Stafford, TX 77477 at (713) 261-5079.

"Lasers have been around for quite some time now. In the medical field surgeons have been using them to cut, burn and vaporize unwanted tissue. Dentists are starting to use lasers instead of mechanical drills. All of these that create enough heat to burn or vaporize tissue are all high energy lasers or what is referred to as High Reactive-Level Laser Therapy (HLLT).

"Lasermedics' unit is different. It doesn't cut, burn or vaporize tissue. It falls under the category of Low Reactive-Level Laser Therapy (LLLT). A little technical background will help you better understand the unique healing ability of LLLT.

"Although I think the following information concerning light is one of the most exciting and useful health topics today, if you're not into details you can skip the next few paragraphs. If you stick with me I promise not to get too technical (When I do I usually end up getting more confused than anybody else).]

"Most of us have a pretty poor understanding of light. Since it's something we can't touch or feel we don't give it much thought. All light is actually electromagnetic waves. The color of the light or whether we even see it or not depends on the length of the wave or wavelength. Any light with a wavelength between 400 nanometers (nm) and 700 nm is visible to the human eye. This is called the visual spectrum. (Nanometers, by the way aren't very long. A meter is 39.37 inches, or a little over a yard. A nanometer is one-billionth of a meter!)

"Generally speaking, the smaller the wavelength the greater its ability to penetrate tissue. In the chart to the left you can see that ultraviolet rays, x-rays, gamma and cosmic rays all fall below visible light on the electromagnetic spectrum. But infrared rays, microwaves, television, FM and AM radio waves have much longer wavelengths.

"What most people don't understand is that light and all electromagnetic energy travels as bundles of energy called photons. (This is where things start to get a little difficult.)

"If you recall anything from your high school chemistry class you may remember that the center or nucleus of an atom contains neutrons and protons. The nucleus is surrounded by electrons moving in specific orbits. Energy in the form of photons are released when the electrons change orbits. It is these weightless bundles of energy called photons that trigger biological changes within the body.

"While random photons from ordinary light sources are constantly bombarding the surface of our skin, lasers have the ability to "concentrate" these photons. Photons from ordinary light are emitted in all different directions. In contrast most of the photons emitted from a laser are in perfect order and follow the same path. The effects of the energy released from a laser depend on several factors. The wavelength and the wattage output of the laser are two of these factors.

"Some high energy lasers are absorbed by water within the skin, making their penetration very shallow. Others will penetrate several hundredths of an inch and vaporize any tissue in their path. And low energy laser devices are designed to penetrate deep within tissues (by utilizing a different wavelength) without causing any heat or tissue damage (by operating at very low power settings).

"Lasermedics' device operates at 830 nanometers and at the low energy output of only 30 milliwatts. This allows the photons to penetrate over an inch deep (3 centimeters) without any danger of tissue damage or destruction. If you've stayed with me so far, you're probably wondering: 'Who cares? What good are these worthless little bags of energy called photons anyway?' "

The Magic of Photons

"All life on this planet is dependent upon light energy (photons) derived from the sun. The sun's energy is first captured when the chlorophyll molecules in plants absorb photons. This energy is then used in the process of photosynthesis to create glucose and oxygen.

"Through the consumption of plants, animals (this includes all humans, not just wild apes, wildebeests and your in-laws) are able to release the energy stored in glucose.

"We also receive energy directly from the sun, independent of our food supply. And even though the amount we receive is far less than that which comes from food, it is essential for good health.

"The sun's photons, which strike the skin directly, convert a form of cholesterol into vitamin D. Studies have shown that vitamin D deficiencies lead to osteoporosis and result in increased fractures of the hip and spine. Dr. Holik of Tufts University found that 30% of the elderly who experience hip fractures are deficient in vitamin D. And 50% of those evaluated in New England nursing homes were deficient in vitamin D during the winter months.

"Low levels of vitamin D have also been linked to increased rates of both breast and colon cancer (Med Trib 89;30:[30]1).

"Photons also enter the body through the eye. These are absorbed by several different light-sensitive chemicals like rhodopsin. Rhodopsin transfers these power bundles to the crucial little energy factories inside cells called mitochondria. Through an intricate pathway this energy is transferred to the pineal gland—a small pine cone shaped structure located exactly in the center of the head.

"The pineal gland is the "master gland" of the body. Based on both the amount of light energy absorbed by the body and the particular cyclic pattern of the Earth's magnetic field, the pineal functions as our biological clock and regulates the operations of all the other glands in the body. We now know it controls other glands by releasing dozens of regulating chemical substances plus several major neuro-hormones like dopamine, melatonin and serotonin. Understandably, an imbalance in the amount and intensity of light energy reaching the body can lead to disastrous effects."

What Photons Do Inside the Body

"Before photons (light energy) can produce any effect they must be absorbed into the body. Then, regardless of how they were absorbed, three events can take place when their energy is released.

"1. Heat can be generated. The more energy liberated, the higher our body temperature becomes. Any increase in activity, such as exercise, requires the release of additional energy which warms the body. (On the other hand, drinking beer while watching television conserves energy, but it makes your feet get cold.)

"2. Another photon with less energy can be released. Our bodies aren't 100% efficient in their use of energy (no living organisms are). As such, some of the energy escapes. This leakage of energy is continuous and contributes to the energy field that surrounds all living organisms. This energy field has also been referred to as the aura.

"3. Photons can trigger a long list of cellular changes which fall under the heading of photobiostimulation. The ability to place these photons exactly where they're needed and elicit these cellular changes will make laser therapy one of the most advanced forms of healing ever discovered.

"I need to make one thing clear before I continue. Keep in mind that whenever I mention laser therapy (or more precisely Low Reactive-Level Laser Therapy or LLLT), it's actually photons I'm talking about. Lasers are simply tools that create photons. Next time you see your doctor and mention you've become interested in photon therapy he or she will probably have no idea what you're talking about. On the other hand, while most doctors don't know about LLLT, they have heard of lasers.

"When I first started checking into LLLT, I was very skeptical. From the reports I was receiving it appeared to cure almost everything. And it's been my experience that when a therapy or product reportedly cures everything, it generally cures nothing. LLLT is a noted exception.

"From first hand experience, I can tell you LLLT is a miraculous healing tool that on the surface seems contradictory. It can alleviate the sensation of pain, but it can also bring back a sense of feeling in areas that have gone numb. It can remove overgrown scar tissue or it can stimulate tissue growth. It can remove excess pigment, but it also restores pigment in areas where needed. It can activate healing components within the immune system, but also decrease the body's sometimes harmful inflammation response. The beauty of LLLT is that its photons normalize tissue. Photons do this by activating enzymes.

"Enzymes are molecules that speed up the chemical reactions among other substances without itself being destroyed or used up in the process. By directly triggering enzymes the power of photons is multiplied by thousands through a domino-type effect. One photon can activate a single enzyme which in turn triggers a chemical reaction, which triggers another and another, etc.

"And with LLLT there have been no adverse side-effects noted. It apparently has no effect on normal tissue. It seems to act much like a nutrient. Photons will only be absorbed by the cells that need help. If a cell is functioning normally, no benefit will be observed from LLLT."

Specific Conditions Being Treated

"The full FDA approval process for Lasermedics' **MicroLight 830** is expected to be completed in the near future. Safety trials have already been completed and the LLLT has been found to have no adverse effects. Selected doctors around the country are now allowed to use these units for treatment to determine the breadth of their effectiveness. These trials under an investigative license from the FDA. If you are interested in this treatment contact one of these physicians to see if your problem falls into the parameters of this program. (We at the Healing Research Center are now an official investigator for this therapy.)

"I have personally had the opportunity to use Lasermedics' portable laser unit, the **MicroLight 830**,.for several weeks. I have seen chronic arthritic joint pain (duration of three years) disappear after one 3 minute treatment period. The same results have been achieved with shoulder, neck, knee and lower back pain.

"I have also conducted interviews with several of the doctors who have been testing these units in their practices for the last year or so. Each of the doctors I've spoken with had nothing but the most glowing reports for LLLT.

"Dentists have used the instrument for dry socket problems, gum disease and temporal mandibular joint (TMJ) disorders. Others have used it on keloids and scar tissue, torn knee cartilage, 2nd and 3rd degree burns, surgical and open wounds, damaged nerves, headaches, sinus problems, strains, sprains and athletic injuries.

"One of the fastest growing complaints in this country today, carpal tunnel syndrome (CTS), responds to the laser as well. CTS is caused by repetitive motion and trauma to the median nerve passing through the wrist. Assembly line workers are particularly prone to the problem. The automotive giant General Motors has found that 25% of its workers' compensation cost is from repetitive stress injuries like CTS. The standard medical treatment for CTS is still surgery, which has a dismal success rate of less than 10%. Dr. Wayne Good, the plant physician at General Motors' Flint Assembly, has treated close to 600 patients with LLLT and achieved positive results in over 70% of the patients. He is in the process of submitting his results for publication as further studies continue.

"Photobiotherapy will become one of the premiere healing tools of our future. It will eliminate the need for many of today's common surgical procedures. I can see the day when every household in this country will have an LLLT unit on hand. When used properly, it is a safe, effective, natural therapy for a wide variety of health problems. Until this happens I wanted you to be aware of an extremely effective therapy that, in many cases, could very well eliminate the necessity of surgery and the dangers associated with it.

"Photobiotherapy is nothing new. It is as old as the sun itself. Harnessing and refining this therapy through the use of "tuned" lasers is new, and can enhance, rather than oppose, the body's own innate healing powers."

The Invisible Healing Light

"About a year and a half ago, I covered a therapy that I considered to be a real breakthrough in natural healing: Low Reactive-Level Laser Therapy (LLLT). Based on research at that time, I was surprised that the national media hadn't picked up on the story and alerted the public. Even more surprising is the fact that LLLT still remains practically unknown among health professionals, despite continuing evidence of its effectiveness in a wide range of health problems. Numerous readers have reported getting excellent results using LLLT and hundreds of others have been asking for an update. I can tell you, since I last reported, a lot has been happening with LLLT.

"In that earlier report, I thought the FDA would quickly approve the use and sale of the **MicroLight 830**, the laser unit being tested and manufactured by Lasermedics. Although the FDA has approved its use, they haven't yet given the manufacturer the go ahead to market it freely. Let me share some of the latest research involving this unique apparatus.

"I originally referred to LLLT as Star Trek medicine. This was a reference to the almost magical healing properties of a small, playing-card sized device used on the television show Star Trek. By simply holding this device over a wound or injured body part, the patient would

112

experience almost immediate healing. The more we learn about LLLT the more it seems to work like the Star Trek device.

"I'm not going to go through the detailed explanation of exactly what LLLT is or how it appears to work, since I covered that earlier. Suffice it to say that LLLT involves a device that focuses light energy in the form of photons. It delivers them to cells and organs over an inch or so below the skin without any tissue damage whatsoever. These photons have the unique ability to stimulate healing in damaged cells."

An Effective Treatment For Carpal Tunnel Syndrome

"Much of the original work with LLLT involved its usefulness in treating the condition called carpal tunnel syndrome (CTS). CTS is a condition involving the inflammation of the median nerve in the wrist. It is a type of repetitive motion injury. In other words, certain wrist movements that are performed over and over can irritate the tendons and nerves that pass through the bony tunnel of the wrist. Once the nerve becomes inflamed, symptoms like pain, numbness, tingling or a complete loss of feeling in the fingers, hand and arm are not uncommon.

"CTS is just one of many problems low reactive-level laser therapy (LLLT) treats effectively. I've seen it eliminate chronic muscle and joint pain in a matter of minutes. It can dramatically speed up the healing of wounds, strains, sprains, burns, athletic injuries, headaches, chronic skin ulcers and gum disease. Dentists are using the instrument to treat dry socket and temporal mandibular joint (TMJ) disorders. Researchers at St. Joseph Hospital in Houston, Texas, have even used the laser unit to treat Peyronie's disease."

New Hope For Peyronie's Disease

"Peyronie's disease is an inflammatory reaction, accompanied by the formation of hard fibrous tissue, that occurs in the penis. It results in painful erections and often times, a severe distortion of the penis. Standard medical therapies like surgery, or steroid or hormone injections, are generally unsuccessful. When treated with LLLT, however, eight of the eleven patients in a recent study showed significant improvement. The patients were only treated for a period of five weeks. Following that, many of the patients' problems began to return. Considering the nature of the problem, it might be necessary to continue the treatment for longer periods of time. The fact that any improvement at all was achieved is in itself remarkable. I don't know of any other therapy that has shown such positive results in that high of a percentage of Peyronie's patients.

"Studies are also underway by members of the Harvard University orthopedic department at Massachusetts General Hospital to determine the effects of LLLT on damaged cartilage cells. Early information indicates that LLLT appears to stimulate the regeneration of cartilage cells. Currently, tests are being conducted in vitro, using cartilage cells from cattle. In the next four to six months, these researchers hope to be conducting those same tests involving human cells. If the preliminary results are any indication of what will happen in human cells, LLLT could revolutionize the way arthritis is treated. The ability to regenerate cartilage would be an unparalleled medical breakthrough. Rest assured, I'll keep you up to date as we receive additional information.

"Using a special dental attachment on the laser, researchers at the famous Beckman Laser Institute, in California, have been able to prevent mucositis in radiation-treated cancer patients. Dr. Petra Wildersmith, who heads the study, will be reporting the results early next year. Laser therapy was given to twelve patients prior to their undergoing radiation therapy to the head and neck area. In all but two patients, the therapy prevented the patients from developing mucositis. Mucositis is a painful, severe inflammation of the membranes lining the mouth and throat. The problem which stems from the radiation therapy interferes with the patient's ability to eat or drink. The discovery that laser therapy can prevent the problem will be a godsend to thousands of cancer patients worldwide."

Lasers and Human Energy Fields

"In my first report, I gave a pretty detailed explanation of how light energy, in the form of energy packets called photons, promotes healing in the body. The ideas I presented have been well researched and documented; however, the idea that an invisible light can promote healing still mystifies most people. This is especially true in the Western cultures.

"In the Far East, it is common knowledge that living cells emit a form of energy or life force. For hundreds of years, acupuncturists have treated all kinds of diseases by balancing and harmonizing this energy. Many Westerners, however, continued to doubt the existence of this so-called "Life force" until the 1960's, when newer technology enabled researchers to demonstrate that living cells emit coherent light energy called Biophotons." (Popp FA, Electromagnetic Bio-Information. Baltimore, MD: Urban and Schwarzenberg: 1989.)

"When a group of cells are functioning in harmony, they emit biophotons (light energy) at the same wavelength and rhythm. When there is damage or disease, this harmony is lost. This phenomenon has been observed and recorded by individuals "sensitive" to these subtle en-

114

ergies throughout history.

"These biophotons or packets of light, have been referred to as "Ch'i" or "Qi" by the Chinese. Acupuncturists balance "life force" or the yin and the yang. Jewish theosophy refers to the energy as Astral lights. Christian paintings often portray Jesus and other religious figures surrounded by a light energy. Native Americans and other cultures around the world have reported observing these energy fields. Count Wilhelm Von Reichenbach called it the "odic" force. Wilhelm Reich named it the "orgone." Under a cloak of secrecy, the Russians conducted a considerable amount of research on the subject of subtle energies. Many of their findings are just now being released to the scientific community. In a future issue I hope to go into more detail concerning their work. For purposes of this report, suffice it to say that they have clearly demonstrated that the human body releases energy from its "biofield" at frequencies between 300 and 2,000 nanometers.

"What makes this energy even more interesting, is the fact that it conforms to two laws of physics: sympathetic resonance and harmonic inductance. If this sounds too technical, bear with me. It's really not. You've probably seen these laws of physics demonstrated with tuning forks. After you strike a tuning fork, other tuning forks in close proximity will begin to vibrate at the same frequency and give off the same sound. In much the same way, diseased tissue or unbalanced groups of cells in your body can be brought back into harmony when exposed to the proper wavelength of energy.

"The MicroLight 830 laser unit emits photons at a frequency of 830 nanometers, which is apparently an effective wavelength for balancing the abnormal energy patterns associated with several conditions. These photons have been shown to activate enzymes, but only in cells in need of help (apparently those sending out energy at abnormal wavelengths). An enzyme, as you probably recall from high school chemistry, is a special molecule that remains totally intact, yet has the ability to speed up chemical reactions between other substances. Once an enzyme is activated, it starts a chain reaction of events. In the case of LLLT, the activated enzymes promote the repair and healing of damaged tissue in the area. The researchers involved in the General Motors study demonstrated that in addition to initiating the healing process, LLLT therapy also increased blood flow to the areas involved. (They thought even greater changes would be noticeable if there were a better method of monitoring blood flow at the microvascular and cellular levels.)

"LLLT is undoubtedly only one of many techniques that can be used to stimulate healing by balancing cellular energy. I suspect in the

115

future we'll discover that certain types of music, homeopathy, acupuncture, massage, color therapy and a long list of other therapies work in much the same way. (Most of the therapies now used here at the Healing Research Center are used to create the same or similar effect.) For now, however, LLLT is on the forefront of modern, noninvasive therapy. It truly is the beginning of Star Trek medicine. The user doesn't have to have special abilities, talents or extensive training. It's safe. And most importantly, consistent results can be achieved by anyone using the proper equipment."

Star Trek Generation Doctors

"In my initial article on LLLT, I predicted that everyone would someday have one of these units in their home. Instead of running to the medicine cabinet for aspirin at the first sign of a headache or pain, the laser will be the first choice of treatment. After using the unit for close to two years now, I'll stick with that prediction. It seems like every day we're getting a little closer to realizing that subtle energies, like those emitted from these laser units, can have a profound effect on stimulating healing within the body. It's only a matter of time before physicians and the general public learn about LLLT and just how beneficial it can be.

"Low Reactive-Level Laser Therapy (LLLT) is alive and well. And while it is still far too expensive for the average consumer to own a unit, after using it for the last couple of years, I can't imagine a doctor's office without one. It's a therapy whose time has come. If you suffer from carpal tunnel syndrome, TMJ disorders, damaged nerves or any of the other conditions I've mentioned above, I would highly recommend seeking out a doctor who uses LLLT. In the large majority of these cases, it could very well eliminate the problem without the use of drugs or surgery."

In our experience, we have had very few patients who have not received benefit from the **MicroLight 830** and many have received truly outstanding help for conditions that had previously defied all other therapies.

The instructions that come with the device include protocols for the following: healing of open wounds; dermatitis; eczema; lack of granulation tissue formation (thus retarding wound healing); overcoming and softening scar tissue formation; fistulas; edema; cysts; bursitis; muscle inflammation, contusions, ruptures, atrophy and contractures; neuritis; neuralgia; nerve injuries; atrophy of nerves; paresis; paralysis; prolapsed disc disease; spondylitis; periostis; spondylosis; bone fractures and fissures; arthritis, both rheumatoid and osteoarthritis; arthrosis; strains and sprains; dislocations (following reduction); tendonitis; epicondylitis; tendon strains and contusions; tendon ruptures and following tendon surgery; hematoma; tissue infiltration of blood after blood taking or injection.

Since the **MicroLight 830** is stated to penetrate the tissues up to 30 mm (a little over one inch), we have used it over various ailing organs that we felt we could reach by this penetration. These include the liver, celiac nerve plexus (Solar Plexus), urinary bladder, inguinal hernia and prostate. Preliminary results of these efforts are very promising.

In the future we expect to find many new and fascinating uses for this little wonder. If you have a problem not very well served by previous treatments feel free to ask your Healing Research Center physician about the **MicroLight 830**. It might well be the answer you have been searching for.

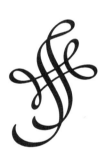

Chapter VIII
Colon Therapy

Therapies that relate to the large intestine, or bowel (colon), have always been the stepchildren of medicine. From the inception of medical treatment, complaints related to colon activity have been prevalent. The use of cathartics and laxatives dates from time immemorial and the enema in various forms was described in humanity's very earliest therapeutic writings. Yet to this day, very few doctors are anxious to do any constructive work on this poor, maligned and misunderstood part of the body.

Medical advice and consensus constantly fluctuates on this subject. Some physicians tell us that we are overly concerned about defecation (movement of our bowels) and that if they move once a week this is sufficient. However, others assure us that unless the bowels move at least three times a day we are constipated and our body is being destroyed by constant absorption of unremoved fecal material. Some practitioners are convinced that practically all our colon problems come from wrong thinking and that if we stop worrying the problems go away. But when they don't go away, still other physicians tell us that the only practical therapy is to cut the colon out and then bring the end of the small intestine out through a hole in the abdomen (colostomy). After all these centuries of attention to this part of our system, there should be some consensus, but this isn't the case. In fact, more people are probably troubled by colon problems today than ever before and it is to be wondered if our modern recommendations are any more efficacious than those of our illustrious ancestors. We are attempting to present here a thoughtful, rational program and therapy for these problems.

It is a rare person who doesn't have some difficulty with the colon at some time in his life. If these problems are met and corrected early, they will not assume the severe characteristics of the diseases that can afflict the large bowel.

The organs of elimination, particularly those for the discharge of urine and feces, have always been regarded as dirty or unclean and weren't to be discussed in polite company. I have often thought that if fecal matter had a delicate odor and a good commercial use, the colon and its attendant difficulties might be viewed in an entirely different light. Our Creator apparently was of a somewhat different opinion. Therefore, since it doesn't seem possible to change the nature of the colon's product, we should attempt to do the next best thing: change our view of this whole process of the elimination of the body's solid waste.

There are many misconceptions about the nature of fecal matter and some understanding of this substance is necessary to discover the best methods of keeping the colon functioning normally. I find that most patients believe that fecal matter is what remains of ingested food by the time it reaches this portion of the gut. This is basically untrue. Only the parts of food that because of their consistency or construction move through the digestive tract unaffected by the digestive juices become a part of the fecal mass. These substances consist almost entirely of various forms of undigestible cellulose. Though readily handled by the digestive systems of the various ruminating animals, cellulose is not broken down to an assimilable form by the human digestive apparatus. Most of other food components are broken down and absorbed in the small intestine. The normal feces consist mainly of cellulose products that have passed through the system undigested and bacteria that have been carried to the large intestine, which contains a medium facilitating their growth and multiplication.

No known digestive enzymes are secreted in the large bowel. It is generally held that even enzymes that may be carried from the small intestine are usually exhausted by the time they reach the colon. There is, however, some bacterial activity on undigested food in the large bowel. Some cellulose components are acted on by the colon bacteria and are broken down into their simpler parts. If the digestion has been relatively normal up to this point and the bowel is properly functioning, the acid-forming colon bacteria break down what is left of the food and relatively normal colon physiologic processes occur. This action tends to produce stable peristaltic movements of the bowel; there is very little gas formation and a healthy condition of this area is assured. If bacteria other than the endemic colon bacilli inhabit and multiply in the bowel, this happy picture can change rapidly. Because the proper function of the colon depends on the bacterial activity within its lumen (tubular cavity), this activity is discussed here at length.

Fermentation and Putrefaction

Bacterial action on food in the large bowel may be divided into two types—fermentation and putrefaction. Fermentation is the action of bacteria on starches or carbohydrates. By this action, the gases methane, hydrogen, and carbon dioxide are produced. Also organic acids, such as butyric, acetic and lactic acid are formed. If the degree of fermentation is minor, there is little or no distress or knowledge by the individual of this process. On the other hand, if the circumstances are such that there is excessive fermentation, large amounts of gas are formed which may cause distention of the large bowel. This excessive gas formation causes either pain in the more severe cases or at least the passing of the objectionable gas. Where digestion is weak, or where the individual has a digestive idiosyncrasy, certain foods tend to cause more fermentation than others. The common offenders are the various types of beans, onions, peanuts, cabbage, cucumbers, and dried fruits.

The second type of bacterial breakdown occurring in the large bowel is putrefaction. This is the bacterial disintegration of proteins resulting in the formation of the gases hydrogen sulfide and ammonia and the so-called aromatic substances skatole, indole, phenol and creosol. These substances are responsible for most of the foul odor in flatulence. The basic fermentation gases—methane, hydrogen and carbon dioxide—are odorless. In general, offensive bowel gas is due to putrefaction; that which is odorless, though perhaps abundant, results from fermentation.

Some degree of bacterial action in the lower bowel is beneficial since the bacteria can split foods into the same products as those created by the digestive enzymes. (1) They disintegrate the cellulose and thus liberate the enclosed food for its proper digestion; (2) they may transform complex proteins into simpler compounds; (3) they change fats into fatty acid and glycerol; and (4) they change disaccharides to monosaccharides. However, if this bacterial decomposition goes still further, the action becomes wasteful and compounds (such as indole and skatole) may be formed that are toxic when absorbed. Against this contingency the body has two lines of defense: (1) the intestinal wall bars entrance of these compounds into the bloodstream to a large extent and (2) the liver detoxifies the compounds.

All material absorbed from the intestine is carried to the liver by the portal vein. The liver then exercises a selective action on the material seeking entrance into the body. When putrefactive compounds arrive at the liver, they are, to a great extent, taken out of the circulation and transformed into less toxic substances. These are then put back into the circulation and excreted by the kidneys. For example, indole absorbed from the intestine unites, in the liver, with acid potassium sulfate to form a compound called indican and as such it is excreted in the urine.

From the foregoing discussion, we can draw two important conclusions vital to our thinking concerning the health of the colon. First, we should do what we can to see that bacterial decomposition in the large bowel is regulated and doesn't have an opportunity to go beyond its more useful stages. Second, we can readily see the importance of a properly functioning liver in all problems concerning the lower bowel.

In summarizing we can safely state that the large bowel is not a garbage can. It is a functioning organ in which controlled bacterial actions occur to properly complete the last stages of food breakdown. It is obvious that much of the distress that commonly occurs in the colon is due to a malfunctioning of this bacterial process and that any therapy designed to correct abnormalities in this process would be most efficacious in improving the health of the colon. Such therapies are usually designed to remove intruding bacteria (those not needed for normal bowel functioning) that may inhabit the colon and to replace them with the normal acid-forming bowel bacteria.

Water Absorption and Stool Formation

In addition to offering the proper medium for bacterial food processing, another major function of the colon is to absorb excess liquid from the mass of substance that comes from the small intestine and to transport this mass to the rectum, where it can be discharged (defecation) at regular intervals. Material is moved along in the large bowel by mass peristalsis, which is generally initiated by the entrance of food into the stomach or duodenum (the first part of the small intestine). This is called the *gastric colic reflex*. Powerful waves of peristalsis (rhythmic contraction of muscles) pass from the cecum (blind pouch in which the colon begins) over the entire length of the colon. In this manner the contents are gradually worked toward the sigmoid flexure (s-shaped curve of colon above rectum) and rectum. This peristalsis may occur two or three times a day, depending generally on the patient's eating habits. Various emotions may inhibit this reflex in some people and in other susceptible people the emotions may have a stimulatory effect, as in the many forms of colitis.

The rectum is the lowest four to five inches of the large intestine and the anus (opening that lies at the lowest end) is guarded by two muscles, one called the internal sphincter and the other called the external sphincter (fig. 10). The internal sphincter (circular muscle) is involuntary, that is, not generally under the individual's control. The external sphincter is voluntary and can function at the will of the individual unless some damage to the spinal cord causes a loss of control. Surprisingly, the rectum is normally empty until the bowels are ready to move. At this time, peristalsis forces some of the fecal matter from the descending colon and sigmoid (portion of the lower bowel just above the rectum) into the rectal area. Nerve endings in the rectum are then stimulated by this distention and the desire to defecate occurs.

When this reflex mechanism is inhibited for various reasons, constipation occurs. This stagnation most invariably occurs in the lower part

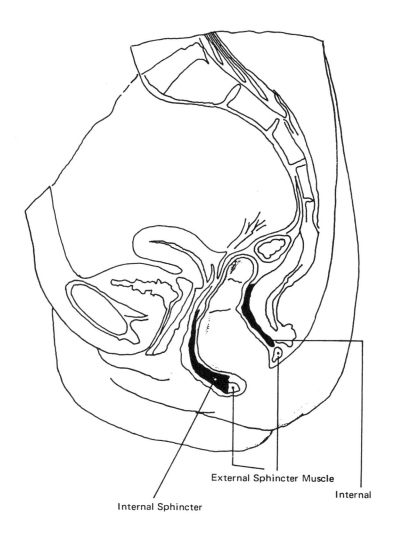

External Sphincter Muscle

Internal

Internal Sphincter

Figure 10

123

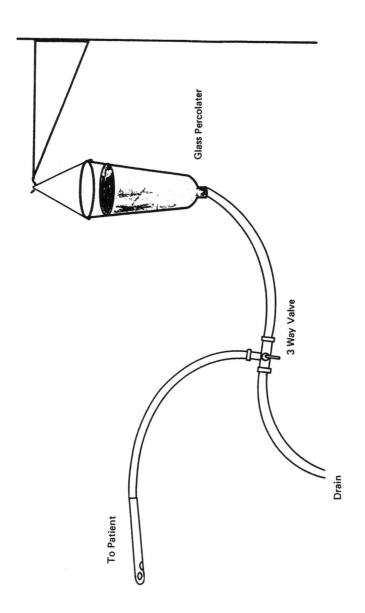

Glass Percolater

3 Way Valve

Drain

To Patient

Figure 11

124

of the bowel. Tuttle and Schottelius (in their text book of physiology) state that constipation is a disease of civilization and is most usually due to: (1) the failure to eat food leaving a sufficient residue (ballast) in the colon; (2) sedentary habits; (3) emotional states such as nervous tension, worry and anxiety that inhibit peristalsis and the relaxation of the anal sphincters; and (4) the failure to establish or maintain habitual regularity.

When I examine a patient rectally and can not palpate (touch) a fecal mass, I know the rectal reflex is still functioning, at least partially, and there is a good chance for a rapid cure. On the other hand, if, during such an examination, a large fecal mass is found settled into the rectum and the patient has no urge to defecate, I know that the normal rectal reflex is all but gone and I must revitalize the nerve and muscle activity of this patient before normal bowel functioning can be reestablished.

The normal stimulus for a bowel movement is distention of the rectal walls by fecal bulk. This is best supplied by the indigestible cellulose of vegetable foods. Therefore, a diet containing a proper amount of these foods is one of the best preventatives of constipation. Such foods include practically all fresh vegetables, all fruits except bananas and whole grain products, such as bran, whole-wheat flour and oatmeal. These foods, by their stimulative nature, tend to hasten or quicken peristalsis. This leaves the fecal material somewhat more moist, making defecation easier.

To prevent constipation, nothing should be allowed to interfere with the all-important rectal reflex. When fecal matter reaches the sensitive part of the rectum and the desire to defecate is initiated, every effort should be made to fulfill this desire as promptly as possible. If this is not done, the reflex will gradually lose its effectiveness and the fecal matter will remain in the large bowel longer than it should. Since the colon, by its nature, absorbs moisture, the longer the material remains, the more water is absorbed, thus causing the fecal mass to become hard and dry, making subsequent elimination more difficult and painful. When this overloading of the lower colon continues over a long period, the muscles gradually lose their tone and classic constipation occurs.

Such constipation can in turn lead to many other related conditions, not the least of which is hemorrhoids (piles). The hemorrhoidal veins, which drain the blood from the rectal area and adjacent parts, are not supplied with valves as are many other veins. They are therefore subject to enlargement, even to the point of breakage, which causes bleeding piles. Congestion of these veins is often caused by the prolonged straining to defecate in constipation. Constipation thus often leads to hemorrhoids and because of the pain and difficulty in defecating, hemorrhoids tend to aggravate the preexisting constipation.

Diseases of the Colon and Their Treatment

Some conditions of the large bowel call for surgical treatment; some are of such a nature that the lay person can do little to assist with either the diagnosis or treatment. These diseases are not discussed here. In most early colon conditions however, the patient can do much to help bring the therapy to a satisfactory conclusion.

Chronic conditions that affect the large bowel can be divided into those that produce constipation, congestion, and stagnation; and those that manifest symptoms of over activity such as rumbling, frequent loose stools and frank watery diarrhea. In the natural therapy used to correct these symptom patterns, there are many similarities because in our methods we attempt to restore normal bowel function, which in turn corrects the condition. Specific therapy for each separate condition must also be used, of course; this is adjusted to the needs of each patient.

Herbal Colonic Therapy

The most useful specific treatment used in our Centers for problems of this nature is the herbal colonic instillation. The so called "colonic" has been used by the natural healing profession for many years and although it can be useful I believe it must be used cautiously and with a full understanding of its possible consequences. In my medical school days, the colonic room was unceremoniously referred to as the "gut laundry." I always had deep reservations about its general effectiveness, particularly in the form in which it was administered at that time. In the type of apparatus then used, gallons of warm water were made to circulate in the large bowel in an attempt to remove retained and impacted fecal material. After even a few such treatments, I noticed that many of my patients seemed to be physically weakened, owing either to the somewhat abnormal sluicing of these rather delicate membranes or to certain physiologic effects caused by so much plain water in the large bowel. Sometimes this type of colonic may prove useful for long-impacted fecal matter, though experience has convinced me that continued use of such treatment can be detrimental in all but the most robust subject.

While still in medical school, Dr. Henry Linke, a man trained in the Swedish school of treatment, showed me a method that changed my opinions regarding the colonic. Dr. Linke had developed a type of colonic irrigation that seemed far superior to those normally used at that time.

The type of apparatus Dr. Linke developed was considerably different from that normally used in colonic irrigation (Fig. 11). The solution

126

to be instilled is placed in a simple glass percolator kept two feet above the patient. A tube from the bottom of the percolator is attached to a special three-way valve. From this valve, one nipple is connected to the outlet drain while the other is connected to a rubber tube that is used to transfer the percolator contents into the patient. When the three-way valve is turned to operating position, the solution in the percolator passes through the rubber tube into the patient; when the valve is turned to the drain position , the solution, gas, and bowel matter will pass from the patient into the drainage system.

This simple technique was used exclusively at the Clymer Health Clinic for twenty years, in preference to those using more complicated equipment. When this method is properly utilized, it is possible to thoroughly cleanse the colon, although this isn't the major objective. This therapy is used most productively to instill various herbal solutions into the large bowel to aid in healing, detoxifying and in establishing normal muscular tone.

The herbs used in this treatment are in powdered form because we can then instill the greatest amount of active herb with the least possible distress. Were we to use teas, decoctions, or tinctures, the amount of active agent we could use would be limited because of the lack of concentration in this form. Powdered herbs do present one serious problem, however, which we circumvent by the use of our simple system. Powdered herbs are very sticky and inclined to block the small orifices and regulating mechanisms that are an integral part of the more complex colonic machines. They pass easily through the three-way valve, however. Thus, we find that our simple apparatus is in this way superior to the most expensive and complicated alternatives. Experience has so convinced me of the superiority of the powdered herb instillation to other forms of direct colon treatment that I have retained this rather uncomplicated equipment ever since my earliest years of practice.

Our simple equipment also enables us to manually adjust the amount and pressure of the solution as it enters the colon. By simply pinching the rubber colon tube, at a position a few inches before it enters the anus, the physician can regulate the inward flow from a few drops at a time all the way to a full open tube, which enables a quart to enter the colon in just a few seconds. This degree of regulation is absolutely essential to managing the great variety of conditions for which we use this treatment. Such delicate control it is not available in most commercial equipment.

Perhaps the value of this therapy can best be demonstrated by going through a usual colonic treatment as might be given by one of the specialists at our Center. After disinfecting the equipment thoroughly, the percolator is filled with our own well water heated to the specific temperature. This temperature usually varies anywhere from body heat to 110° (100° to 105° is the most common range). The specific powdered herbal mixture is then prepared for the intended patient and mixed with water in a special container to disperse the powders as completely as possible. The patient is properly draped and made comfortable on the colonic table. The three-way valve is then turned so that water passes through the colon tube. As soon as water appears in the openings of the colon tube, the three-way valve is turned back to stand-by. This procedure eliminates any gas or air that might be trapped in the colon tube. The colon tube is lubricated and gently inserted into the rectum, far enough for the side hole on the tube to adequately clear the internal sphincter and other structures that might obstruct the ready flow of liquid into and out of this tube. Once the tube is inserted, the patient lies on his back with his knees bent and his feet flat on the table. The herbs are now placed in the percolator and the physician turns the three way valve, allowing the solution to enter the patient. When the solution first fills the rectal area, the patient usually experiences a desire to defecate. The valve is reversed and the fluid allowed to drain until this feeling has passed. The physician then alternates between instilling the solution and draining it, all the time using his free hand to massage the bowel ahead of the ascending solution to help work the herbs into all the small crevices of the colon. In the normal person, this is an easy matter and the water passes freely with only a minor degree of spasm. In most patients, it is a simple matter to instill the solution throughout the entire large bowel. The patient with a normal colon usually requires less than the full amount for a complete instillation. In certain diseases, however, it may take several treatments before the ascending colon and cecum are properly reached and treated.

Patient response during the treatment helps guide the physician in making his final diagnosis. The information gained during the herbal colonic indicates much about the pathologic condition of the colon. Therefore, we find this form of treatment not only a useful therapy, but also a great aid in diagnosis, particularly when the problem does not yet show obvious pathologic signs in X-rays or other orthodox methods of diagnosis.

Once the solution has become exhausted, the patient is allowed to drain, the tube is removed, and the patient is sent to the adjoining lavatory, remaining there long enough for the colon to empty.

Although this completes the normal treatment, there is a bit of technique I discovered accidentally that may prove of interest to those familiar with this type of therapy. In my early days, I operated my office without an assistant and I had a patient to whom I had given three or four of these colon therapies without reaching the cecum with healing solution. One day while I was about half through with the treatment, my phone rang. I turned the valve to drain and assured the patient that no water would be going in her until I got back. The phone call was from a long winded patient. Finally after 10 minutes, I was able to end the conversation and return to my patient patient. She didn't seem any the worse for wear, so I again started the solution to finish the therapy. As soon as I placed my hand on her abdomen, I knew something had happened. Previously her abdomen had always been hard and spastic; now it was soft and supple. I found that the solution had worked its way into the cecum and my job had been done for me while I was talking on the telephone. Further investigation substantiated that for a difficult patient, a rest about half way through the colon treatment is frequently beneficial. The desensitizing effect of the herbs, plus the fact that the patient is better able to relax knowing that no one is around, apparently enables the solution to move into the spastic areas, which were resistant to more active treatment.

Herbal colon therapy is the cornerstone of much of our treatment for bowel conditions in the same way that endonasal therapy is the cornerstone for the treatment of ear, nose and throat diseases. Not all patients, however, require or can tolerate herbal colon therapy; where it is indicated and readily accepted, it is able to hasten improvement to such a degree that it would be folly not to use it. In many spastic colon conditions, even those of many years standing, relief is achieved in just one or two treatments and apparent complete recovery can take place in a matter of weeks. It is necessary, however, that these patients adhere to specific diets, take nutrient elements that benefit their problem and are willing to help us by establishing the proper mental and emotional outlook necessary for a complete resolution of their difficulty.

Spastic Colitis

Spastic (mucous) colitis (now known as irritable bowel syndrome)* is, next to constipation, perhaps the most common colon disorder.

Opinions vary regarding its cause, but most physicians agree on a few points. The effect of the emotions on the colon is generally accepted

---

*I have personally always been suspicious of conditions whose name is constantly being changed by the establishment. To me it indicates that they really know little of the true nature of the condition.

in spastic colitis. This does not necessarily mean that the patient with this problem is openly nervous or emotional. Very often he will seem to be a calm, quiet, withdrawn person who almost never shows nervous tendencies. In this instance, the feelings may be held in, only to manifest in a physical manner as spastic colitis.

Many believe that improper food plays an important part in this condition and certain vitamins, particularly those of the B family, can be beneficial to the proper nervous functioning of the bowel and are frequently given in this condition.

I personally have found that a hereditary influence also plays a strong part in this form of colitis. Some people, no matter how careful they are with their emotions or diet, seem to be readily affected by this disorder, whereas others can eat atrociously and have severe emotional difficulties but yet remain free from this condition.

In practice, the herbal colon therapy has proved to be almost a specific for spastic colitis. The irritation that accompanies this condition is usually stopped by the first or second treatment and an almost complete abatement of symptoms can be assured within a few weeks. We do of course, treat these patients as a whole, and depending on the severity of the condition, they are placed on specific corrective diets. Only in the most severe cases, however, do we use the classic bland diet. Because we believe that the consumption of too many refined and devitalized foods often aggravates this condition, we stress the use of raw fresh vegetable juices, fruit juices that can be accepted and other natural whole foods as rapidly as the progress of the condition allows. We do not fanatically adhere to any one dietary regimen, however, and each case is individualized. In the very sensitive patient, we use our new nutritional analysis and advanced allergy testing methods to ascertain a patient's sensitivity to various foods. Then a specific diet is arranged that is correctly constituted for his individual body chemistry.

All our spastic colitis patients are given supplemental nutritional agents that have proven their value. These vary somewhat, depending on the actual needs of the individual patient but a general idea of their nature can be discussed. Most spastic colitis patients have an imbalance in the acid/alkaline makeup of the colon and products are given to help reimplant the normal acid forming bacteria following removal of the foreign bacteria by herbal colon therapy. Usually products such as acidophilus culture (either liquid or tablets) and lactic acid yeast are used. Occasionally, in a difficult case, the liquid culture may be instilled by the colon therapy apparatus in place of the usual herbal medication. In this way, many patients have been helped who were resistant to all previous therapies. There has been of late much evidence to show that many of these implantation compounds do not have active bacterial activity by the time the patient purchases them. Therefore, we ask our patients to please consult with us before obtaining such products so that we can supply you with a product that does what it is supposed to do.

Various types of natural B complex are also used. We like to use high biological low potency products since we find them far more beneficial in the long run than the high potency low biological products usually available.

Most patients with a spastic colon require more concentrated nutrition than others due to the fact that the food passes through them so rapidly that it usually is not well absorbed. Their diet and supplementation must take this fact into consideration. All such patients need to discuss these items with their physician at our Centers.

Patients with spastic colitis and emotional difficulties are divided into two groups—patients who may have had past emotional difficulties that are now conquered and patients presently under an emotional stress that is continuing without abatement.

The first group is usually easy to treat. Even though the previous emotional stress may have had an important part in causing their colitis, these patients respond very well to the standard therapy I have outlined. For example, a woman may be saddled with a drunken husband. Her constant concern and worry about him can readily help initiate spastic colitis. But if he dies, or if she gets a divorce, she can continue her life without the previous anxiety. Even without the stress, however, spastic colitis usually doesn't automatically go away. It may improve, but it usually persists until the physical components are corrected by therapy such as that described here. Following such treatment, since there is now nothing to perpetuate the condition, the improvement usually is permanent, unless the patient finds herself again in a situation of great emotional turmoil.

For the second group of patients, however, the problem is much more difficult. In these patients, it is usually necessary to institute supportive psychologic therapy along with the usual natural treatment measures. Such psychologic therapy must be individualized to the situation at hand. Usually, it is directed in one of two paths—either we try to help the patient change the situation causing the emotional stress or, if this is impractical, we aid him in changing his outlook concerning the situation, so that while the stress may not be removed, it can be prevented from causing psychologic injury.

131

Ulcerative Colitis

Ulcerative colitis is sometimes mistaken for spastic colitis. Unfortunately, ulcerative colitis is an entirely different condition. It doesn't respond well to any known conservative therapy, including the herbal colonic. In fact, I rarely use herbal colonic therapy in treating ulcerative colitis.

In ulcerative colitis, gaping ulcers occur throughout the large bowel. Blood and pus from these ulcers may be detected in the stool. The condition usually attacks those in their 20s or 30s, and it seems to be more common in women than in men. Many theories have been advanced regarding its cause. Some believe it is an allergic reaction; some, that it is perhaps due to a hormonal imbalance. Many assert that it is purely psychologic and some in my own field are certain that it is a nutritionally oriented problem. In my own experience, I have seen where all these factors could play some part, but I can't say that any one specific factor consistently overpowers the others in this somewhat dreaded disease.

Because of its inflammatory nature, it is frequently treated with cortisone or other sterols. However, it isn't generally cured by this therapy and many of these patients go on to have a colostomy in which all, or a portion, of colon is removed.

At present, I still find ulcerative colitis enigmatic. Almost every case has had characteristics different from all other cases I have treated. I have seen patients I was not treating personally, but who were under my observation, change from a well controlled to a very severe, desperate situation within a matter of days and these patients may perish even though the most heroic medical measures were used without avail.

On the other hand, many cases have progressed extremely well under natural therapies. Some patients sent to us by other physicians to have their health built up so that they could go through a colostomy were found on later examination to be free of ulcers and the operation was unnecessary. I have also seen these same patients, apparently because of emotional stress, revert to their previous condition within an extremely short period.

In summary, while there is no specific cure I know of, frequently considerable help can be offered ulcerative colitis patients through natural methods. This help must at times be given in conjunction with the sterols and other orthodox medication, though in many instances it can be used in place of such medication. I treat each patient as an individual and not as a disease, for I have yet to see two patients respond exactly alike. Herbal colonic irrigation doesn't seem to be practical in most of these patients, and it can possibly do harm during certain stages of the disease. In almost every instance, all efforts must be made to reduce to a minimum the degree of physical and emotional stress under which these patients live. When all these factors are watched carefully, we have good results in treating ulcerative colitis at our Healing Research Center. These patients, however, must be watched much more closely than the general run of patient.

Many of these patients respond to pulsed electro-magnetic therapy (Magnatherm) and to manual reduction of the abdominal tension. Recently we have been using the new Low Level Laser Therapy on these patients and the early results are promising.

Diverticulosis and Diverticulitis

Another troublesome condition of the large bowel is diverticulosis. A diverticulum is a small pocket (invagination) occurring along the surface of the bowel. Some patients may have two or three of these diverticula; some will have nearly a hundred covering the whole surface of the bowel. If these little pockets become inflamed or infected, they can cause considerable distress. This condition is then called diverticulitis (the "itis" indicating that the diverticula are inflamed).

The frequency of diverticulosis seems to be growing. It occurs generally in the middle-aged to elderly patient and while certainly not on the order of ulcerative colitis, it is generally more troublesome than simple spastic colon. For years, medical authorities disagreed about the cause of diverticulosis. However in recent years, more credence has been given the theory that it is caused by foods that are too soft and mushy, therefore do not produce sufficient stimulation of the colon walls to induce proper colon muscle tone. From this a weakness occurs in the walls and a blowout or distention of the weak wall occurs, producing the pocket or diverticulum.

We in the natural therapeutic field received this information from the medical authorities with rather mixed feelings, for although it does substantiate a hypothesis we have expounded for many years, no credit has ever been given us for our early work in this condition.

Unfortunately, once a patient has diverticulosis, he must be careful about his diet. Once the pockets develop, it is possible for certain stimulative foods to irritate them to the point of inflammation, producing diverticulitis.

Both diverticulitis and diverticulosis, if not too far advanced, respond well to herbal colon therapy and its allied natural therapeutic measures. The pain and irritation that often accompany these disorders usually abate rapidly with the herbal instillations. After a few treatments, it is generally possible to place the patient on a slightly modified basic maintenance diet. In this way, we can usually prevent further diverticula from forming by strengthening the bowel wall.

Diverticulosis usually doesn't have a particular emotional component, although it is certainly possible that a patient may have both diverticulosis and a spastic colon at the same time— in which case the two treatments can be combined. However, most uncomplicated diverticulosis cases respond well without psychologic therapy.

The nutritional therapy is quite important and it is essential that the patient is well-supplied with the elements that help rebuild and sustain the tone of the smooth muscle fibers.

Because an actual pathologic change occurs in diverticulosis, it is not often possible to speak of a definitive cure. Most of our patients are brought to a state in which they are comfortable and symptom-free. To maintain them in this condition, we implement certain maintenance measures, consisting of corrective diet and specific nutrient supplements on their part, and of the occasional use of herbal colon therapy on ours. Most patients so maintained have little trouble with their diverticulosis and they live entirely normal lives.

Intestinal Flu

This disease, which afflicts us all at one time or another, responds well to herbal therapy. After a bout with intestinal flu, the colon is often left denuded of its normal bacteria. If we are unlucky, gas-forming or putrefying bacteria take their place. In these instances, the cramp-like pains so common in acute stomach flu don't leave entirely, or the diarrhea may persist even after the fever and aches have left. In some patients, this situation may persist for weeks and even months after the original infection. An herbal colonic usually brings almost instant relief for these patients. At times only one such treatment is required, and rarely are more than two necessary.

Intestinal Problems due to Antibiotics

A state similar to that found in flu may occur in patients treated with oral antibiotics. Most broad-spectrum antibiotics tend to sterilize the colon rapidly and the bowel may then become inhabited by harmful bacteria.

My first contact with herbal colon therapy, and Dr. Linke, arose from this situation, when one of our fellow medical school students was recovering from lobar pneumonia treated by broad-spectrum antibiotics. A few days after he was discharged from the hospital, he began to have severe abdominal cramps. His teachers were not sure what to do with him, but Dr. Linke gave him a series of three herbal colonic irrigations and acidophilus bacillus capsules by mouth for bacterial reimplantation. The cramps began to abate after the first treatment and by the time the third was finished the student had fully recovered.

It is possible for a person to take oral antibiotics without this problem occurring, but it happens often enough to be mentioned here. With the present universal use of oral antibiotics, this condition is undoubtedly one we must consider whenever unexplained bowel pains occur.

Constipation

To the uninitiated it might seem that the most obvious reason for the herbal colonic treatment would be for correcting constipation. Although used for constipation, herbal colonic therapy is much more specific in mucous colitis, diverticulosis, various forms of idiopathic diarrheas and other conditions in which the bowel is irritated or overly sensitive. At best, colon irrigation (enema) is only a temporary cure for constipation. To be of lasting help in constipation, the treatment must always be directed toward establishing normal bowel function. To this end, it is important that we try to stimulate the mass peristaltic wave if this has been diminished. It is also particularly important that we correct any malfunctioning of the rectal reflex, which alone institutes the mechanism and the desire for defecation. To do this, in the early stages of treatment herbal colonic therapy is useful. Once we free the rectum of impacted material, it is possible for the herbs to rebuild the natural tone of the rectal muscles and to reestablish the integrity of the sensitive sensory nerve endings that have so long been dulled. The practitioner who uses this treatment must always keep in mind that it is his purpose to rebuild and stimulate the natural functioning of the body, not to do the work the body should do for itself.

In our colon work, we use a tube of small diameter instead of the large tubes used with most commercial colonic machines. We don't attempt to bring the fecal matter out through the tube, as is done with most of these machines. We only try to stimulate the normal nerve-muscle mechanism so that when the urge to defecate comes to our patient, we can stop the treatment and send him into the adjoining bathroom, thereby producing a constructive habit pattern for the weakened bowel.

For our treatment of constipation, we use special a four pad sine-wave machine that alternates the current from one pad to the next in a circular fashion. These pads are placed on the patient's abdomen in such a way that they simulate normal peristaltic wave. The circular activity of this muscle contractility has proven a great aid in initiating the normal reflex defecatory mechanism of the colon. We have also found this machine (the Myoflex) to be very helpful even in cases of visceroptosis (prolapse of the abdominal organs) a common condition in older patients.

Although authorities accept that such sine-wave stimulation affects the abdominal skeletal muscles, they may not agree that it can affect the slower smooth muscles of the colon itself. I really don't know if it works on the smooth muscles or not, but I do know that it works. We have patients come from great distances to obtain its therapeutic effects and some of our constipation patients desire and need no other treatment. I'm sure someday some bright researcher will discover a reflex center in the skeletal muscles that affects certain centers in the smooth muscles and that by controlling one, the other is affected. Then I may have a real answer to why my sine-wave machine alleviates constipation. If we wait until that time to use this treatment, however, many of our patients would suffer unnecessarily from constipation.

Many authorities believe that the first cause of constipation is failure to eat food leaving a sufficient residue in the colon. I also find this a problem that must be corrected if there is to be any lasting help in most constipation cases. Unfortunately, constipation often occurs in the elderly, who frequently have dental problems and find it difficult to chew raw cellulose foods adequately. We place these patients on a bulk substance such as psyllium seed or karaya gum compound. Both work effectively, although they differ in consistency. The psyllium seed is tough and stringy and will eventually pull anything through the bowel. Unfortunately, it can be more irritating than the karaya gum in certain spastic conditions. Karaya gum produces a soft gelatinous type of bulk that, though not as effective in many instances as psyllium seed, is not as irritative and it is preferred in certain cases. One of the great advantages of prescribing a bulk substance is that a certain amount of water must be taken for the bulk to function properly and this water intake may have just as beneficial an effect on the constipation as the bulk substance does.

Laxatives

In the beginning treatment of most chronic constipation, it is necessary that the patient be kept on some type of stimulant until normal or near normal reflex actions can be instituted. Products in this category are generally called laxatives and they were one of the first medications used by man. Unfortunately, most lay persons are confused about these agents. The most common error I find concerns the use of the word "herbal" or "natural." Often a patient will tell me, "Oh, I'm taking a natural laxative." Their assumption is that if it's natural, it can't be harmful or habit-forming. This is not true. The most used laxatives the world over are natural and herbal and still they can be habit-forming and harmful if misused. One laxative that was used in ancient Egypt is the Aloe plant; it's still used today. If used in small amounts, it's not likely to cause any harm, but it is still basically an irritant; if its use is prolonged, it is habit-forming and tends to weaken the normal reflex mechanisms of the large bowel. Senna is used in some of the best-selling laxatives, but it too is a stimulant and can in time produce the same adverse effect. The only herbal remedy I know that works exclusively on the large bowel is Cascara Sagrada; although it is a stimulant, its effects are more controlled than the others. Cascara is probably the most practical laxative in most cases that can't be controlled without stimulants.

The various salts and physiologic laxatives—such as the fleet enemas, disodium phosphates and the various other mineral laxatives—all have their place, but they must be used carefully. Those high in sodium should not be used in patients with high blood pressure or heart disease.

In our own Centers, we use several laxatives. In the beginning of our therapy, we give the laxative with the weakest possible action that will be effective in a specific patient. We therefore have laxatives that range from the gentlest nudge to pure dynamite. A selection of laxatives is kept on hand because in many patients the laxative action of a compound is exhausted shortly. Laxatives must therefore be changed frequently to keep the bowels functioning until normal activity can be restored by our usual therapeutic measures.

The colon walls are an acid medium and this state helps support and in turn is sustained by the acid-forming colon bacillus. In constipation, the bowel frequently becomes alkaline and putrefaction or fermentation organisms predominate. This alkaline state may inhibit the normal colon movements. Many cases of mild constipation can be cured completely by the use of measures to change the bowel "soil" and implant acidophilus or lactic acid organisms. Even chronic conditions are helped by these measures, although much more must usually be done for a thorough cure.

The early chiropractors and men like Albert Abrams, with his spondylotherapy, treated constipation by stimulating the spinal nerve centers. These methods are still used at our Centers. These methods are quite useful in treating severely chronic constipation. These chronic cases require all the tricks of natural therapy to encourage the bowel back to reasonable activity.

In some constipation cases, we find that carefully applied rectal dilatation, in which the tissues around the coccyx and ganglion impar are gently stretched and freed from spasm, often is the difference between success and failure. As in all such nerve rebuilding, the patient must be taught to respond whenever the urge to defecate is felt. The way to build a weakened nerve reflex is to respond to it as rapidly as possible whenever it manifests. If the patient attempts to defecate whenever he feels the desire, it will aid greatly in rebuilding this important reflex. On the other hand, if he attempts to wait until the reflex is stronger, the reflex will probably never gain the necessary strength.

Exercise is also of great importance in treating constipation. The best exercise usually is walking. Walking at a good arm swinging pace productively stimulates more organs of the body than almost any other exercise. It is particularly useful for the digestive system, especially the liver and gallbladder. It is difficult for a case of constipation to really become entrenched unless the liver is sluggish. The liver, via the gallbladder, puts into the alimentary canal substances that are natural laxatives. If through the absorption of toxic substances or dietary habits that cause liver congestion these substances are not adequately produced, constipation can result. Natural remedies are useful in establishing the normal function of the liver. Please speak to your Center physician if you are interested in liver cleansing.

In summary, I offer these thoughts: Constipation can be corrected and the earlier the treatment is begun, the quicker and the more thorough the cure can be. The worst action you can take for constipation is to accept it; once you accept constipation, the disorder will become entrenched. However, just keeping the bowels moving by the use of laxatives is not treating constipation. It is simply a resignation to it. The bowels should function without such stimulation. Read again what I have said in this section. If constipation is your problem, don't give up. Tell us about it and together we will correct it.

Hemorrhoids

Hemorrhoids are a most disagreeable condition that is often treated by surgery. Recovery from such surgery can be extremely painful; even then, the condition may return later. Many cases of hemorrhoids, if caught in the early stages, can be treated successfully by natural means. At our healing Centers, we first treat hemorrhoids by correcting the constipation that so often causes them. At the same time, we analyze liver function and, if needed, take measures to decongest this organ. Besides the remedies given to the patient to correct constipation and to decongest the liver, specific remedies are useful for hemorrhagic venous engorgement. The herbs collinsonia and hamamelis have proven most efficacious over the years; rutin, vitamin C, and vitamin E are also of great use.

In milder cases, the most successful local treatment has been garlic inserted into the rectum each night. To do this properly, a clove of garlic is separated from the bulb, and small scratches are made in its surface with a razor blade or paring knife. The clove is then inserted into the rectum just before bedtime, as far as it can be pushed by the index finger. It will pass out with the stool the next morning. At first there may be some burning when the garlic is inserted. However, this sensation soon disappears and after its use for only a few nights the burning ceases. The hemorrhoids are usually much improved in short order.

Another useful local treatment, though not quite as convenient as garlic, is to insert a small amount of unpasteurized honey into the rectum each night. This isn't too difficult if the honey is warmed slightly to thin it, sucked up into a baby syringe, and then injected into the rectum. In many cases, the alternate use of honey one night and garlic the next proves the most beneficial. Some patients like to dip the garlic in the honey and then insert this into the rectum, thus effectively combining the two treatments.

Diet is very important in hemorrhoids, because the two basic causes of hemorrhoids are liver congestion and constipation. Both problems tend to be caused by a diet that is too rich, soft and complicated by the use of alcoholic beverages. Those who would be free of their hemorrhoids should choose a diet rich in fruits and vegetables, fish, cottage cheese and nonfat milk products such as yogurt. They should stay away from red meats for awhile, alcoholic beverages, particularly wines, fatty foods and foods high in refined sugars. The whole-grain cereals can be useful in overcoming hemorrhoids, because they help correct constipation.

Bowel conditions plague many of us. We at the Beverly Hall Corporation Healing Research Center have devoted many years of effort and research toward curing these cantankerous diseases. This experience has proven to us time and again that natural methods produce the best cures. If you are troubled with a bowel disorder, I encourage you to give natural therapy a fair trial.

Chapter IX
The Electromagnetic Nature of Life: Magnatherm

Since the beginning of man's existence on earth, he has pondered the nature of life itself. Even with all our great scientific advances, there is still no CONSENSUS on the basic nature of the life within us and other animate beings. The most generally accepted theories are based on the chemical and/or stimulative-inhibitive theory of existence. The most we can get from most authorities is that it may be of some value to regard life as the sum total of the properties and activities of a highly organized aggregate of various chemical compounds that we call protoplasm.

Among these properties they have called attention to irritability as a diagnostic property of a living body. Upon this Herbert Spencer based his classic definition: "Life is the continuous adjustment of internal relations to external relations." Observation teaches us that this adjustment to environmental changes is possible only within narrow physiologic limits. For example, the human body can adjust itself to changes in external temperature only when these changes are very moderate.

Viewed from this angle, they hold that life is the interplay between the organism and its environment by which the organism either adjusts itself to the environment or adjusts the environment to itself.

I believe that such a definition is what our young people call a "cop-out." It tells only what life does; it doesn't tell what life is. Unfortunately, such an attitude has frequently been the nature of science since its inception. When a scientist is incapable of explaining something, he describes what he sees, makes up a few Latin or Greek names for the rest to impress us and then goes on to something else. This is particularly true in medicine, where most of the tongue-twisting disease names have nothing whatsoever to do with the cause or true nature of the disease but are only the description of its most obvious symptoms in Latin or Greek.

Some researchers haven't been satisfied with such smug descriptions of the nature of life. Some have listened to the voice of their conscience when contemplating the usual theories on the nature of life and have been able to see through the usual inane double talk couched in Latin and Greek, which all too often passes for scientific thought. They realize that much of the phenomena we encounter in living can't be explained readily by the stimulus/response theory of life as put forth by their orthodox colleagues.

Surprisingly, many of these researchers have developed concepts simi-

141

lar to each other, even though their work has been accomplished without knowledge of their fellow investigators. All these studies have gone beyond the chemical or mechanical basis of life and have been carried into the molecular and atomic structure of matter. From this effort first developed an electrical, then an electronic, and finally a vibratory, or wave concept, of life and the activities carried out by the living subject.

Some of the most well-known researchers in this field were Dr. Georges Lakhovsky, Professor Jacques d'Arsonval (the discoverer of the meter movement that goes under his name), Dr. George W. Crile, Dr. Albert Abrams, Nicola Tesla and Ivan G. McDaniel (who advanced this theory into the psychologic, mental, and spiritual spheres of human activity).

In Dr. Lakhovsky's book, *The Secret of Life,** the basic theories of the vibratory nature of cellular activity is clearly and thoroughly documented. Lakhovsky hypothesized that every living bit of protoplasm emits radiations. He taught that each cell in the human body emits electromagnetic radiations similar to those from a radio station and that these radiations are of different frequencies, which act and interact, producing the normal functioning of the human body. Disease, on the other hand, was held to be something that interferes or changes these radiations. To overcome disease, therefore, it is only necessary to upgrade or bring these radiations back to their normal pattern. Abrams, although approaching the subject from a different point of view, arrives at almost an identical conclusion.

Dr. George Crile, in his book *A Bipolar Theory of Living Processes,*** approached this subject from yet another point of view. The similarity between his conclusions and those of the other researchers in this field, however, is startling. For instance, Crile wrote, "It is clear that cellular radiation produces the electric current which operates adaptively the organism as a whole, producing memory, reason, imagination, emotion, special senses, secretions, muscular action, response to infection, normal growth and the growth of benign tumors and cancers—all of which are governed adaptively by the electrical charges that are generated by the short wave or ionizing radiation in the protoplasm."

In *Lamp of the Soul,**** Ivan G. McDaniel speaks of biologic wave

---

*Lakhovsky, Georges: *The Secret of Life.* Rustington, Sussex, England. True Health Publishing Co.. 1963.
**Crile, George W.: *A Bipolar Theory of Living Processes.* New York, Mac Millan, 1926.
***McDaniel, Ivan G.: *The Lamp of the Soul.* Quakertown, Pa., Philosophical Publishing Co.. 1942.

142

systems that are vibratory interconnecting systems, that tend to hold a part or organ together for a specific functioning purpose. All this is based on the principle that the cell is an electromagnetic radiating entity. Concerning life on earth McDaniel says, "We may therefore picture life on earth as beginning with simple spores, or cells, which were built up by organizing wave systems when earth's conditions were suitable for life to express in that manner. As conditions changed, the fertilized genes were incorporated into the cells, bringing physical and mental growth. When a new gene and its corresponding wave system is introduced into an organism, we would expect to find the new biological wave competing with the older wave for the same cell material, and this may explain the peculiar combination of plant and animal sometimes found in the earlier species. The balance of the activating hormone between the old and the new biological wave systems may flow back and forth until one gains control and eliminates the effect of the other by absorbing all the vitality."

I've gone into this somewhat extensive background because one must understand the basic theory of cellular vibratory activity before the different treating modalities discussed here can be properly understood. Because the nature of this work is somewhat revolutionary, I didn't want my readers to assume that any part of this theory was original, or that the treatment devices I am about to describe are based on fanciful dreams. Also, I have described the scientific character of cellular radiation because of the attitude of many in the Food and Drug Administration. This bureau, a useful watchdog at times, has among its administrators many who seem to be adherents of the chemical theories of human existence, probably stemming from their drug company-oriented and subsidized educations. Whatever the cause, they have been unsympathetic to any type of therapy that purports to function at the level of cellular electrical activity. I therefore wanted to give reasonable evidence about the scientific soundness of the discussion to follow.

Electromagnetic Theory of Cellular Activity

The human cell, as all matter in the universe, is composed of oscillating components known as atoms, which in turn are composed of particles called protons, electrons, neutrons, and positrons, among others. All these particles are in constant movement. The movement of the electron is especially great, as it rapidly circles this central mass of the atom in various bands, or orbits. The atomic structure is analogous to our own solar system, in which the sun represents the central nuclear mass and the various planets the encircling electrons.

Any motion tends to produce pressures in a circulating fluid around a moving object, producing effects known as compression and rarefaction. The effect of such compression and rarefaction is to set up wave motions similar to the waves produced when a ball on the end of a string is whirled around one's head. The whistling sound given off by the ball is due to sound waves produced by this movement. If we make our ball move faster, if we use a smaller or larger ball, or if we add more balls, the pitch of the whistling would change. Any variation in the compression/rarefaction pattern in the air changes the nature of the sound waves emitted. Thus, matter of all kinds gives off a vibratory wave that is specific to itself. Because the combination of atoms in any matter is unique, this combination produces a wave structure that is unique, which could in turn be differentiated from all other forms of matter if we had apparatus sufficiently delicate enough to measure the wave or vibratory rates. Such apparatus has been constructed, though its practical usefulness is still debatable.

Because all matter is made up of atoms, the world is nothing more than a mass of structures vibrating at different frequencies and intensities.

Lakhovsky and Crile expanded on this idea in their work on the living cell. Lakhovsky hypothesized that the nucleus of the living cell is so constructed that it acts as an oscillating electrical circuit, giving off not only atomic vibrations, but also waves of electromagnetic origin, similar to those generated by a radio or TV station.

Owing to the minute dimensions of the cells, the frequency of these waves is very high. He stated that the electromagnetic waves given off by the various organs are separate and distinctive, and it is the nature of these waves that enables the differentiation of fetal tissues. Each specific gene in the fertilizing cells has a characteristic wave pattern, and as growth and maturity take place, this electromagnetic pattern is gradually developed until the organ and/or personality trait is completed, somewhat like a tape-recorded program that is broadcast over the ether from a radio station.

Not only is growth under the control of these electromagnetic wave patterns, but also tissue repair. Therefore, as long as the vibratory rates in the cells remain normal; there should be no disease. If, however, these electromagnetic waves are altered, the cellular structure and its basic functioning must then subtly change and disease, of one form or another, can begin in the system. This state Lakhovsky used to refer to as oscillatory disequilibrium. Many factors can produce this oscillatory disequilibrium and it was experimentally shown by Lakhovsky, and others, that the disease producing effects of poor diet, bacterial invasions, overindulgence in alcohol or other toxic substances, stress, anxiety, lack of sleep, and similar assaults on the system can be shown to produce their effects by producing oscillatory disequilibrium.

Lakhovsky believed that what we know as infection was but a vying of the various electromagnetic oscillatory rates between the human cell and the bacterium for dominance. He theorized that the electrom agnetic wave structure of the pathologic bacterium tends to interfere with the normal wave patterns of the infected organ or part and that if the body is successful in overcoming the infection, it indicates that the body's wave mechanism is sufficiently powerful to overcome that of the bacterium. If the opposite is the case, it is a sign that the bacterial vibratory patterns are sufficient to so disorient those of the body that the body cells can't function as a unit any longer and that death must ensue.

The work of these men is highly documented and very extensive. Although books on this specific matter haven't been published recently, there have been a couple of very interesting correlated researches. One is entitled *The Secret Life of Plants* by Peter Tompkins and Christopher Bird,* in which the authors describe the various effects of human thought waves and emotions on plant structure. They discuss experiments showing that plants respond very adversely to human anger, hatred and condemnation. If these emotions are only feigned, there is no response whatsoever on the part of the plant. In this fascinating and authorative work, we find further support for the vibratory theory of cellular life. To me these experiments show that the electromagnetic wave energy put out by human feelings and emotions can radiate for some distance, affecting the vibratory structures of other living organisms. That feigned hatred and anger had no effect on these plants shows that it is neither the sound nor fury that produces these effects, but the effect of electromagnetic vibrations produced only by the factual and not contrived emotions.

A new type of photography called Kirlian photography has been used recently to demonstrate strange emanations that come from living matter, both animal and plant. These emanations seem to me to be a visualization of the electromagnetic waves that are a part of all living structures.

Therapeutic Devices Based on These Principles

Because of the complicated nature of this subject, I suggest you read and even re-read the previous section carefully before attempting to understand the following therapies.

*Tomkins, Peter. and Bird. Christopher: *The Secret Life of Plants*. New York. Harper & Row. 1973.

In considering the following therapeutic devices, two questions must be asked. First, is the theory on which the modality is based sound? Second, is the specific instrument capable of delivering the benefits of the espoused theoretical method? Specifically we are asking, "Is the cellular electromagnetic wave principle of health and disease practical and does the instrument we're using perform according to the theory and to the benefit of the patients?"

My own experience in healing has constantly confirmed the validity of the electromagnetic theory of life. Whether all the specific details described by Crile, Abrams and Lakhovsky are correct doesn't particularly interest me. It isn't essential to know exactly how these wave structures are produced or specifically interact to help a patient. Future research may somewhat modify exact findings of the early work done on this subject, but I'd be surprised if future investigation were able to invalidate the fundamental hypothesis involved. Therefore, in my own mind, treatment by electromagnetic means resolves itself down to one fundamental question. Does the instrument I am using help to normalize the electromagnetic structures of the body and to overcome the oscillatory disequilibrium, which we call disease?

Abrams' Radionic Treating Devices and the Depolar Ray

Abrams, in his work on cellular radiation, developed two types of instruments to test his theoretical work. One was a diagnostic instrument designed to detect and classify the normal electromagnetic vibrations of tissues and of the different disease entities in the body. Due to lack of sufficiently sensitive detectors, this instrument could function only through the use of the human nerve reflex and thus its true scientific nature was difficult to verify, since the effectiveness varied with each operator. Such diagnostic instruments were tested at our Center in years past but the results were not consistent. Attempts are now being made to utilize new sensitive electronic means to determine the electromagnetic wave structures of the different organs and tissues. Until these attempts are successful, we feel, this piece of apparatus must remain only a curiosity.

The other type of instrument produced by Abrams was for treating and it used very low-power oscillating currents to produce electromagnetic waves similar to those of the human cells. The last machines of this sort, to my knowledge, were produced by the now defunct Electro-medical Company of San Francisco, headed by Fred Hart. These instruments produced various wavelengths to treat different conditions; in some, these wavelengths were applied one after the other in succession to the treating organs. This last pattern was similar to a circuit known as the Knight circuit, which was somewhat similar to Lakhovsky's multiple wave oscillator, though his instrument was based on the spark-gap principle rather than on the wave production of the triode tube used in the Knight circuit.

The energy from the Abrams machines was applied by a variety of electrodes, generally four, which were placed over various parts of the body to produce the desired effects in specific diseases. These treating machines flourished for a time in the 30's and 40's, but today, it is our understanding that they are being produced only in England for the home market.

The Fred Hart Company also produced an instrument called the Depolar Ray, which wasn't much more than a large coil of copper wire through which an alternating electrical current circulated. The basic circuit was identical to that of a "degaussing agent," an instrument used to demagnetize objects inadvertently magnetized. In the opinion of the Fred Hart Company, this alternating electromagnetic unit helped overcome problems present in congested tissue. It was originally recommended for a variety of athletic injuries, though I find the usual ice pack treatment superior. The Depolar Ray did have a valid use, however, in the benign prostatic enlargements of middle-aged men and in simple cases of hemorrhoids.

There were other types of machines based on the Abrams theories, but in general they were all variations of those just described. I know of none manufactured today in our country and more research and scientific evaluation is needed before this type of instrument is manufactured in the United States again.

The Diapulse and Magnatherm

Some time after the work of Abrams, Lakhovsky, and Crile, Dr. Goldberg of New York City observed what he considered unusual effects on patients under treatment with orthodox diathermy apparatus. The diathermy machine uses a form of electromagnetic energy to radiate heat deep into the tissues. As the electromagnetic energy from the diathermy machine passes through the tissues of the body, a combination effect of hysteresis and eddy currents is produced causing thermal activity in the tissues proportional to their density and the magnitude of the electromagnetic wave. In other words, as the diathermy wave passes through the body, a sort of electrical friction is set up in the denser tissues that produces heat. The stronger the wave put through the body, the greater the friction formed and the greater the heat produced.

Dr. Goldberg detected benefits, that his patients attributed to the diathermy treatment he was giving, that couldn't be accounted for from the use of internal heat alone. Goldberg eventually assumed that another form of energy besides heat was imparted to the tissues by the electromagnetic wave of the diathermy machine. Further investigation led him to believe that the aptitude (strength) of the electromagnetic wave in the standard diathermy was too weak for the investigation he had in mind, so, to further examine his new effect, he had built a machine that had a much greater power than those then available. Unfortunately, the increased strength of the electromagnetic wave also increased the heat in the tissues. Because this heat was already at the maximum allowable without injuring the patient in the standard machine, it was necessary for Goldberg to find a way of increasing the strength of the electromagnetic energy without increasing the heat. To do this, he designed a machine that later became known as the **Diapulse** machine. The electromagnetic waves in this instrument were pulsed instead of constant. Because of this pulsing, heat did not build up in the tissues; thus, a much greater electromagnetic force could be applied than before. Goldberg could thus concentrate on the pure electromagnetic effects of the diathermy energy and his results were published in many professional journals.

The **Diapulse** machine was eventually produced commercially as an auxiliary aid in many diseases. It was used in many hospitals and by physicians of all the health professions. It was originally produced by Sperry Remington Rand Company and later by the Diapulse Company of America, which claimed it was useful in approximately 150 conditions. The FDA took the company to court to see if it could prove these claims. The final decision of the court was that the company could prove approximately half the claims, but the court didn't think the other half were adequately proven and they therefore could not be listed in the company's literature. Later, the FDA thought the company was still making claims that hadn't been substantiated and sought and obtained an order stopping the interstate sale of the machines. A later decision by an FDA administrator (not a court of law as we understand it) stated that the machines, in his opinion, were worthless, and he therefore ordered their destruction or confiscation. The Clymer Health Clinic was using five **Diapulse** machines at this time and we believed that such a completely arbitrary and unlawful decision was entirely counter to our Constitutional rights and so we did what we could to prevent confiscation and destruction of our machines. However, it is usually impossible to fight government agencies over such confiscation, and finally all our **Diapulse** machines were subsequently unceremoniously destroyed.

(This was the status of this matter when I wrote the first edition of this book. However, in the ensuing years the Diapulse Corporation took the government to court and finally won their case. They are now allowed to sell the **Diapulse** once again. Now that it was determined that the FDA had destroyed tens of thousands of dollars of our Clinic's equipment without legal cause, you might think that the government would be forced to reimburse us for the loss. That did not happen. We did not even get a "We're sorry.")

A pulsed electromagnetic generator such as the **Diapulse** is basically little different from the orthodox diathermy machine. If the pulses are fast enough and the power great enough, it will produce tissue heat similar to that encountered in ordinary diathermy. Therefore, it would be possible for a manufacturer to produce an instrument based on the principles of the **Diapulse** that could put out sufficient heat energy to function as a diathermy machine. If such a machine were produced without any claims other than those made for normal short-wave diathermy, it should not rouse the ire of the FDA.

The International Medical Electronics Company of Kansas City has produced such an instrument—the **Magnatherm**. Besides being a much more sophisticated instrument than the original **Diapulse**, the **Magnatherm** has also been especially helpful in our busy Centers because each unit has two separate treating heads, rather than the single one on the **Diapulse**. Because of this, we are able to treat our patients in half the time required for a **Diapulse** treatment. The **Magnatherm** is truly a space-age instrument. Its controls are all digital readout modular units and it even has a built-in oscilloscope so that the rate and aptitude of the wave being administered can be visually analyzed. We have several of these instruments in heavy use at both Woodlands Medical Center and the Beverly Hall Corporation Healing Research Center, and as far as I know, we are the only establishment with such an array anywhere in the country.

The use of the **Diapulse**, and now the **Magnatherm**, has been one of the backbones of the healing methods used at the Centers. Our patients well know the high regard we have for these instruments. However, it is not the **Diapulse**, **Magnatherm**, or any other such instrument that makes the patient well. These instruments are but the tools of our physicians. The tool doesn't produce the final product; only the skill of the physician can do that. We could perform our cures without the **Diapulse** or **Magnatherm**, but it would be a slower and more arduous task. These machines have proven to be fine, but not indispensable, tools.

What the Magnatherm Does*

The electromagnetic wave pulses produced by the Magnatherm machine are used in our Centers to regenerate various organs or systems of the body directly at the cellular level. In acute conditions—those of an infectious or an inflammatory nature—the energy is used to hasten and support the body's reactive ability. In combination with other forms of natural treatment, this therapy has proven most efficacious. Experience has shown me that when properly used the Magnatherm activates the reticuloendothelial system of the body, thereby hastening healing in acute disorders.

Treatment of Chronic Diseases.

It is in chronic conditions that the Magnatherm plays its major role at our Centers; in these conditions, natural therapy easily outshines its competition. To understand the reason for this success, one must first understand the nature of a chronic condition.

All acute conditions are self-limiting in that the patient either recovers and returns to his normal state, or he dies. Colds, flu, boils and pneumonia are all examples of such acute conditions.

In chronic conditions, the healing process of the body is not sufficient to cast off the offending problem, nor is the afflicting ailment strong enough or of such a nature as to destroy the vital functions of the body. We thus have a stalemate in which neither the disease nor the body defenses conquer one another. The patient thus continues to suffer until he either dies or by some means the body is finally able to overcome the disease.

Orthodox medical science has been relatively successful in the last fifty to sixty years in overcoming many acute disorders. They have, however, made little headway in dispelling chronic disease. Although some of the symptoms of these disorders may be relieved by drugs, at least temporarily, little curative help is offered for these increasingly common disorders.

The usual chronic condition must be overcome from within, not from without. The general therapeutic method most useful to us at our Centers is that which stimulates and revitalizes the body repair

---

*This discussion is not based on generally accepted medical opinion. Anything I say here concerning the Magnatherm must he taken as my own opinion, arrived at from my own extensive clinical work with this method of therapy and I don't want to imply that the manufacturer of the Magnatherm in any way substantiates my opinions or conclusions.

mechanisms so that this innate system can overcome the chronic ailment. To do this, we generally apply the following five techniques:

1. All known toxic substances are removed from the patient's internal and external environment. For instance, if a patient is working, we check his job environment for any form of poisonous or toxic substances he may be breathing, ingesting, or in any way contacting during his employment. His foods are also carefully selected to reduce additives and pesticide residues. His home environment is investigated to find and correct any factors that may be causing toxic reactions.

2. The patient is placed on a diet carefully adapted to him with which we hope to supply a good balance of the elements generally needed and an abundance of the elements particularly important to his specific disorder.

3. Every effort is made to establish a constructive, optimistic mental and emotional attitude to prevent the adverse effects of antagonistic vibrations that result from negative and destructive emotions .

4. Specific nutrient substances designed to act as builders of normal cell functioning are prescribed. These are carefully chosen after tests indicate the special needs of the patient.

5. Electromagnetic treatments are given to mildly stimulate the parts of the system that have become sluggish and inactive and that thereby may have enhanced the disease. In regard to this last technique, one may consider the person with a chronic ailment as someone in whom there is disorder and general sluggishness in some of the organ structures. If we can mildly stimulate these organs to aid in their regeneration, we can gradually direct their activity toward more normal function. To accomplish this fully, however, it is usually necessary to see that our first four techniques of the treatment of chronic disorders are also met.

In our own Clinic, we use electromagnetic energy in chronic disorders in both a specific and general fashion. When we are striving for a general encouragement and regeneration of glandular and body function, we treat the liver, spleen, pancreas and adrenals. Where some specific organ is involved other than the kidneys, which will receive the electromagnetic radiation on the adrenal setting, a separate setting is also made on this part. For more specific treatment, the **Magnatherm** may be placed directly over the offending part, such as the knee or hips in osteoarthritis, or over the face in sinusitis.

Great care must be used in the beginning treatment of chronic cases. An old professor from medical school used to say, "You can't take these old chronic cases and try to push them to health. You must take them by the hand, and very gently lead them to health." His words have repeatedly come to mind over the years and without exception his advice has proven sound. The worse a case is, the gentler we must proceed.

The electromagnetic energy of the **Magnatherm**, or of the regular diathermy machine, has a potent stimulating effect on cellular activity and must be carefully used if the desired result is to be obtained. Almost any form of electromagnetic or vibratory therapy can have vastly different effects on the treated part, depending on its intensity, character and the length of time applied. For instance, if we take an electromagnetic wave and apply it at a low rate and intensity for a reasonably short time, we can produce a relaxing effect on a nerve. If we take this same electromagnetic energy, increase its frequency, or increase its strength or time, that same nerve may be stimulated. If we continue to increase the frequency aptitude and time, it is eventually possible to reach a point at which the nerve is destroyed. This is done, for instance, when the short-wave diathermy is used as a cautery unit. It is easy to see why I have stressed the physician's skill and not the machine's ability in overcoming disease. If a nerve needs to be relaxed but the practitioner operates his instrument so that a stimulative treatment is given, the patient will certainly not exhibit the desired effect. On the other hand, if a relaxing treatment is given in chronic ailments where a stimulative effect is needed to start body healing, the patient may feel somewhat better for a short time but his condition never will be structurally improved. The competent therapist must use his machines as a musician plays his instrument. He must be able to evoke in the cells and organs of the patient the exact effect needed at the time of treatment.

Almost any form of body dysfunction can be helped by a careful and judicious use of the electro-magnetic force. It is really not a mysterious treating method but simply a way to produce on specific organs or other parts of the system relaxing or stimulative effects needed at that point in the progress of the disorder. This is no more irrational or mystical than the medical practitioner who gives a diuretic to stimulate the kidneys, digitalis to stimulate the heart, or belladonna to inhibit alimentary canal muscles. One is a chemical stimulation-inhibition method; the other is electromagnetic. It is our experience that the electromagnetic method is somewhat weaker, but much safer and without the side effects all too common to chemotherapy.

In many of the disorders for which we use electromagnetic therapy, there are no generally recognized acceptable chemical alternatives. When the disease is of long duration, the treatment may seem to be overly long, leading some patients to complain that while natural methods are safe, they take longer than orthodox medical methods. Actually, the opposite is true. Because most medical treatment of chronic disorders with drugs is only palliative (symptoms are controlled, but no cure takes place), little time is involved, but if we attempt to cure, much time and effort must be expended. The true cure of a chronic disease is effected more rapidly through natural therapy than by any other means.

Conclusion

In summary, many accomplished physicians and scientists believe the cells of the body can produce and are affected by specific electromagnetic waves. Methods have been developed to measure and categorize these waves in both sickness and disease, but there is as yet no conclusive scientific evidence that these methods are entirely accurate or repeatable. Many treating modalities have been developed to make use of changing the disease wave forms into healthy tissue wave forms by electrom agnetic means. Owing to the nature of the machines and of the diseases they purport to treat, it is difficult to assess these devices on an impartial, scientific basis. We have sufficient interest in several, however, to use them in research projects at our Clinic. The machines we have in daily use are generally available to the medical profession and are fully authorized by the FDA. It is the manner in which these machines are used by us that produces our desired effect and not some mysterious characteristic of the instrument itself.

Chapter X
Natural Therapy Of
Gynecologic Problems

While not personally a zealot for the Women's Liberation Movement, I do think that men have taken advantage of the fair sex in the field of gynecology and obstetrics. Women's bodies for years have been fair play for almost every kind of surgery the fertile mind of man could invent.

The professor who taught me natural gynecologic methods used to say, "As soon as an ovary becomes inflamed, the physician is all too eager to remove it. But, on the other hand, I have seen many men with very severely swollen and inflamed testicles, but I have never seen one of them cut off yet." Apparently it bothers these physicians very little that they may produce psychologic and physiologic traumatic effects on their patients that are all too often completely unnecessary.

Dr. Ralph Wiser, who specialized in gynecology by natural methods, used to say, "Cutting into a woman's sexual organs is like cutting into her brain." What he meant, of course, is that the emotional nature of a woman is so integrally entwined with her sexual structures that one must assume that any surgery on these organs may have farreaching and unforeseen effects. This doesn't mean that surgery should never be performed on these organs, but if it is to be performed, one should be sure that it is the only answer. Many natural nonsurgical methods of treating disorders of female organs are available to be tried first.

If surgery is a necessity, its extent should be limited. Often, it is necessary only to remove the uterus or just one ovary. Some surgeons are all too inclined to remove far more than the patient desires or is necessary. At our Centers we have come across many case histories of patients subjected to complete hysterectomies for simple uterine fibroids without any substantial justification other than the surgeon's whim. I have known cases in which such women were subsequently placed in mental institutions for lengthy periods because of the traumatic shock induced by such surgery. We have seen others who have previously been healthy develop a variety of physical conditions that specialists certified were, in their opinion, caused by unnecessary removal of the female organs.

Surgery is not necessary for many of the female disorders for which it is now often used. Many of these disorders can be treated successfully by the use of drugless therapeutics, especially if seen at an early stage. The causes of female problems are generally simple; if proper precautions are taken or treatments given in time, rarely will a hysterectomy be necessary.

Menstrual Difficulties

Most female problems are directly related to the patient's function as a woman. The first problems encountered usually occur with the beginning of a girl's menstrual cycle. While such a cycle is uneventful in many women, as it should be, some women have great discomfort. Most of these women can be helped readily by natural methods. If no structural abnormalities are present, which must be checked for, most of these difficulties are due either to an imbalance in hormones or abnormal enervation.

Our usual treatment, which has proven most effective, is to place these women on a supplement of raw wheat germ oil extract, relieve nerve tension in the pelvic area by chiropractic adjustment and correct imbalances by the use of electromagnetic energy (Magnatherm). We have found only certain wheat germ oils to be effective. It isn't the vitamin E content of these oils that is helpful, but rather some undiscovered compound(s) that must be present in the natural product. This oil is processed below body temperature to preserve such activity; oil not so produced doesn't seem to be effective.

At times we also use oil-soluble chlorophyll pearls. These seem to function similarly to wheat-germ oil. Although either oil is sufficient for most, an occasional patient requires both types.

Chiropractic adjustments that correct lesions in the lumbar and sacral spinal areas are usually necessary and are a routine part of our therapy for this condition. Many of these young women have pelvic torsion or sacroiliac syndrome (See Chapter III). When this is corrected, the menstrual periods improve greatly.

Our patients also receive specific electromagnetic regeneration treatments of the gland structures involved.

Prenatal Care

The next most important group of disorders that usually affect young women are those connected with childbirth. There is no other condition in which natural therapy has been more discussed than that of childbirth, and in our profession, we find this very interesting and heartening. Little credit, however, has ever been given to the natural healers who have developed and practiced this art long before Dr. Ralph Read or any of the other latecomers had even considered such methods. Long before thalidomide or any of the other drugs that were found to cause congenital defects, we admonished our patients to refrain from medications and

156

X-rays during pregnancy. Because there are many excellent books about childbirth, I mention here only a few special factors that I have not seen before in general circulation and that I believe are helpful for mothers-to-be.

We give our pregnant patients a mixture we call "Mother's Cordial," which is a combination of various herbs noted for their salutary effect before, during, and after delivery. This mixture consists of two parts Mitchella repens (partridgeberry), one part Viburnum opulus, one part Leonurus cardiaca (motherwort) and half part of Hydrastis canadensis (goldenseal). To this formula may be added other herbs that the individual patient may need. This remedy should be continued through lactation to assure a good supply of breast milk.

Besides the foregoing, Dr. R. Swinburne Clymer always recommended an adequate supply of iodine during pregnancy, and for some patients suggested the use of thyroid substance. He held that many cases of mental retardation were caused by subclinical under activity of the mother's thyroid gland during pregnancy.

We also prescribe a good natural vitamin-mineral formula designed especially for the mother-to be. If you want the best ask your physician at our Centers. Remember, we are the ones who specialize in good nutrition and it is our job to know the best of all supplements for each specific condition. Wheat-germ oil pearls are given for their normalizing action on the hormonal production. It is also important to make certain that the mother-to-be has sufficient folic acid in order to assure proper neural tube closing. Here again we have always insisted on the use of this nutrient while the FDA, for many years, specifically restricted its use in supplements to prevent it from masking the symptoms of pernicious anemia. While orthodox medicine now recommends folic acid for pregnant women, one cannot help but wonder how much pain and suffering could have been avoided if the FDA had not restricted in use in supplements previously. Such is the nature of things when men presume to control the lives of others.

One of the most common discomforts of pregnancy is the low backache. Most patients are told by their doctors that this is just an expected part of their pregnancy and nothing can be done for it. We find that most of these backaches respond very readily to mild chiropractic adjustments of the pelvis and lower spine. The type of adjustment used doesn't require the patient to lie on her stomach and no pressure is put on the abdomen or fetus. Such treatments can be used up to the time of delivery. (See chapter III)

At Woodlands Medical Center we are now building a maternity

live-in section where those who desire natural childbirth will have all the advantages available in a home delivery plus equipment on hand to take care of unforeseen medical difficulties.

Natural Treatment of Problems Arising From Childbirth

After delivery, several difficulties can develop that if corrected in time are of little consequence, but if left uncorrected can sow the seeds of much future discontent. The disorders that occur most frequently are vaginal constriction, cervical erosion, misplacement of the uterus and ovaries (usually due to a lack of tone in the broad ligament and other associated structures), and boggy uterus.

Episiotomy and Vaginal Constriction

During most first deliveries, some form of cutting and repair (episiotomy) is required. Although such surgery theoretically shouldn't be necessary in a woman who is properly prepared for childbirth and who has conscientious care during delivery nevertheless such a minor operation is invariably essential. I think this procedure is necessary because we have deviated so far from the natural ways of living that the tissues of most women are insufficiently elastic to enable the first birth to occur without some form of surgical relief. Such an operation isn't required in all cases, however, and the conscientious physician truly skilled in his craft will wait until the child's head fully crowns, or seats itself in the perineum, ready for delivery, before he makes his decision to cut. As the head moves slowly forward distending the vaginal opening, he can watch carefully for signs of strain on the tissues between this opening and the anus because this is where tearing generally occurs. If the physician sees that the head can't pass through without tearing these tissues, he can make a simple clean cut of just sufficient size to enable the head to emerge without further injury to the mother. If the episiotomy is done in this manner, it is always beneficial because here it is used only as an alternative to tearing and a ragged, torn perineum is much more difficult to repair and heal than a clean, smooth-edged incision. If this procedure is properly followed, it will be found that there are those, even with their first child, who do have sufficient elasticity to deliver without perineal injury. These can then be allowed to deliver without the necessity of surgical intervention .

When episiotomy is necessary, the suturing must be carefully done if future difficulties for the mother are to be avoided. Dr. Wiser used to teach that a few separate sutures, not too tightly sewn, was the best possible form of episiotomy repair. Although such a procedure doesn't look particularly neat at the time, it does provide for ample drainage during the healing process and allows for the normal swelling and contraction that take place when such a wound heals. If the incision is sewn tightly to begin with, by the time the wound is healed the opening will be more constricted than normal and later intercourse will be painful.

The all too common form of episiotomy repair used by many obstetricians is what is known as a continuous, or basket, stitch. This produces a neat, professional looking wound closure that unfortunately can be painful during the healing process, because it doesn't provide for tissue expansion. Even more important, however, is that once healing is completed, the wife and husband often find that the scarring has left her with a vaginal opening that is smaller than before and very sensitive to distention. If this contracture is slight, dilation will occur with normal intercourse. In time, the vaginal opening will resume its normal size and sensitivity. Unfortunately, not all patients are so lucky and we find many women so repaired who continue to have severe vaginal constriction pain on intercourse for long periods after the original delivery. Probably because of residual Victorian attitudes, these women rarely seek medical advice for their problem or discuss the difficulty with their husbands. They simply suffer and, because intercourse is painful, they usually find excuses to keep sexual activity to a minimum. Their husbands, not understanding the true cause of their difficulty, may assume that they are merely growing cold. Thus are sewn the seeds of much marital discord.

In some instances, with subsequent children, the condition may be corrected by a more understanding and knowledgeable obstetrician. Unfortunately, once nerve reflexes are produced that relate sexual intercourse to pain, they are difficult to eliminate, even though the original cause is corrected. If a woman has gone through several years of unpleasant sexual experiences, she will begin to relate the unpleasantness with intercourse itself, not with the poor technique of her obstetrician. When we correct these physical contractures at our Centers, we generally must do a considerable amount of emotional and psychologic retraining before these women can once again become truly loving, responsive marital partners.

Although the mishandled episiotomy is one of the most common causes of vaginal constriction, it isn't the only one. This problem is also found in widows who may remarry after some years without sexual relations. When the vaginal tract of the middle-aged woman is not used for sexual relations, the tissues surrounding the outer opening will often gradually contract. This constriction may become so severe that it is not possible to insert more than an index finger without causing severe pain.

If such women remarry, intercourse is practically impossible until corrective measures are taken.

This problem may occasionally develop in married women where sexual intercourse must be suspended for a time because of an illness of either party, or perhaps because of a job that keeps the husband away from home for long periods. Still other cases seem to occur simply because of advancing age. When some women reach late middle life, their tissues surrounding the vaginal opening undergo a natural progressive constriction. As this process continues, intercourse becomes gradually more and more distressing. These women also tend to find increasing excuses for not having intercourse. Few seek medical advice; most are content to let their husbands assume they are growing cold or old and in time intercourse between them becomes only a memory. If the husband is still sexually vigorous, he may seek other women. The woman often tends to become neurotic—going from one doctor to another with a variety of conditions that resist even the most competent care.

It may seem that I am overstating the consequences of such a seemingly simple difficulty. The difficulty is definitely simple, but the consequences can be far greater than I have intimated. I know of women who have committed suicide because of this condition. The far-reaching consequences it can produce when not corrected are due to the ignorance of both women and physicians regarding the true nature of the woman's emotional system and of its interrelation with her sexual structures. Any problem that affects the proper functioning of a woman's reproductive or sexual nature is serious. No one can truly foretell its complete consequences. Therefore, we believe it absolutely necessary that every possible attempt be made to remove and correct any problem or difficulty that might affect the proper functioning of a woman's reproductive or sexual apparatus.

Treatment

The treatment of such vaginal constrictions is simple, but it may be accomplished with a high degree of art and care by one who knows all the factors. In our Centers, treatment consists of gentle manual dilation of these tissues at weekly or biweekly intervals, depending on the nature and severity of the condition. In this method, the physician simply inserts the first two fingers of a well-lubricated gloved hand into the vaginal opening. If scar tissue is present, as after episiotomy repair, this must be done with exquisite care at first; with persistence, even the most resistant case can soon be corrected and the woman may once again resume her normal role in marriage.

Where the condition, particularly in the middle-aged woman, has been a problem for some time, gentle but definite reassurance about the value of her true role as a woman and the possibility of reawakening her somewhat dulled sexual sensitivities must be effected. If the physician is willing to accept the role, he may become a true psychologic evangelist. These women often believe the once-pleasurable aspects of sexual intercourse have passed them by and that they must content themselves with only the more mundane activities of life. While the doctor removes the physical obstructions, he must also work hard to remove these emotional and psychologic obstructions. If he doesn't, he is not truly performing his task as a healer.

You women readers should never allow any physical discomfort to rob you of the pleasures of your sexual and loving nature. If there are problems, seek professional attention.

Cervical Erosion

The mouth of the womb (cervix) is one of the areas most commonly subject to pathologic conditions in a woman. Next to the breast, it is the most common sight of sex organ cancer and it is from this area that we take our samples for the well known Pap (Papanicolaou) test. The cervix is an interesting structure, in that while it may be susceptible to many pathologic conditions, it has no real amount of sensory or pain nerve endings. Therefore, very little direct pain is experienced from cervical diseases and many cervical conditions may go unnoticed and untreated for years.

The lack of sensitive nerve endings in this area is essential to the conduction of normal childbirth. It is necessary for the cervix to stretch many times its normal size during delivery. If it contained many sensory nerve endings, such dilation would produce unendurable pain. Although such a lack of nerve fibers is a physiologic necessity, it makes it imperative for a woman to be examined in this area at least once a year during her childbearing years and at least every other year thereafter. Cervical disease does not give the warning symptoms that other diseases may.

The portion of the cervix visible through the physician's vaginal speculum is covered by tissue that is inherently resistant to vaginal secretions and to substances introduced by the penis. Within the os (the part of the cervix from its opening to its entrance into the uterus) is a different type of tissue, which isn't generally subjected to such substances and which has no natural defenses against them. During delivery, the cervix must dilate from a diameter of a couple of millimeters to the normal head size of a hundred millimeters or more. Shortly after the passage of the child, the cervix must again return to its shape and condition before this dilation. Often in this process, small portions of the inner tissue of the os are left exposed and are subject to the various effects of the environment of the vaginal canal. These tissues, bereft of natural defenses, tend to break down and form a type of lesion (sore) known as cervical erosion. Cervical erosions can range all the way from a small amount of tissue that remains slightly inflamed but without other apparent abnormalities, to a state in which bacterial invasion may occur, cystic formation follow and the entire cervical area become an angry pathologic problem. Although cervical erosion can occur at almost any age, it is most common during the childbearing years. It is the obstetrician's duty to detect such a problem at the six weeks check-up and to correct it so that it doesn't progress from the uncomplicated form to the more severe variety.

Although the cervix doesn't have pain nerve endings as such, it does have nerves that can cause reflex patterns, which may cause backache, vague abdominal aches and even such unrelated problems as headaches and nervous tension.

The milder forms of cervical erosion are often ignored by the gynecologist. When they become severe, he often performs a procedure known as cautery, in which an instrument is inserted into the cervical erosion area and the offending tissue is burnt off. This treatment usually causes a discharge, a certain amount of discomfort and even more important, a definite degree of scar formation (cicatrix). This scar formation can make dilation of the cervix more difficult in future deliveries. If the woman doesn't plan to have more children, cautery might be more rationally considered as a form of therapy. However, I have found in these patients that the resultant scarring can often so constrict the normal cervical opening that future menstruation is made difficult and painful. Most erosions can be treated best by natural methods without such searing, so these difficulties following cautery don't have to be accepted.

These milder forms of cervical erosion are usually left untreated by the thoughtful gynecologist. His reasoning is honest, though not entirely practical. He is all too familiar with the possible consequences of cautery and he may reason that mild cervical erosion is probably less problematic than the scarring effects resulting from the surgical method. The only difficulty is that a small cervical erosion left untreated usually progresses to a state in which some form of treatment is necessary and the physician is thus brought to use cautery whether he wishes to or not.

In treating these patients by natural therapy, we can institute treatment on even the simplest forms of erosion and cure them rapidly so they don't progress to the more severe types. There are also natural methods of treating the most severe of these cervical erosions without the use of cautery and its resulting cicatrix (scarring).

Cervical Erosion Treatment

For our treatment to be successful, we must take into consideration the basic physiology of the area. The vagina is normally slightly acid, and this acidity helps protect this area from the invasion of pathologic organisms. In the normal vagina, an organism called the Doederlein bacillus is found. This is a lactic-acid-producing bacillus whose end products produce the necessary acidity to keep the vaginal tract clean and normal. If as often happens after delivery, small portions of the cervical os remain exposed to vaginal secretions, these tissues won't become pathologic as long as the vaginal secretions are normal. Under such normal conditions the tissues change to a more resistive type of tissue similar to that normally found on the exposed portion of the cervix. Generally, only when the cervical secretions are abnormal and parasitic organisms inhabit the vagina does distressing cervical erosion occur. It is thus imperative that the gynecologist using natural therapy make every effort to keep the vaginal secretions normal during the first three to six months after delivery. If this is done and the cervix is carefully watched during this period, it should return to a near-normal state, thus avoiding the ravages of cervical erosion.

The most physiologic method to accomplish this end is the daily douche with a dilute lactic acid solution, followed by the insertion of a lactic acid yeast tablet. The douche, which helps to eliminate all organisms that are unable to live in its acid medium, leaves the physiologic lactic acid as a residue rather than the unnatural acetic acid left by the commonly suggested vinegar douches. The lactic acid yeast tablet provides an ideal growth medium for the normal Doederlein bacillus. When a properly growing Doederlein bacillus culture is established, it will eliminate all foreign organisms, producing the acid pH needed for the natural restoration of the cervix.

When the erosion has advanced beyond the simple stage, the treatment just mentioned is usually not sufficient for complete healing. It is usually necessary that the inflamed and diseased tissue first be removed and then the physiologic treatment be instituted to complete the cure. Although this morbid tissue can be removed by cautery, I think the scarring inherent in this method is too great a price to pay when less damaging and superior methods are available. We use a variety of herbal packs with mild astringent and escharotic properties that first draw out

163

the inflammation and then encourage a proliferation of healing granulation tissue. This is accomplished over a period of several treatments and in such a way that scar tissue formation is not stimulated. When the treatment with these packs is finished, the cervix should look completely normal, with its normal elasticity entirely intact. When properly used, these packs often produce in a middle-aged woman a cervix that looks as if it belongs to a much younger woman. Once the treatment with the packs is completed, an occasional lactic-acid douche and bi-yearly checkups are recommended to be sure that nothing causes a recurrence of the difficulty .

I also must mention that a common complication of this difficulty comes from the use of the "pill." Oral contraceptives often cause an imbalance, breaking down the normal tissues in the cervix. This not only causes a certain form of cervical erosion, but also often causes a cystic degeneration of the cervix. We have yet to discover a satisfactory cure unless the contraceptive pill is discontinued. When the pill is discontinued and a nonchemical form of birth control is used, these patients respond rapidly to herbal pack therapy.

Displacements of the Uterus and Ovaries

A considerable number of female disorders begin because of malpositions of the uterus and ovaries. These malpositions are usually caused by an incomplete reinstatement of these structures after childbirth. During fetal growth the uterus must enlarge many times and the ovaries are pulled from their normal position by the growth and extension of the related structures. The broad ligaments that connect the uterus and ovaries are much stretched during pregnancy. After delivery, these organs must return to their pre-delivery positions for the normal function of the female sexual and regenerative system. Often, these organs don't completely return to these positions and one or the other of the organs becomes malaligned, causing considerable distress in the future.

The most common problems encountered are those caused by a weakness in the ligaments that control the position of the uterus and ovaries. A forward-bending (anteroflexed) uterus or a backward-bending (retroflexed) uterus is the most common result of these weakened ligaments. Such abnormal positions put unusual stresses on the pelvic structures and can cause a variety of symptoms. The most common of these are backache, bearing down pains, vague aches and discomforts in the lower abdomen, headaches and exhaustion and tiredness after standing for some time.

Some gynecologists believe that it is possible for malposition disorders to cause congestion in the organs and lack of proper nerve conductivity and blood flow so that conditions such as menstrual pain, hormonal irregularities, certain types of cystic involvement, fibroid tumors and even cancer could be produced.

Many operations are done to correct problems that might have been prevented had uterine and ovarian malpositions been taken care of when they occurred. I find there are few mothers who don't have some sort of pelvic malalignment due to childbirth, which, if corrected early, should definitely decrease the flood of hysterectomies.

The most important factor in treatment is the physical replacement (through manipulation) of the malaligned organ. Owing to the stretched and weakened ligaments, it may be necessary that this replacement and corrective tone-building treatments be given several times before the organ will retain its proper position. However, Dr. Wiser, one of the first men to work in this rewarding field, said that in more than 40 years of practice he never had seen an organ that couldn't eventually be corrected. The measures used in treating these conditions are akin to an older therapy known as bloodless surgery, in that the various organs are nudged and coaxed into proper alignment while adhesions are stretched and blood and nerve supply freed so that they might again initiate proper activity to these organs.

Because muscle tone is generally low in these cases, the patient is encouraged to eat as many natural foods as possible, supplemented by nutritional additives to increase the tone of the normal supporting structures attendant to these organs.

After the manipulative therapy has begun to have effect, specific exercises are prescribed to aid directly in promoting the good results of the office treatment.

One of the happiest and most satisfying experiences our practice offers comes when we can assure a woman that a suggested operation on her sexual organs is not necessary and that our constructive manipulative method of treating these conditions will help her. Such work may sound somewhat dull, but it is deeply rewarding. It not only helps prevent unnecessary surgery, but it also helps sustain a woman's belief in herself and preserve her being as a woman. No matter what philosophic words we use to console her or what masculine scientific rationale we preach, no woman divested of her "female" organs can help but feel less than that which God created.

The Boggy Uterus

After childbirth, the uterus may not return to its normal compact shape and size, remaining large and soft—the boggy uterus. This condition is usually accompanied by a retroflexed or anteroflexed uterus, perhaps because the size and weight of the uterus are such that, even with normal ligamentous tone, it can't be held in its normal position.

Treatment of the boggy uterus is similar to that of uterine and ovarian misplacement—that is, general pelvic manipulative therapy, toning exercises and nutritional and supplemental therapy. To these, other natural methods such as electromagnetic-wave energy and sine-wave therapy may be added to aid in strengthening the general muscle tone of the area. In addition the various herbs give good results in these cases. Vibernun, Mitchella, and Leonorus as used in the "Mother's Cordial" often are of great value in the boggy uterus. In fact, where these herbs are used during pregnancy and for at least three months afterwards the boggy uterus is rarely found.

The Middle Years and Menopause

If a woman passes through childbirth with her female organs functioning properly, there is usually little to concern her until she nears menopause. However, the fibroid tumor, the ovarian cyst and cancer may occur at almost any time.

The Fibroid Tumor

The fibroid tumor is a hard, benign (noncancerous) tumor that generally occurs in the uterine wall. It usually has no toxic effects on the body and causes problems only if it grows large enough to physically encroach on vital structures. If such tumors are present in the uterus as the woman approaches menopause, they may produce abnormal menstrual bleeding. At times this bleeding can be controlled only by removing the uterus. Luckily, in many cases, much less extreme measures are satisfactory. The cause of fibroid tumors remains unproven though there are many theories. Researchers in the natural field believe they may be due to certain trace mineral deficiencies. The specific trace minerals involved, however, have not been adequately verified. The ovarian hormones must play some part in their formation because as a woman goes through menopause, the fibroids present frequently retrogress and atrophy along with the normal shrinking of the uterus.

We usually follow a conservative treatment of fibroid tumors at both our Centers. Many patients—especially when the tumors are in the early stages or are small—respond well to the use of certain homeopathic medications and trace mineral supplementation. Because the effects of specific trace minerals are not well understood, we use a supplementation containing a broad spectrum of trace minerals. The supplementation, combined with manipulative therapy (both chiropractic and the internal manipulation of the female organs) and the use of electromagnetic energy, has proven very satisfactory in many patients.

If the patient is nearing menopause and the tumors are small and not causing abnormal bleeding, usually no treatment is given unless the patient requests it. In these instances, the tumors usually retrogress with menopause and no external therapy is necessary. If the tumors cause bleeding, our regular therapy is instituted and specific measures are taken to control the bleeding. To accomplish this, we use Geranium (the herb); supplements such as ionizable calcium; chlorophyll pearls for its vitamin K activity; and protein supplementation usually in the form of unflavored gelatin. This combined therapy is effective in most patients. In the few in whom the bleeding can't be controlled or in those in whom the tumor is so large that the vital organs are detrimentally affected, we usually suggest that the patient undergo surgery for removal. When surgery is necessary, we try to arrange it with a surgeon who will remove only the fibroids involved, leaving as much of the uterus and cervical structures as possible. If the whole uterus must go, we make sure that the ovaries are not removed unless so affected by disease that their presence would endanger the future welfare of the patient.

Regarding surgery for fibroid tumors, time and again we hear of a surgeon who removes healthy ovaries during the fibroid operation simply because the woman wanted no more children or he believes that the ovaries might later become diseased. Such action should be cause for criminal prosecution of the surgeon; I believe that if a few of these surgeons were prosecuted, this despicable practice would soon stop.

Ovarian Cysts

Ovarian cysts are of many types. Some are innocuous—only sacs filled with sterile fluid, which often break by themselves and are self-curing. Some can be dangerous. The normal medical procedure is surgical removal. We find that many cysts respond to constructive internal manipulative therapy. Once the circulation is promoted and the congestion removed, the cyst is often reduced and even disappears entirely. This can't be assured in every patient, however, and we send some of our severe cyst cases for surgical removal. Here, as with the fibroid tumor, however, we are very conservative with ovarian tissue and we insist that the surgeon remove only the tissues that are definitely abnormal and beyond the help of our general reparative methods. Here, as with fibroids, we seldom find indications for the complete removal of the ovaries. I can't remember a case of our own in which complete removal of both ovaries was necessary because of cystic involvement. Most surgeons are not particularly happy when we insist on these restrictions. However, those that have worked with us for some time find that our patients recover much more rapidly than most of their patients and have many fewer complaints after surgery. Some of these surgeons have even made our requirements part of their own general procedure. I only hope that in time all gynecologic surgery can be so influenced.

Cancer

Cervical cancer can usually be detected by using the Pap (Papanicolaou) smear. The smear is a harmless and simple method that can be used to find cancer in an early state, when correction is usually successful. We recommend that our patients get a Pap smear at least once a year and if there is any problem, more frequently. If definite trouble is found, we usually recommend removal of the uterus, for although many natural therapies can be used, there is none that is absolutely 100 per cent certain. The safest method known is removal of the uterus. However, when the results of the Pap test are suspect but not obviously positive for cancer, we use various natural methods to build up the resistance of the tissues to overcome the precancerous condition. According to subsequent smears, we are successful in many cases. We are careful not to fall back on past laurels, however, and these patients are constantly checked to ensure that such improvement is truly permanent. If the state of the cervix ever becomes what we consider dangerous, we insist on surgery.

Breast Cancer

The most common site of cancer in women is the breast. Because the female breast is such an integral part of femininity and its removal such an obvious blow to this femininity, breast cancer produces greater fear in most woman than almost any other cancer. This fear is not unfounded because breast cancer has a very high incidence. In fact, some physicians have even suggested that the woman whose mother or other close female relatives have had breast cancer should have their breasts removed in their youth to prevent the possibility of development. I don't advocate this and consider it an extreme form of therapy. However, the mere fact that it could be suggested gives us some insight into the prevalence of this disorder.

As common as breast cancer is, no one has adequately explained why this organ should be so affected. My naturopathic training teaches me to examine any abnormal condition that may be present in the breasts that may stimulate the development of this disease. For surely God in all

168

his wisdom did not mean to plant in this organ—one of the most beautiful forms of his handiwork—the seeds of its own self-destruction. Surely, something we have done causes our women this grave problem.

Many of the substances we take into our bodies today may be carcinogenic (cancer-forming). One factor, however, might alone have affected the breast—the changeover from almost universal breast-feeding to almost universal bottle-feeding. Through propaganda from physicians and the milk companies, women were told that it was indelicate to put a baby to their breast. Therefore, the breast that usually produced milk after delivery was unceremoniously forced to cease its production, usually by means of hormone therapy given the mothers. Isn't it possible that when we don't allow an organ to fulfill its purpose, we create abnormalities that may plague us later? I haven't seen statistics on breast cancer related to breast-feeding or non-breast-feeding, or to the use of the hormones for drying up the milk. Such statistics probably don't exist; thus I can't substantiate this argument. I just suggest at this time that this is a possibility. Happily, this trend is now being reversed, with increasingly more women being encouraged by orthodox physicians to once again nurse their offspring.

The diagnosis of breast cancer has often proven a fertile ground for the greed of certain physicians. I am appalled at the authoritarian approach of many surgeons, who upon discovering any palpable abnormality in the female breast insist that it promptly be removed for examination. The character of breast cancer is relatively distinct from the ordinary lymphatic swellings and cystic disorders common to the female breast. Any physician can easily and convincingly differentiate a mild lymphatic enlargement from a cancerous growth in the breast, without creating the fear produced by surgical biopsy. Most physicians on the West Coast, where I practiced for thirteen years, were very practical and constructive in their breast examinations; they requested a biopsy only when there was doubt about the nature of a breast abnormality. In eastern Pennsylvania, where I have practiced for the last twenty-seven years, I find physicians much more eager to slash into this lovely piece of feminine anatomy.

Fortunately in the last few years, two new methods of diagnosis have been perfected that should greatly aid in preventing unnecessary surgery. Mammography (now Xeroxmammography) is a new method of breast X-ray that enables the physician to rapidly distinguish between most benign enlargements and true breast cancer.

The other new diagnostic measure is thermography, using a heat-detecting electronic instrument (thermograph) that records changes in tissue temperature and displays them on a television tube. These pictures can be photographed by a camera (usually Polaroid) and a permanent record kept of the woman's breast skin temperatures. If a mammary carcinoma is present, a change in the skin temperatures will show up on the thermograph reading. These new methods of diagnosis make it possible to decide accurately whether the lump in the breast is a cancer without surgery. (This method was gaining popularity in 1975 when the first edition of this work was published but we have heard little of it lately. I feel that this is a pity since it was effective and without the possible damage of X-ray.)

Once breast cancer is diagnosed, the physician must decide whether radical or sub-radical removal is best. There is much controversy on this point. Many recent reports show that if the lymph nodes are removed—especially the ones under the arm— the body's defense mechanism for stopping any further cancer growth is reduced. If any cancer cells are left after surgery, they thus can spread rapidly because one of the body's main lines of defense against such cancer activity has been removed. Recent reports again validate the evidence that simple lumpectomy (just removing the cancerous lump) is just as successful as removing the entire breast in most instances. So the argument rages on. Whatever the outcome, it is at least good to know that some physicians are challenging orthodox concepts.

If the tumor is detected early, breast cancer can be successfully treated surgically. The rate of recovery in these cases is high, certainly far better than any of the other internal cancers.

Many cancers are detected too late for surgery, either from ignorance on the part of the patient or from fear of breast removal. In the past, we recommended surgery for some of these patients in the hope that a chance of success still was possible. They all died miserable deaths. On the other hand, those who did not undergo surgery but were treated by natural means are still alive and comfortable, some as long as eight to twelve years after we first started therapy. I don't want to indicate that we have a specific treatment for breast cancers. I only want to state that some breast cancers, if not treated by surgical means, are often very slow in their growth and the patient can often live a considerable time before succumbing to the disease. On the other hand, most breast cancer patients that are operated on unsuccessfully usually don't survive longer than a year.

This knowledge has made me very cautious in advising a woman in whom we suspect breast cancer. The problem facing us is this: If the patient is operated on, there is some chance that she may be cured. There

170

is also a chance, even if the operation is seemingly successful, that she will die in six months to a year. If the patient is not operated on, she may survive several years, but with the possibility of gradual increasing distress from the breast cancer. There is always the hope, however, that medical science or our own natural therapists will discover a method other than surgery of correcting and controlling the cancer.

I carefully weigh my words in speaking to these patients but I must be honest in telling them what chances I believe they have with such surgery. I generally never advise any form of therapy to my breast cancer patients, but I believe it is my duty as an honest physician to tell them the truth as I see it. I make every attempt to explain as clearly as possible the percentages of success with the various treatments, enabling the patient and her family to make the choice.

In recent years I am beginning to place all breast cancer patients into one of two simple categories. Those whose cancer is systemic and those whose cancer is not systemic. If it is systemic, surgery will have little to offer except a small hiatus period before it returns with a vengeance to metastasize all over the body. If it is not systemic it has little tendency to metastasize and surgery is almost always successful. In these latter patients the growth of the tumor is such that even not removing the growth may have little adverse effect on the life span or life quality of the patient. In the patient with systemic cancer, as mentioned above, they may well live a longer and more contented life if the tumor were left undisturbed.

If my conclusions are correct (obviously they are not shared by the vast majority of the medical professions) then we would do well to develop tests to determine just which of the types of cancer a woman has. Let us pray that such will be soon forthcoming.

Noncancerous Breast Diseases

Fortunately, most lumps in the breast are not cancerous. The most common type of nodule is usually caused by an imbalance of female hormones or the ingestion of caffeine and caffeine like substances. This imbalance may often be readily corrected by the same procedures suggested for the treatment of menstrual difficulties—the use of the raw, unrefined wheat-germ oil; oil-soluble chlorophyll; and manipulative therapy of the thoracic and pelvic structures. To this general therapy, I usually add specific homeopathic remedies indicated in the specific case and some of the herbal remedies such as **Mitchella** or **Caulophyllum**. Occasionally, the specific hormones involved are given, but generally I find them very difficult to use, more satisfactory results usually being

171

obtained by using the nutritional substances.

Lymphatic congestion of the breast is also a common cause of lumps. For treating this condition, we institute general measures to encourage a normal flow of the lymphatic fluid. This, along with specific lymphatic DNA substance and the homeopathic remedy Conium, is often successful in controlling these lymphatic enlargements.

The chronic cystic breast is very difficult to treat. The best therapy is to do all one can to improve the general health of the patient, then using the selected herbs and homeopathic remedies to make the specific changes desired in each patient. Although patients usually can be helped, no single definitive treatment is successful for all of them.

Of late, many physicians are convinced that caffeine in any form can cause or at least aggravate cystic breasts. Therefore, it is imperative to avoid anything containing caffeine in the treatment of this condition.

We are also using the Low Level Laser on this condition. At the time this is being written the results are still inconclusive.

Breast Size

Next to cancer, the greatest concern women have about the breast is its size. Although I have occasionally been asked if I can reduce an oversized breast, the usual request is for a natural therapy to enlarge the breast. I wish I could hold out a great deal of hope, but I know of no natural form of therapy consistently useful in enlarging the breast.

Breast structure is usually determined by heredity and it generally isn't possible to change this by any natural form of therapy. On the other hand, the deflation of the breast that occurs after childbirth and nursing may be minimized by certain measures. A properly designed supporting bra during pregnancy and lactation can help retain good breast function and structure. A diet high in nutritive elements and supplemental additions where necessary helps improve the tone of the various muscles and ligaments connected with the breast. Exercises that include the arms and the chest improve the muscle and ligament tone, and thus provide more support for the breast.

Menopause

In addition to several conditions already described in this chapter that may occur at menopause, several problems are unique to this period. To some, menopause is nothing but a name. They pass through it so easily and smoothly that they can't understand the concern of most women approaching this time. Fifteen per cent of women pass through this period without any recognizable difficulties. Thus, to eighty-five per cent of women, menopause can be characterized by anything from mild inconvenience to an almost hellish torment. Much of her difficulty during this period depends on a woman's own attitude and on the type of medical advice and care she receives.

Menopause begins anywhere from the mid-30s to the early 50s and beyond. It can last anywhere from a few weeks to many years. Most of its effects are due to the irregular production of the female hormones. It is not the mere lack of female hormones that produces most of the distressing menopausal effects but their sporadic appearance. In the early stages of menopause, in which the estrogen levels vary from day to day, hormone therapy is recommended to even out these variations. We usually suggest the minimum dosage of natural conjugated estrogens (though of late we are beginning to use more sophisticated natural products for this purpose), which will control the symptoms. While, the most common symptom is hot flashes (irregular changes of body temperature), menopause is also characterized by many other symptoms, particularly those of an emotional nature. These generally aren't recognized by the woman herself and it is much easier to use her hot flashes as a guide in therapy than to use any of the other manifestations of menopause. In early menopause, a woman may have periods of several weeks, even months, when her hormone output is level. At this time, it isn't necessary for her to continue hormone therapy. However, we always make sure that a woman has hormones available if the hot flashes return.

Many women are afraid of hormone therapy because they have heard that it causes cancer; some physicians fear its use for the same reason. I believe when natural hormones are used such an attitude is overly protective. The body already produces, and has for many years produced, hormones identical to the ones we use. We only attempt to balance a production that has long been active. We don't put a foreign substance into the body. We only supplement the severely erratic hormone production that occurs at various times during early menopause. In forty years, I have yet to see cancer in any one of my patients—nor have I heard of it from any of my colleagues—that was related to natural hormones used in treating menopause. Until such evidence is forthcoming, we shall continue to give help to these women in the form of natural hormone therapy.

Besides hot flashes, menopause can cause many neurologic symptoms. I've known women to go into extreme states of hysteria, and, true cases of psychosis may even occur at this time. Such cases are rare, however, and most untreated women become merely peevish and generally "bitchy," as they say themselves. Heart palpitations may occur, leading many women to imagine all kinds of diseases. Most of these symptoms disappear with a little considerate treatment, understanding and a rational use of hormone therapy. It is understandable that the busy physician may dislike taking time to talk to a woman going through menopause when he has other more serious cases to treat, but most of these women require only a small amount of time and understanding, if it is given early and factually. I personally enjoy talking to these patients and find them full of gratitude for all the care given them. Only rarely do I find them irrational or overly demanding once proper therapy is instituted.

One common mistake many physicians make in treating menopause is to attribute too many symptoms to it. Women often develop other conditions at this time and a symptom of uncertain source may not be related to menopause. At the Beverly Hall Corporation Healing Research Center, we take great care in listening to and checking every complaint of our menopause patients. If we don't do this, many conditions may be overlooked, causing potentially serious problems.

The adrenal glands must take over much of the work previously done by the ovaries, which atrophy during menopause. If the adrenals are strong and healthy, few or no difficulties are encountered. If the integrity of the adrenal glands is only marginal, the patient may become hypoadrenal owing to the stress of menopause. These patients must be treated for hypoadrenalism (see Chapter II), as well as for menopause. Many of our patients previously under treatment by other physicians using hormone therapy for menopause without success have responded nicely when the adrenal was also treated.

Those women who, because of previous cancer or fears, can't or won't be treated with natural hormones can usually be treated successfully with specific nutritional and herbal support. More time is usually required, however, to obtain the proper combination than for those on hormonal treatment.

No woman should suffer physically, mentally or emotionally from menopause. With proper hormone therapy, natural foods and herbs, psychotherapy, and nerve-and muscle-relaxing methods (see Chapter XI), we can readily overcome the difficulties involved in menopause. Properly managed, menopause can be as constructive a time in a woman's life as any other. If your present physician doesn't agree, keep searching until you find one willing to treat you in the manner you deserve.

Chapter XI
Tissue Sludge

In my early days of practice, a young woman patient of mine didn't respond to her treatment. She had had pains in her shoulder, neck, and arm for some time that resisted the best work of several fine physicians and that also didn't respond to my own chiropractic manipulations. One day as I was treating her she started crying softly. In answer to my query about the cause, she replied, "Doctor, I'm the only one in my family who believes in natural methods and they all think I'm crazy for coming here. I want so much to show them all that your methods are right, but this arm of mine really isn't getting any better and everybody knows it because they can all see how much pain I'm in and how difficult it is for me to use it. I'm so upset about the whole thing, I just don't know what to do."

I really didn't know what to do either. I had thoroughly examined and X-rayed her and given her the best chiropractic manipulations and modalities that I knew, and yet still she didn't improve. What was I to do? In desperation I put her face-down on my treatment table once again; using my thumbs I went over her affected areas, pressing here and there. "Does this hurt?," I said. "No." "Does this hurt, then?" "Oh yes, very much."

Whenever she said an area was painful, I dug in with my thumbs. "Oh please don't, doctor, that hurts too much," she would exclaim. "I know," I said, feigning as much assurance as I could, "the more it hurts, the faster it will improve." I really didn't know why I was doing this. I just didn't know what else to do. Actually, I was frustrated and upset at my failure with this patient and was probably taking out my aggression on this poor woman by assaulting her sore areas. But, relentlessly, I continued to prod all her irritated nerve and muscle areas I could find around her shoulder girdle.

When I thought she couldn't stand any more, I stopped and let her dress. "Let's see what happens now, Donna," I said, "Make an appointment for Friday." To myself I thought, "Well, that's the last I'll see of Donna. I sure hope somebody can help her; she really needs it."

To my great surprise, Donna did show on Friday. Not only did she show up, but also for the first time since I had begun treating her she came in smiling. I rather reluctantly asked her how she felt. "You were right about that treatment, doctor," she said, "That's the first real relief I've received in six weeks. Let's get on with another one." Well, I was

175

kind of in a fix now, for I had made up that treatment on the spot and really wasn't sure that I could duplicate it. Ever willing to try, however, I started checking and working over the inflamed shoulder areas. To my surprise, I found these areas were much less sore than they had been.

There was still some soreness left however, so I again began my deep prodding, this time with sincere scientific interest. After a while, I was able to work out much of the soreness in these areas. I stopped the treatment and let her dress. After three or four more treatments, Donna's shoulder problem was entirely cured and when I left the Seattle area some eight years later, it never had returned. She was more than overjoyed, and her relatives were somewhat chagrined to find that this small town "quack" had corrected a condition that the best of their big city MDs couldn't touch.

The results in this case had been so dramatic that I began to check more and more of my patients for this same type of muscle-nerve-fibrous tissue inflammation. I discovered that such difficulties were present in sixty to seventy per cent of the patients that I was then treating. Although few of the disorders were as severe as Donna's, all were considerably improved by the prodding treatment of these muscle-nervefibrous reflex areas.

Further research over the years has demonstrated that such nerve-muscle-fibrous reflex difficulties are so common that one of the first examinations I make on any new patient is to check for such problems. I believe that no patient with musculo-skeletal pain is adequately diagnosed or treated unless these reflexes are sought for and, if found, properly corrected. This research also led me to an explanation of the reason for the effectiveness of this method.

When the body is placed in a situation of stress (similar to that described in Chapter II), it is common for certain muscles to exhibit tension and eventual spasm. When such a muscle goes into spasm, the spasm usually irritates adjacent nerves and other soft-tissue structures. In time, this irritation can cause enough inflammation to aggravate the muscle again, causing more spasm. From this process a congested area is formed because of the sluggish exchanges of nutrients by the cells, and by irregular areas of vascular dilation and constriction. This process can, in time, even produce a substance I call *tissue sludge*. This tissue sludge can be felt by the physician's fingers as he works over these nerve-muscle areas. The flesh feels granular or nodular and has at times a doughy consistency instead of the soft smooth elastic feel of normal connective tissue and muscle.

One of the most common areas for these deposits to occur is around

176

the scapula (shoulder bone) and upper spine. I place my patients face down and with my thumbs gently examine the tissues over the scapula, around its edges, particularly the area between the scapula and the spine, then I work into the shoulder tissues themselves and finally I work along the nape of the neck up into the cervical area of the spine. Some patients are so sensitive in these areas that the gentlest touch causes them to cry out in pain. Before my examination, many have no idea that they are sensitive in these areas. We therefore find it is possible for these tissue-sludge areas to be present causing reflex symptoms without the patient having experienced any previous pain or discomfort in the offending part.

With problems in the lower part of the body, similar reflexes, though nowhere nearly as sensitive, are usually found over the buttocks and in the large muscles on either side of the lower (lumbar) spine.

The tissue-sludge areas described for both the upper and lower parts of the body are general areas of inflammation and do not alone tell the treating physician what type of difficulty is involved. Almost any disease or nervous affliction that affects the upper portion of the body causes reflex irritation in the tissues around the scapula. This is particularly true of nervous disorders. I can't remember a patient with a nervous or emotional disorder who did not have inflamed scapular tissues. In like fashion, almost any disorder of the lower portion of the body affects tissues along the lower spine and buttocks. This is particularly true of old chronic pelvic torsions (Chapter III) and disc lesions of the lower back (Chapter IV).

In my many years of treating, I have found that no matter what other treatment is used, unless some help is given to reduce the inflammation in these reflex areas, other treatments will never be entirely successful. The patient will either never reach an optimum state of health, or if he does reach it for a short time, he will tend to retrogress continually until the tissue sludge is removed.

This treatment is not a massage, as thought by so many of my patients. Although massage of this area soothes the condition temporarily, it doesn't eliminate the basic inflammation. Many patients, before our care, have had long series of massage treatments, but I still find in them as high a percentage of muscle-nerve inflammatory states as in my ordinary cases. Ordinary massage doesn't eliminate this problem; only the specific muscle-nerve prodding can dispel the sludge deposits.

One might ask, if it is not massage, just what is this so-called muscle-nerve prodding. Let me describe just how it is performed. When I examine a patient, I first gently pass my thumb over all the usual reflex areas. If they seem to be not too severely inflamed, I repeat this procedure, but with increasing pressure. With this increased pressure, certain areas usually indicate sensitivity. The tissues in these areas also feel different to the knowledgeable hand from those of the adjacent areas. There may be a lumpy or hard doughy consistency to some; there is a nodular or granular feel to others. The patient is well aware when I find these areas and lets me know because he is generally exquisitely sensitive to the prodding. At this time, I concentrate my efforts on these offending areas. If the patient tenses, I back off just enough so the patient is comfortable while I still retain sufficient force to feel the tissue give properly under my touch. When the proper technique is used, the doughy or granular areas gradually give way and a more normal tissue feel is reinstated. The length of treatment depends entirely on the need and the ability of the patient to accept the therapy, but an average treatment lasts five to ten minutes.

I always work so that the patient has little adverse reaction from any of these treatments. The first and perhaps second treatments may produce a mild stiffness or soreness in the treated areas, but after these first few treatments there is enough general improvement to more than make up for the mild discomfort. Usually after the third or fourth treatment, there is no adverse reaction and the patient feels so much improvement that he is amazed at his own progress.

Once the tissue sludge and inflammation are corrected, we usually suggest an occasional maintenance treatment, the frequency of which depends on the severity of the original condition—usually from once a month to two or three times a year.

Let Me Summarize What I've Discussed Thus Far:

1. Most patients, from living in our stressful modern society, have in specific parts of their back, particularly in the tissues around the scapula, a certain degree of muscle and nerve inflammation of which they may be entirely unaware. This inflammatory condition can cause or aggravate many apparently unrelated conditions.

2. This common inflammatory condition can be readily corrected by a series of treatments utilizing specific deep manual prodding and manipulation of the substances produced by this inflammation—*tissue sludge.*

178

3. When inflammation is reduced, many related conditions also improve.

4. If tissue sludge exists and is not treated at the same time that other conditions in the body are treated, optimum improvement generally won't be achieved.

5. The conditions that respond most rapidly to this treatment are of a nervous or emotional nature. The nervous conditions that so frequently accompany menopause, hypoglycemia and hypoadrenalism (Chronic Fatigue and Fibromyalgia) are helped rapidly by this therapy.

6. Once the inflammation is brought under control, it is readily controlled by an occasional maintenance treatment, and it shouldn't return if the patient is faithful in this therapy.

No other treatment in our Clinic has been so personally satisfying because it helps establish a successful physical and emotional rapport between physician and patient. Because of the simplicity of this therapy, I have had great difficulty interesting other physicians in the method.

Acupuncture

The therapies known as acupuncture and acupressure use various forms of pressure on nerves and other elements of the body to produce beneficial effects. I have been asked by many patients if the tissue-sludge method is a style of acupuncture or acupressure. In general, I'd have to say no. In these Oriental techniques, a specific pressure is held over an area to produce a reflex action; in my method, I work not to produce a reflex action but to change a local physical tissue congestion. I don't disparage acupuncture and acupressure. They have a definite place in natural therapeutics, but they are based on principles different from mine.

In addition to the previously mentioned area, tissue sludge may occur almost anywhere in the body—in the deltoid muscles of the upper arm, the wrists, knees, calf, and thigh. Most deposits in the extremities come from some form of injury or malalignment of the bony structures. In treatment, the bony malalignments are first corrected; if rapid recovery doesn't take place, I search for inflamed tissue areas in the affected part. When such areas are found, I again use the prodding procedure. I dig into the affected areas, gradually working out the tension and spasms resulting from the injury. With this treatment it is possible to correct the after effects of injuries in a few days or weeks, which might otherwise take months to heal without specific therapy.

179

Now that we have the new **MicroLight 830** low level laser, we have added it to our tissue sludge work. It has proven to be an invaluable aid in all these efforts. LLLT (Low Level Laser Therapy) is used on all the same areas as we use tissue sludge. This therapy helps to reduce the inflammation in short order. Often remarkably. It also has one great advantage over our tissue sludge alone—no discomfort.

Chapter XII
Bloodless Surgery

By bloodless surgery, I mean a treatment that changes or alters the position or placement of bodily parts without actually cutting the skin itself. Most bloodless surgery is performed on the abdomen, because the physician's fingers can most advantageously work in this area. Many forms of internal distress respond to this classic but little known therapy—pyloric spasm, nervous indigestion, gastritis, adhesions due to surgery, constipation and certain types of spastic colitis often give way to this therapy.

Long before I became a physician, I read an article in the *Readers Digest* entitled "The Man with the Miraculous Hands," which described a doctor Felix Kersten, who lived in Germany during World War II. Kersten had the reputation of being able to correct many abdominal disorders without surgery by using certain manipulations performed on the abdomen. Heinrich Himmler, then in charge of the S.S. in Germany and one of that country's most powerful and feared men, was afflicted with occasional severe attacks of abdominal pain that were beyond the ability of Germany's best physicians to alleviate. Himmler had heard of this so-called "Doctor with the miracle hands," and had his storm troopers bring him to his headquarters.

When Kersten arrived, he examined Himmler and declared that he could alleviate the abdominal cramps. Kersten would take no pay for his work, but requested that certain people then held in custody by Himmler be freed. Himmler responded characteristically by threatening to torture Kersten if he didn't help him. Kersten admitted that Himmler could do this if he so desired, but of course if he were tortured or killed, Himmler would never obtain help for his condition. This answer increased Himmler's rage, which also increased the severity of his abdominal distress.

In desperation, Himmler agreed to free the hostages, but only if the doctor's treatments were successful. Kersten accepted the challenge and set to work. After a few minutes of manipulative therapy on Himmler's abdomen, the pain disappeared. The Nazi was so elated that he ordered the prisoners released. His condition returned at various times during the ensuing years, however. Whenever it did, Himmler immediately sent for Kersten. Each time he was called, Kersten requested the same fee, and each time Himmler relented and certain "enemies of the Reich" were released.

After I became a physician, I ruminated on two aspects of this story that had originally interested me. First, that functional abdominal pain could be severe enough to cause even a fanatic such as Himmler to meet demands directly opposed to his interests. Second, I conjectured that if Kersten could correct such severe abdominal pain by simple manipulation, why couldn't I do the same?

In my early practice, I encountered patients with problems similar to those of Himmler. Because there was often no ready medical answer to some of their difficulties, I began experimental manipulations of the abdomen. In most patients, I found tension directly over the solar plexus (the section just below the ribs and above the navel). By careful palpation of this area, I often found hard nodular accumulations beneath the upper fatty layer of tissue. With gentle manipulation of these areas, I found I could reduce this tension and encourage the hard knots to disappear.

As the knots disappeared, my patients' difficulties also disappeared. In time, I felt that I had discovered many of Kersten's secrets. I later found that the methods I had developed were related to a technique known as bloodless surgery and they had been used in one form or another by physicians in the natural field for more than seventy years. While the relaxing work just described usually creates its beneficial effects through reflex influence of the solar plexus (a large autonomic nerve center behind the stomach also known as the abdominal brain of celiac plexus), many other types of movements are utilized in the full breadth of bloodless surgery.

Pyloric Spasm and Nervous Stomach

A common problem encountered in digestive disorders is a spasm of the pylorus part of the stomach (Distal end). This area of the stomach has several circular muscles that must contract and relax to enable the proper release of food into the small intestine after it has been thoroughly digested by the stomach. In some patients this stressed muscle will become spastic, causing a disorderly release of the stomach contents. This in turn can produce symptoms very similar to those of a gastric ulcer. Upon X-ray examination, if no ulcer is found, the diagnosis of a nervous stomach is made and tranquilizers or antispasmodics are given. Sometimes, these drugs are effective, but all too often the pyloric spasm is not affected by their action. However, a pyloric spasm usually responds well to bloodless surgery. In treating this condition, we generally use a deep penetrating twist directly over the pylorus, performed using both hands simultaneously. This usually breaks the immediate spasm. After this movement, the solar plexus treatment is given as previously described.

In some patients this treatment may need to be repeated several times before complete recovery is assured. However, it is a rare pylorus that doesn't eventually succumb to this therapy. This is another treatment given us by the prolific Dr. Linke.

The so-called nervous stomach may or may not be a true nervous stomach, because pyloric spasm is often diagnosed as such. A true nervous stomach usually responds well to the basic solar plexus therapy.

Adhesions

Adhesions are fibrous bands of tissues that can form from fluids that develop during almost any type of surgery. Adhesions most commonly develop in the abdomen and when not too tenacious or thick, can often be stretched or even freed from their attachments by the proper use of bloodless surgery.

In this type of treatment, the physician first palpates the abdomen to determine if there is a lack of proper movement of the various parts. If he finds a restriction, he can usually be certain that there are adhesions in this area. If he is knowledgeable in anatomy and bloodless surgery, he can find the attachments of the adhesions and calculate what forces are needed to either stretch or free them from these attachments. I usually work toward stretching adhesions because I find it very difficult even by bloodless surgery to break an adhesion. Even if one can be broken, the damage caused by this action might produce more adhesions that could be more troublesome than the original problem. Because the major difficulty caused by adhesions is their tendency to prevent parts and organs from moving freely, thereby interfering with their normal blood and nerve supply, the stretching of adhesions to provide more normal movement for parts and organs usually produces results as beneficial as those gained by adhesion removal.

When the adhesions are old and thick, poor results are to be expected from this method. If the patient tends to form adhesions readily, orthodox surgery is also a poor risk, because there is no way of being sure that surgery for adhesion removal will not cause even more adhesions. For these patients.we usually use a combined therapy of bloodless surgery, herbal colonic therapy and, in women, pelvic manipulative therapy, plus the various modalities that encourage circulation such as surging sine wave, diathermy, and the magnatherm. With this type of therapy, these patients are usually greatly relieved of their previous distress. Although the treatment may need to be repeated occasionally, it is rare that a patient is not satisfied with its usefulness.

Recently we are using the **MicroLight 830** to help these conditions. Preliminary results are encouraging.

183

Manipulation of the Lower Bowel

Manual manipulation of the lower abdomen can often be of great use in treating constipation and colitis. It is one of the few methods I have found that may be of immediate value in ulcerative colitis. Because ulcerative colitis seems to depend greatly on the integrity of the nervous system, the manipulative work on the tissues that reflex to the solar plexus combined with gentle manipulative therapy over the colon itself has proven of great aid. This is not a cure, but it does aid in reducing the irritation and in reversing the adverse emotional effects on the large bowel that are so often present in these patients.

Constipation can be caused by many problems, but the proper use of bloodless surgery can be a real help in revitalizing a poorly functioning colon.

Mucous colitis also responds well to manipulation of the bowel. In general, however, this is carried out at the same time that the herbal colon therapy is given. Thus, with this therapy two types of treatment are given simultaneously. It is perhaps this combination that makes our colon therapy as effective as it is.

Chapter XIII
Natural Pediatrics

Tina's Ear

It all started with a desperate telephone call from a young mother: "My daughter's been sick for three months. At first it seemed she just had a cold and then just as she was getting over one, she'd get another one. No matter what we did, she wouldn't improve. We took her to our medical doctor and he gave her antibiotics that seemed to make her better for a few days, but then it started all over again. He gave her stronger antibiotics and this seemed to help for awhile, but in a short time the problems returned and she again became worse. Not only is she stuffed up and can't breathe at night, but also her ear started to hurt and was running, with thick yellow matter.

"We took her back to the doctor for more antibiotics. The ear has stopped running, but she has never really gotten well. Her eyes look glassy; she is running slight fevers off and on. Her ears are always sore, she doesn't eat well, and I'm becoming frantic. I took her to an eye, ear, nose and throat specialist. He said she was really in a bad way and had to have her tonsils and adenoids out and her ears were so bad that he had to cut the eardrum and put in little plastic draining tubes so that the infection could drain out, otherwise she'd never get well. Can you help me?"

This mother didn't want to go through with the operation. Some friend had told her about our Healing Center and although we were over fifty miles away, she decided to call us in hope of help.

I told her that although I couldn't be positive until I examined the child, I was sure that we could help her and could probably avoid surgery. She brought Tina in the next day and upon examination I found the usual pattern of mistreated (from our point of view) upper respiratory infection that had become so familiar to us. The nasal membranes were swollen, with bloody areas where the mucous membrane had become so inflamed that the surface capillaries had broken through. The tonsils were inflamed and swollen but not actually necrotic (dead tissue) or pus-filled.

Both eardrums were ballooning out, severely inflamed and the surface tissue looked like the wrinkled skin of an old person. The child was running a low grade fever of about 99.5°F, but though somewhat languid and lacking in natural sparkle, she otherwise did not appear to be sick.

I assured the mother that we could help her child. It would be necessary, however, for her to follow my instructions exactly. While I could not yet assure her that ear surgery would be unnecessary (because I had no way of evaluating the child's basic vitality), I nevertheless believed that we had better than a seventy-five per cent chance of preventing such surgery. The mother was overjoyed and, though still somewhat skeptical because of her previous experiences, she carefully followed our instructions and kept up Tina's treatment schedule.

Within two days, Tina's temperature was down to normal. Her ears no longer hurt and she was able to sleep at night without breathing difficulties. Within a week, the eardrum inflammation had been cut in half and the wrinkled appearance was diminishing. I was then able to tell the mother definitely that surgery would not be necessary.

Within two weeks, Tina looked like a different child. She was almost completely free of symptoms. Her ears, though not yet entirely normal, began to look like recognizable structures and she was playing outside with her old vim and vigor.

About this time, some of Tina's playmates came down with bad colds and flu. Her mother was very worried about Tina, and was certain that if Tina came down with the same condition all our work would be undone. I assured her that this would not happen, but mothers being mothers, I could not prevent her from worrying. Within a few days, Tina did, indeed, begin to run a fever and many of her old symptoms began to return. Her mother, again very distraught, called me, wanting to know if she should take Tina to her neighborhood physician for antibiotics. I assured her that if she did this, she then would really undo a great deal of the constructive healing we had accomplished and if she would only double the specific nutritional remedies I had given Tina, her present condition would very quickly abate.

Tina's mother followed my instructions with great trepidation, but she followed them nevertheless. Because it was physically impossible for the mother to bring Tina to my office for about two weeks, to reassure herself about the severity of Tina's condition she took her back to one of the medical doctors that had seen her originally. On examining Tina's ears, he simply shook his head in disbelief. "What have you done to this child?" he exclaimed. The tone of his voice struck fear into Tina's mother. "Oh my goodness," she thought, "what has that crazy quack doctor done to my child? What was wrong with Tina's ears now?" "Why, what's the matter?" she said. "Nothing," said the physician. "These ears are almost perfect. I can't understand it. I remember how bad they were. What did you do?"

Later when Tina's mother called me and described the incident, I asked her what she told the physician. "Oh nothing, doctor," she said,

"Don't worry, I didn't tell him anything about you." I thought to myself, no wonder our methods are so poorly understood when patients are afraid to let their orthodox physicians know of our ability to help patients when they fail.

Tina has by this time made a complete recovery from her condition and as long as her mother follows the simple maintenance schedule I outlined for her, there is every reason to expect she will remain a healthy child with all thought of surgery completely dismissed.

Toby's Stomach

A friend who runs a hi-fi stereo business near Philadelphia called me one day about his daughter Toby. She'd had the stomach flu a few days earlier, but the abdominal cramps hadn't left. In fact, they were becoming worse and he wanted to know if I would see her. After I examined Toby, I thought the problem to be either a residual colitis caused by the virus or possibly acute appendicitis. Our resident osteopath at that time, Dr. Edwin Cook, also examined her and his tentative diagnosis was acute appendicitis. Her temperature was slightly elevated and her white blood cell count was somewhat above normal. While in serious cases of appendicitis we always recommend surgery, in a mildly inflamed appendicitis we have often been able to stop the process short of surgery with various natural remedies and treatments. Knowing that my friend wouldn't want surgery for Toby if it could be avoided, I suggested this mode of therapy, but I insisted that a white cell count be taken at least once a day until we were certain the girl was out of danger. Because they lived some distance from our Center, I suggested that such laboratory work be done at their local hospital and the results reported to me. The next day, although Toby's temperature was still a degree above normal, her white cell count had dropped from 11,600 to 9,500. This was thought to be a safe level by the hospital, so I suggested continuing the natural therapy. Their local pediatrician did not think the condition was appendicitis, but rather just an aftermath of the influenza, though he had no specific treatment to recommend for Toby's rather agonizing cramps.

After further white cell counts showed a slight but steady decrease, although the cramps continued, I too decided that it was not appendicitis but probably an acute spastic colon due to the flu virus. To correct this disorder, I suggested that they bring Toby back for a short series of our herbal colonic treatments. Following these, the condition began to improve—although not as rapidly as we are accustomed. Toby's mother, who was, at that time, not completely sold on natural methods, took the child back to her pediatrician, who conjectured that the disorder might be a urinary tract infection. He therefore gave Toby the rather strong antibiotic Macrodantin.

When her father told me this, I was somewhat surprised, since Toby's examinations had never revealed any symptoms of a urinary condition. Not wishing to cause a family argument, I told him to go ahead with the Macrodantin, but if it didn't clear up in a few days, it should be discontinued because it could have severe after effects on the normal bowel bacteria. If the pediatrician was correct, the pain should abate very quickly after use of this drug. The pain did not abate and so the pediatrician concluded that there was no urinary infection and the Macrodantin was stopped.

He admitted he really didn't know what was bothering Toby, but when he found out that I had recommended various nutritional supplements he convinced Toby's mother that these were possibly causing her distress and suggested that they be discontinued. This was done with the result Toby's difficulties, pain and suffering increased.

At this time, Toby's father brought her to me again. Upon examination, I found the colon still inflamed, though not as much as it had been earlier. I suggested that we try herbal colonic irrigations once again because I thought that the diagnosis of acute spastic colon was correct and that we had discontinued this therapy too soon for the desired recovery. The father agreed and after two further colon treatments and the use of a mild bulk laxative, Toby's abdominal problems ceased and her rather long ordeal was over. In fact, the only problem remaining was an irritating body rash that apparently was a reaction to the Macrodantin. This also responded to natural methods with reasonable rapidity, although it is unfortunate that such treatment was necessary.

The Effectiveness of Natural Treatment in Children

These case histories have been presented because I find that very few people, including many physicians in my own profession, have a complete understanding of the usefulness of natural therapy in the problems of children. I believe there is no field of medicine in which natural methods can show their true wonders as fully and rapidly as in the treatment of common childhood disorders.

When I was first considering a career in healing, I met a young fellow whose interests were about the same as mine. When I told him I was going to be a naturopath and chiropractor, he was very intrigued, but he decided to become a medical doctor. Although he liked the idea of natural methods, he said he didn't "want to spend all his time treating old people." In fact, natural methods are more effective for the young than they are for older persons. This is due to the very nature of natural methods and the way they function in the body.

In almost all acute conditions, which are those most prevalent in children, we attempt to stimulate the disease fighting mechanisms of the body to greater activity. In order to accomplish this, the body must have sufficient inherent vitality so that such methods do not exhaust it—exactly the opposite of what we intend. At times, in the very aged and weak, we must be cautious about the methods we use to stimulate these defense processes, because the patient's body may run out of basic vitality before we can accomplish our purpose. In the older patient, we must therefore often choose a milder and slower-working method that is safer and less heroic in that particular case.* In children, however, this is only rarely necessary. Because their bodies have not yet been subjected for a long time to the ravages of modern living, they can usually be stimulated by active treatment without any great difficulty or fear.

Also, because most children haven't been subjected to the long-term deleterious effects of smoking, refined foods, atmospheric pollution or emotional stress and strain as much as have their parents and older persons, their tissues respond much more readily to the natural elements we give them to encourage healing and repair. Their digestive and metabolic systems function better than those of most older people; therefore, when a product is given, it will usually be digested and assimilated, an assumption that can't be made with any certainty in adults.

Children are much closer to nature than their old contemporaries; they are not yet filled with the gross toxins and poisons characteristic of so much of the grown-up world. Being close to nature (God), their bodies respond well to things that are native to their own creation. In treating childhood disorders, the more closely allied the products we use are to the structures of nature, the more able the child is to accept and utilize them to his own benefit. On the other hand, the more foreign a substance is to a child's chemical structure, the more detriment it is capable of producing. Most modern drugs are complicated, man-created compounds that are structurally light years away from the substances the Creator placed in our world. Who knows what effects these distinctly foreign substances may have in time on all of us.

This isn't to say that there is not a place in pediatric emergencies for even the strongest and most chemically complicated of modern drugs, but they are frequently used where natural, much safer methods would be entirely adequate. In all too many patients, drugs may produce as much or more disorder than they cure. This is not my own conclusion

---

*See Appendix A on the difference between active and passive treatments.

alone, but also that of many reflective and honest pediatricians.

The natural physician looks on disease not as an entity that strikes the body, but as a condition brought about by various deleterious activities that have produced certain physical, chemical or emotional instabilities in the body resulting in the symptoms and manifestations we call disease. To overcome disease, the natural physician seeks to discover the imbalances, deficiencies or abnormalities that exist in the body and then to ascertain what actions have caused these disorders. Once this task is completed he makes every effort to correct these adverse actions and to utilize various natural methods to overcome the original defects and imbalances.

In children, such imbalances are usually mild and easy to detect. The child hasn't had the time, nor the inclination, to develop the bad mental, emotional or physical habits of many of our older patients. Because these imbalances in children are fairly simple, they usually respond to correspondingly mild and simple therapies. Frequently, we only compound the child's difficulties when we attempt to use harsh, nonphysiologic drugs.

Antibodies and Antibiotics

Our bodies contain marvelous agents of defense known as antibodies. When a foreign germ or substance invades the body, a body mechanism (or system) rapidly investigates the nature of this invader. In a way, you might say that this mechanism is like our body's CIA or FBI. This system examines the invader, finds out all his strong and weak points and then produces a specific entity called an antibody, which when it combines with the foreign invader renders it completely harmless.

Let us assume a foreign invader shaped as shown in example (A), Figure 12. The body knows that example B is a harmless substance. Its job then is to produce another substance (C) that when combined with the foreign invader (A) produces the harmless substance (B). When this is done, these (C) substances, which are now antibodies, are a ready and effective defense against the invader (A). If substance (A) ever again invades the body, the antibodies (C) present in the blood and in some of the other organs of the body are instantly drawn to this invader, combine with it and render it into the harmless substance (B), which is then eliminated by one of various body processes. Since antibodies are lost in this procedure, the mechanism functions so that each reinfection re-stimulates further antibody production to replace those lost in the process of neutralization.

At this time, I want to draw attention to two factors involved in

A

B

C

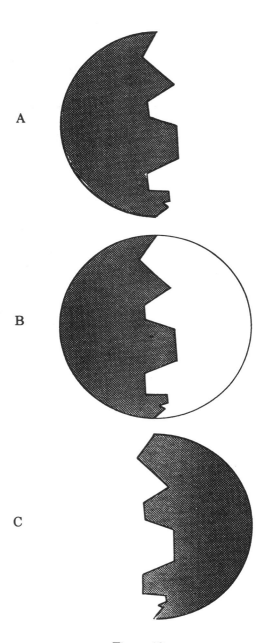

Figure 12

antibody production. First, no antibodies can be formed until an invader first attacks the body. Therefore, during the first infection or invasion, one must depend on something other than antibodies to control and overcome the invading agent. Second, it takes time and the stimulation of the foreign substance to produce antibodies. If anything is done to prevent this natural process from proceeding through its various stages, antibody production is retarded or even stopped entirely.

Although the infant obtains antibody protection from the milk of his mother, assuming he is nursed, he must produce his own antibodies for his proper protection throughout the rest of his life. He also must build a strong first-line defense mechanism, because antibodies are only produced as the first invasion is overcome and it is necessary that the reticuloendothelial system, the white cell phagocytes and the other first-line defenses also function properly.

The common modern medical treatment of children's disease relies heavily on antibiotics. Although these substances are effective, they take over and do the work of the body's defenses, frequently stopping an infection before the body has had a chance to build antibodies. If the child should become reinfected, which is most common in today's world, his body will have no antibodies to stop this infection. Thus, antibiotics are usually used again, further weakening the body's defenses. In time even the first-line defense mechanism is weakened and the child becomes what I call an antibiotic cripple. We do use antibiotics at our Centers, but they are used only when we know that the body's defenses, even with our help, are truly inadequate to protect the patient.

If we take a case of simple tonsillar infection and follow it through with and without antibiotics, the possible damage that can be wrought by these often useful but frequently misused substances should become clear.

An invader attempts to enter the body through the mouth. The tonsils attempt to stop the invader by holding it in their special pockets (crypts) and a battle rapidly ensues. The white blood cells (leukocytes) are drawn to the area, the invader stimulates an inflammatory reaction and the tonsils swell, they become congested with blood bringing more white cells to the area and the body temperature rises. The child feels weak and languid because the energy normally used by his muscles and other tissues is now being used to overcome the invader and to produce antibodies to counteract any such future infections.

In our own treatment of this condition, the young patient is put to bed, to conserve his vitality for the fight. For a day or two he is to have nothing but diluted fruit juices, which give the body necessary elements for its defense and rest the digestive system so its energy can be diverted to the battle. Specific nutritional substances are given to the patient in an easily assimilable form, which provide the body with the raw m aterials needed for the proper function of its defense mechanisms. Certain herbal remedies are prescribed that enhance the body's ability to fight the foe.

If the foregoing program is carefully followed, the body's defense mechanisms are usually readily able to overcome the invasion. The body has adequate time to survey the invading agent and to produce sufficient antibodies to protect the health of the child against further similar insults. This may take several days and in some instances up to two weeks, because antibodies sometimes are produced slowly. The patient is not entirely safe from reinfection until antibody production is well-advanced and the system can use these substances to control the invading agent adequately. If therapy is not continued until sufficient antibodies are produced for complete control, the encouraging results at the beginning of treatment may be followed by recurrence of the ailment within a few days or weeks.

When antibiotics are used, the course of the disease is changed drastically, assuming that the invader is sensitive to the drug. When the proper antibiotic is given, the bacterial invasion and the antibody production stimulated by this invasion are soon brought to a standstill. The child's parents are usually pleased to find that the disease is so rapidly "cured," little realizing that only a small battle has been won, but that the war is being lost because the body's defenses are now weaker than before the disease and not stronger, which would have occurred if natural methods, which allowed proper antibody creation, had been pursued.

If the only difficulty with antibiotics were that they prevent antibody production, we might be able to use them more widely, but they have other adverse effects as well, especially in the young. The first line of body defense—the inflammatory state, the phagocytosis of the white cells, and the fever reaction of the body—is stimulated by use. In other words, when these defenders are allowed to battle a condition to its ultimate successful conclusion, they, like any other army, become more effective as a fighting machine. If, when a young child develops symptoms of infection, the parents rapidly run to have his body saturated with antibiotics, the inherent natural defenses have little chance to develop. All too often, when viral infections (which aren't controlled by antibiotics) attack this child, he has little ability to fight it on his own. Viral conditions that are basically mild in most, can, in these children, become serious. Various overwhelming infections may occur in children whose

193

defense mechanisms haven't been allowed to develop naturally.

Added to all this, we must remember that antibiotics are themselves foreign substances to the body and can trigger reactions which, although usually mild and transitory, have nevertheless been fatal in sensitive children.

I don't mean by this discussion to disparage completely the use of antibiotics. They have a place in overcoming severe infections that are obviously beyond the control of the body's defense mechanisms. Almost every conscientious researcher of pediatric medicine bewails the fact, however, that the average practitioner vastly overuses antibiotics, not only helping to culture a vast army of drug-resistant organisms* because of such constant exposure, but also producing a generation of children that often have great difficulty in overcoming the simplest infections with their own defense mechanisms.

The Character of Childhood Diseases

The first book I read on natural healing, entitled *Nature Cure* and published originally in 1914, was written by Henry Lindlahr, the father of the former radio commentator on health, Victor Lindlahr. I still consider Henry Lindlahr the most dynamic writer I've ever read on this subject. It was this book that first awakened in me the desire to be a doctor of natural medicine. It was also in this book that I first read the rather heretical naturopathic point of view that disease was not necessarily a harmful process, but in fact that certain so-called diseases, properly treated, could be very beneficial to the long-term health of the patient. According to Lindlahr, this was particularly true of acute childhood illnesses and he gave many examples to illustrate his point.

Lindlahr's theory, in a nutshell, is this: When we are born, we bring into the world, as indicated by the Bible, the sins of our father and father's fathers. In other words, Lindlahr believed that the child inherits many disease-producing congestions and toxin-like substances from its parents. He then theorized that many of the various childhood illnesses are an opportunity given to the body, through the action of the acute defense process, to throw off some of this inherited destructive matter. He therefore suggested that little effort be made to isolate our children from such common contagion and if and when it does occur, to treat such a disease by the methods then advised, and still used, by natural therapists. Such treatment should do all it can to stimulate the elimina-

---

*Since we originally wrote these words over twenty years ago even the most conservative of physicians is beginning to be concerned about the possible serious effect of these "Super Bugs."

tion process. In this way the body is given an opportunity to correct many of its congenital weaknesses.

Lindlahr observed, at least in his time, that children who go through their youth with very few childhood ailments often have considerable health problems in later life, whereas those who run the gamut of childhood illnesses successfully and are treated in such a manner that these conditions are not suppressed are often singularly free of disease in later life.

I realize that to talk of congestive or morbid matter in the system in this day and age may bring a smile of contempt from some of my sophisticated readers, but these terms were written originally in 1914, and at that time such words, although not accepted by the orthodox medical profession, were at least understood by the public. From my own experiences, and those of many other physicians in this field, there is a definite consensus that Lindlahr's theory may well be valid. It may not work in the manner in which he hypothesizes, but the beneficial clinical effects are readily demonstrable.

Therefore, to this day, I stress to my patients that whenever an acute disease is present in their children, it is usually to the child's present and certainly ultimate benefit to treat that condition in as natural a manner as possible to enable the inherent body defense mechanisms to function as fully as they can. In this manner we aid the body in performing two vital functions. First, we enable the body to strengthen its own basic defense mechanisms and to develop antibodies to control similar conditions in the future. Second, we give the body the opportunity to utilize the acute reaction to rid itself of other adverse substances that can't readily be eliminated through its normal functions.

I realize that this last conclusion isn't supported by a consensus of medical opinion; yet it doesn't take much research to discover there have been times when the elite of orthodox medicine themselves use this method and use it successfully. In fever therapy, the patient with chronic syphilis has been treated by inducing an artificial temperature or fever, either mechanically or by injecting fever-producing organisms. This feverish state has been used to burn out disease conditions that, though injurious to the body, aren't able to produce a natural fever by themselves. Man devised this method from the simple observation of the way the body itself functions under certain circumstances. My thought, however, is this: if man can create in the body an artificial temperature in order to correct certain disease processes, isn't it just as possible that when the body produces a fever from a natural cause, might it not also use this fever to overcome other disease processes in the body in the same way? It seems that we may almost have a double standard as far as medical theories are concerned. As long as man does something, it's science. When nature does something, it's quackery.

Types of Children's Illnesses

The diseases I discuss here are common to childhood and are successfully treated by natural methods. These can be divided into four basic groups. The first group includes conditions that are mild and commonly encountered in children. The second group comprises those that are more severe, but that have generally been caused by improper or inadequate treatment of the mild conditions. Third, are conditions that are generally congenital; and fourth, are those that stem from inborn hereditary factors.

Most people have difficulty separating congenital from hereditary disorders. A congenital condition is one that may have been caused by some specific situation that occurred while the child was within the mother's womb (uterus) or that may have happened during the delivery. Hereditary conditions are those caused by genetic defects that have been handed down from the child's ancestors and are passed on to the child, even though its term in its mother's womb and delivery were entirely normal. The deformities caused by the tranquilizer thalidomide are examples of congenital defects; sickle cell anemia, which is a genetic disturbance present in the blood cells of many African Americans, is a hereditary defect.

In a child who is relatively free from congenital defects and whose hereditary deficiencies are not severe or overpowering, most of his early illnesses will fall into the first category. These usually consist of upper respiratory infections, chest congestions, tonsil problems, adenoid problems, spinal and other mechanical problems, a variety of infectious diseases, so called childhood diseases, worms, bed-wetting, and other similar conditions. If these conditions are treated by simple natural means, the child usually weathers them successfully and can look forward to a healthy adulthood. On the other hand, if these conditions are inadequately or over zealously treated, they often can give rise to more serious problems that may be the beginning of a lifetime of suffering and medical dependency.

It was an axiom of the early naturopaths that many chronic diseases were the result of acute conditions that had been improperly treated. They believed that if one does not properly treat a mild acute condition, it will worsen and turn into a chronic or permanent condition that is resistant to almost all forms of therapy. My own experience has time and again proven to me that this axiom is well-founded. Therefore, much of the discussion here is about therapy designed to show you, the parent, how you may treat your children's mild conditions so that you will be able to prevent them from developing into more serious or chronic conditions.

Congenital and hereditary conditions can also be treated by natural means. Because of their nature, however, each is an entity unto itself and must be handled by a natural physician well versed in this type of work.

Treating Childhood Diseases by Natural Methods

Acute Catarrh of the Head

As every physician knows, the most common childhood ailment is the upper respiratory infection—the cold, runny nose, inflamed ears, swollen tonsils and adenoid problems. Improperly treated, these can result in chest congestion and the various forms of bronchitis. Many names can be given this ailment, but it all comes from one thing—acute catarrh (mucus congestion) of the head.

The procedures used in treating this condition are basic to practically all infective childhood disorders. I therefore go to some lengths to describe this therapy; when discussing other acute childhood disorders, I will only elaborate on those parts that differ from this basic treatment.

The most common cause of all childhood illness is improper diet. Therefore, the diet must be the first correction made when we attempt to devise a treatment for childhood diseases. In this area the biggest mistake most parents make is to allow their children far too many sugars, starches and dairy products and insufficient amounts of fruits, vegetables, and proteins—the protective foods.

If the child's upper respiratory condition does not elicit a fever, I usually restrict the child's diet to small amounts of lean meat, fish, seafood and plenty of fruits and vegetables. No dairy products (milk, eggs, cheese) or carbohydrates (bread, cakes, pies, cookies, candies) are allowed until the condition is well on the road to recovery. Even then, I recommend that the parents put the child on our Basic Health Maintenance Diet and keep him there to prevent a recurrence of the disorder.

If the child has a fever, I restrict him to a diet of half water and half fruit juices mixed to be given frequently during the day until the temperature returns to normal. Once the temperature is normal, I have the child follow the diet of lean meat, fish, fruits and vegetables until the child's tissues have again returned to normal. At this time, as in the first instance, the child is placed on the Basic Health Maintenance Diet as a general health precaution.

I can't emphasize too much that these dietary recommendations are an absolute must in treating these conditions. All the specific therapy we use is of little value unless the dietary recommendations are followed. I wish to reiterate again most emphatically, most childhood respiratory problems stem from improper diet and it is only by the permanent change of this diet that a true cure can be achieved.

After dietary regulation is assured, we recommend specific herbal and nutritional agents to help our young patients. The most common herbal mixture used is called EMP—Improved. This herbal product is a special mixture of extracts produced in our own laboratory. This grouping of herbs (EMP) has never been known to fail us in these conditions, and yet it is only rarely known to the profession as a whole.

EMP-Improved

This is the most commonly prescribed remedy at our Healing Research Center. Some of the ingredients are proprietary, but those that can be disclosed are described below.

Echinacea: was originally known as an alterative—an old term meaning "that which changes a morbid condition to one of health." An alterative was used to change the nature of a condition—in other words, to start the healing process. It has also been called a blood purifier. I dislike the term because it bespeaks of quackery, and Echinacea is too valuable an herb to have any whisper of quackery connected with it, but the name does describe its clinical effect. Some physicians have called Echinacea a natural antibiotic. I object to this because the action of the herb is entirely unlike that of an antibiotic. Although it controls infections and quickly hastens a return to normal in many, it does not effect its action by stopping the natural processes, as do antibiotics, but by stimulating to greater activity these self same natural processes. Thus, its general action is quite the opposite of that of antibiotics. It is truly a sovereign remedy, however, and is the most frequently used herbal substance at our Centers.

Myrrh: is the same myrrh brought by the Wise Men to the Christ Child. It was used then and now to prevent what has been called "mortification of the flesh"— another way of saying that it prevents abnormal destruction and breakdown of tissues. In this capacity it works happily and synergistically with the Echinacea.

Hydrastis (Golden Seal): is an herb that stimulates the lymphatic system. When the lymph glands are swollen and congested, as often happens in upper respiratory infections, Hydrastis aids in promoting a free and constructive movement of the lymphatic fluids. Hydrastis also acts as a catalyst in any compound containing it. It helps to make all the other herbs function more effectively.

Thuja (Arborivita): is an herb that helps the body rid itself of various toxic substances. It also has been reported to be effective against some viruses that Echinacea may not be able to handle alone.

The EMP-Improved is taken internally, usually in a dose of ten to fifteen drops, three to four times a day in mild congestions and as frequently as every half hour in severe infections with high fevers. It is also specifically effective for sore throats and swollen tonsils. In these instances, the condition is treated directly by swabbing the affected area with a cotton swab dipped in the full strength herbal liquid. This swabbing should be done two to three times a day or more often if the condition is severe. There are no known toxicities from this herbal compound, nor can I even remember a patient who was sensitive to it. It is most certainly one of the great natural therapeutic compounds.

The next therapeutic aid we suggest is a vitamin C preparation. I usually insist on a specific preparation that contains not only vitamin C but also a very high concentration of certain bioflavonoid factors in combination with other natural extracts, some of which have not yet been completely isolated. Although the ordinary vitamin C preparations often give protection in certain persons, the complete tissue repair I desire is not generally accomplished without the more esoteric factors that are part of some specific products available to the Natural Healing professions. Among other things these products now contain various compounds extracted from the Thymus, Adrenal and Spleen. We have found these extracts to be invaluable in all infective diseases, not only those of children.

If the condition is mild and no fever is present, the prescribed diet, and the special Vitamin C preparations usually bring about a very successful recovery. More severe cases and all instances in which fever is present require the addition of more specific and stronger thymus activity. There seem to be in thymic material, properly processed, agents that stimulate body repair mechanisms. Recent researchers have discovered a substance in thymus called interferon, which can destroy viruses. Although it's doubtful that either of the thymic preparations we use has large amounts of interferon, it is possible that they may have precursors that aid the body in making a similar substance that helps control infections. These thymic materials help to control many infections for which antibiotics are apparently worthless. This fact has been verified not only by the members of the natural healing arts but also by an ever-increasing number of medical practitioners who have become disillusioned with the scientific wonders of their own profession and have begun to investigate some of the techniques that we've been using for decades. (This was written twenty years ago and the information is still valid today. The only difference being that we now know much more about the use of Thymic material and it is now available in many new forms including a liquid for the youngest of children.)

In upper respiratory infections that appear resistant to the agents just described, it is sometimes necessary to add fat-soluble chlorophyll capsules. The exact agents present in this fat-soluble chlorophyll compound that help fight infections are unknown, but clinically they are very effective. They are completely harmless and without any counterindications or adverse side effects.

If an upper respiratory infection ends in a tickling cough that doesn't rapidly abate, the body usually needs ionizable calcium, and vitamin F (unsaturated fatty acid substances) to aid in the utilization of the calcium. Several products may serve here. We usually prescribe a phosphorous free calcium and special Vitamin F tablets that rapidly correct this problem.

Other herbal, nutritional, and homeopathic remedies are used in individual cases, but this supplementation regimen usually is adequate in most upper respiratory infections.

The Cleansing Enema

Whenever a young child has a condition that produces a fever and in which diarrhea is not an early symptom, a cleansing enema can be an important part of therapy. This treatment is usually given early in the course of the disease and should consist of one quart of warm water in which has been dissolved half a teaspoon of table salt and half a teaspoon of baking soda. The enema should be given slowly with small amounts of solution being injected followed by a rest period before injecting more. This procedure—injection, rest, injection, and rest—if pursued, will cause less spasticity and cramping in the child and the enema will be accepted with less ruckus. The effectiveness of this treatment can be increased if the mother gently kneads the child's abdomen while the water is being injected to aid in its passage through the various convolutions of the large bowel.

Improvement in the child's condition frequently follows rapidly after the enema. In some cases, the enema must be given daily until the fever is down, but usually one or two enemas are all that are required. If you are in doubt about how to administer the enema or whether one should be administered, it is best to contact your Healing Research Center doctor before attempting this procedure. Some conditions that may be benefitted from this treatment require the careful management of a physician trained in its operation.

Office Treatment

In our office treatment of these conditions, we usually use Magnatherm, treating the affected area and also the general organs of elimination. Chiropractic manipulation also is usually indicated. We generally find that the cervical vertebrae are rotated and a certain amount of fixation is present in most cases. Although a child will recover without a correction of these spinal problems, recovery is more rapid and seemingly more complete when we take these mechanical problems into account.

For the irritated tissues that are such an integral part of these conditions we use Chlorophyll nebulization in the office. This treatment brings almost instant relief to the inflamed tissues of upper respiratory infections.

Antibiotic Therapy

The procedure just outlined, as simple as it seems, adequately corrects most childhood upper respiratory infections, and furthermore it is the cornerstone of treatment for almost all infectious diseases of the young.

Although we make every attempt to refrain from the use of antibiotics in this general treatment, there are two times in which we are more or less forced to contend with antibiotic therapy: first, as often occurs, when a child has been treated by other physicians before we see him and is on antibiotics at the time of his first visit to us; and second when the child is brought to us so late in the progress of the condition that the infection is overwhelming and we think it necessary to use a specific antibiotic to preserve life. In the first instance, we have no control of the doses given; in the second, we try to use as harmless an antibiotic for as short a time as possible, stopping the antibiotic long before the regular practitioner would, because we can depend on natural methods to complete the necessary healing, once the antibiotic has prevented an overwhelming of the body defenses by the infection. When antibiotics have been administered, it is advisable to give some sort of bacterial culture to protect the intestinal flora from the adverse effects of the drug. Acidophilus, Lactic Acid Yeast or even yogurt works in most cases.

Complication of Upper Respiratory Infections

The proper treatment of the simple upper respiratory infection is extremely important in childhood because of its possible rapid extension into nearby areas. The eustachian tube in the child is almost horizontal rather than directed diagonally downward as it is in the adult and it therefore is very easy for upper respiratory infections to pass along this tube into the middle ear of the child. Otitis media (middle ear infection) is very common in this age group. If the aforementioned therapy is begun early in the upper respiratory infection, such extension can usually be prevented. However, if it should occur, more specific therapy is needed. Magnatherm treatment of the ears given daily, when used in conjunction with the standard therapy, has proven most satisfactory in treating otitis media. If, however, the condition has been allowed to deteriorate considerably and if pressure in the middle ear is such that the eardrum is in danger of rupture, it may be necessary to use endonasal therapy. Such treatment, by cleaning out the congestion at the opening of the eustachian tube, usually brings prompt relief, and subsequent Magnatherm therapy will stimulate rapid recovery.

If sinus complications occur, our chlorophyll-oxygen nebulization therapy mentioned above proves most effective, along with magnatherm or diathermy treatment of the sinuses. Of late we are also using the Low Level Laser Therapy to good effect on these sinus complications.

Pharyngitis, laryngitis, and tonsil disorders usually respond well to our general therapy for infectious diseases. In these various throat infections, local applications of EMP are often greeted by rapid recovery if the treatment is begun early.

Laryngitis (loss of voice) is not particularly painful, but it can be rather upsetting to a child. I recommend two procedures: Some patients find great relief by rubbing Capsolin (a capsicum based rubefacient. Your health food store may have a similar item under another name.) into the throat; others use turpentine for this same purpose. I often suggest a heating throat compress in which a long, narrow strip of cloth, such as sheeting material, is soaked in cold water and then wrapped around the throat. Over this is pinned a dry turkish towel to exclude all air from reaching the moist strip. This healing compress can be left on for twenty minutes to half an hour and repeated two or three times a day if desired. It usually draws out the inflammation in the larynx rapidly, the voice usually returning soon. During recovery, the patient must refrain from using his voice as much as possible because if the vocal cords are used before fully recovered, this recovery is prolonged. The **MicroLight 830** low level laser is proving effective here as well sometimes bringing a near miraculous recovery.

Lower Respiratory Infections

Usually, if we properly take care of upper respiratory infections in our young patients, we won't be plagued with those of the lower tract. However, because our patients are often brought to us with the condition already advanced to the bronchial tubes, it is necessary that we know how to treat these conditions. Also, some patients have a definite weakness in these areas. Often a condition will begin in the bronchial tubes and ascend into the upper respiratory tract in certain of these susceptible persons. Many children also are susceptible to asthmatic or bronchial problems, and in these children almost any upper respiratory infection rapidly descends into the lower respiratory tract and must be treated as such.

Our dietary suggestions for lower tract respiratory infections are usually the same as those for upper respiratory infections. We are more specific about such recommendations, however, and must be adamant with the parent to be sure that these diets are followed to the letter, because lower respiratory conditions can become more dangerous than those of the upper respiratory tract.

Our general supplemental therapy is again pursued but with the addition of special nutritional agents specific to this area. These remedies are so effective that we advise all our parents to tell us early on in the treatment of their child if there is any tendency of upper respiratory problems rapidly descending into the bronchials. If there is such a tendency, we begin the child on the special remedies for the lower tract at the onset of the upper tract condition to ward off this tendency. This effort is successful in most of our young patients.

In lower respiratory infections, the temperature must be watched carefully. If it rises suddenly to 104° or 105° and the patient experiences sharp pains in the chest and great difficulty in breathing, the patient may be developing lobar pneumonia. In this instance, we consider antibiotic therapy the only practical treatment and we would send such patients immediately to the hospital under the care of one of the medical or osteopathic physicians. We say "would" because our treatment work has been sufficiently successful that we haven't had to do so for the last twenty seven years that I have been connected with our Healing Centers.

If the child's temperature remains below 102°, we consider the disorder to be either a minor chest congestion or at worst a viral pneumonia that can be treated at home with the proper attention of one of our Centers' physicians. In our office, in addition to the treatments mentioned above, we treat these congestions with short wave diathermy treatments directly through the chest. If this is properly regulated, it is one of the most satisfactory and beneficial therapies for this type of chest problem we have ever seen. By creating a high local temperature in the lungs and bronchials it seems that this treatment is able to augment the body's efforts to heal these troublesome conditions.

Modern medical investigation has shown that chest problems, especially bronchial disorders, are much more common in children who have had their tonsils removed. Therefore, in our young patients, we make every effort to see that the tonsils are properly treated and retained. In more than forty years of practice, where natural healing methods were followed by the parents, I have not had to send even one of my young patients for a tonsillectomy. The tonsils act as filters preventing dangerous organisms from passing down into the bronchial tree. Therefore, to take out tonsils, without very strong reasons, is criminal indeed. It's like disconnecting the bell of an alarm system so it won't wake you up while you're sleeping. You may sleep well, but your house could be robbed.

Asthma

Unfortunately asthma in children is far more common than we would like. Usually, the tendency is inherited. It is possible for a child to develop asthma, even though the parents don't have asthmatic symptoms. At least one of the parents, however, usually manifests other allergic reactions and the child inherits this tendency. Asthma is usually an allergic disorder. Although severe attacks respond to our basic therapy, one usually must check the metabolic problems, such as low blood sugar and functional hypoadrenalism, to find the true cause of the condition and thereby give the most complete aid to the child. Our Woodlands Medical Center specializes in the detection and correction of the allergies that may be a causative agent in asthma. If your child (or yourself) is susceptible to this condition please let your Center physician know and he will give you further information on the allergy correction procedures available at the Woodlands Medical Center.(See Chapter 23)

Influenza

Luckily, every doctor knows that influenza is caused by a virus and that antibiotics are of no use against viruses. Therefore, only the most irrational doctor recommends antibiotics for influenza. The usual recommendation is bed rest, the drinking of lots of fluids and possibly the use of aspirin for aches and pains. **Kaopectate** or some similar substance might be prescribed for the diarrhea that sometimes accompanies it, but generally little other medication is recommended. Such treatment has much to recommend it, and it isn't unlike that used by all natural physicians. It is, however, a negative treatment and although often adequate, it isn't always sufficient to keep a child from developing some after effects from the condition itself. By negative treatment, I mean that the physician simply gives the body the chance to heal itself, though he does little in a positive way to aid the body. Often, this is all the body requires. I'm sure that if most physicians would only do this more often, the number of chronic ailments in this country would diminish considerably.

It is possible to recommend a certain amount of constructive therapy in influenza; in particular, after the acute stage has passed, methods can be used to prevent the possible devitalization of the body so commonly a part of the disorder.

During acute influenza with gastritis, it is difficult for the patient to keep anything in his stomach, so it is generally impractical to suggest specific food or nutritional supplementation. However, Homeopathic remedies can be used since they do not enter the stomach but are absorbed directly into the capillaries under the tongue. Your Center physician can give you further information on these remedies.

When the patient is constantly vomiting, it is very helpful to have him suck an ice cube. There seems to be some reflex from this ice cube sucking that gives liquid to his body and yet tends to inhibit the vomiting reflex. Because the patient is not hungry we have very little worry about him overeating—most are placed, by Nature, on a therapeutic fast at this time.

The cramps and diarrhea often caused by this condition can be relieved by hot, moist packs put over the abdomen.

After the acute symptoms have passed, natural therapy can be of great aid in preventing some of the distressful aftereffects of this debilitating ailment. As in the case of Toby, mentioned at the beginning of this chapter, the intestinal irritation doesn't always leave spontaneously, but it usually yields rapidly to herbal colon therapy. In general, two treatments at most are all that are necessary. Very rarely do we encounter a case as resistant as Toby's.

The most prevalent after effect of influenza in children and in adults is adrenal exhaustion. This is best treated by the use of the remedies discussed in Chapter II.

Magnatherm, spinal adjustments, and other natural therapies are often required. The method isn't as important as the objective—which is to be sure that the child is returned to vibrant health. We never like to release a patient on the unproven assumption that he will get better later on his own. This isn't an assumption one can readily make. If the child is not returned to full vibrant health before we release him for school, he may be more susceptible to the next infection that comes along, and this infection could in turn leave him weaker. This process can continue until the child is seriously affected by what might otherwise be a relatively mild disorder.

The So-Called Childhood Diseases

Most childhood diseases—measles, mumps, chicken pox, whooping cough—are virus infections, producing antibodies to the infection that usually provide lifetime immunity. Childhood illnesses shouldn't be treated lightly. Properly handled, they are not serious. But it is important that the child be given sufficient time for his body to build up the proper amount of antibodies before he is sent back to school or is allowed to participate in his regular activities after one of these diseases. It isn't unusual for mothers, eager to resume their personal agenda again, to send a youngster back to school before his body has had adequate time to build proper antibody protection. When this is done, the ailment may recur, though this is rare. What usually happens is that the youngster remains below par for some time. While the body slowly builds the antibodies, and because of his low resistance, he is susceptible to other infectious diseases. In general, a full ten days to two weeks should be allowed for complete recovery from any childhood disease, and some of the more severe cases may even require longer.

In treating childhood diseases, the general therapy for upper respiratory conditions can usually be followed with excellent success. Specific treatments, however, may prove extremely useful in individual diseases.

Mumps

Fresh carrots, ground in a meat grinder, placed in a bag or wrap made out of old sheeting, and applied directly over the swollen glands usually stops the pain almost immediately and aids greatly in reducing the swelling. Once the pack becomes dry, it should be replaced with a fresh one. If this treatment is used for only a couple of days, the disorder is usually miraculously helped.

Measles

Suspected measles, both regular and German, can usually be brought out to the rash stage by a hot bath. If the eruption itself is itchy or irritating, the full body wet sheet pack is a great aid in relieving this distress and also in speeding recovery.

206

The wet sheet pack is prepared by placing two spread-out woolen blankets over a bed. A single bed sheet of ordinary size is soaked in cold water, wrung out and spread out on top of the blankets. The young patient is then placed nude on top of the sheet, with only his head above the top edge of the wet sheeting. The sheet is rapidly wrapped around his entire body, mummy fashion, eliminating as much air between the sheet and body as possible. Then the dry woolen blankets are also rapidly wrapped around in the same fashion as the sheet, first one, and then the other. The blankets should be so wrapped that no air is allowed to reach the wet pack. If properly applied, the pack may seem cold at first, but will very rapidly warm up and the young patient will get almost instant relief from his itching and discomfort. The pack may be left on anywhere from twenty minutes to two hours. As soon as it is removed, the patient should be rapidly sponged off with cool water and sent directly to a warm bed. This pack was originally designed by the early naturopaths to draw out toxic substances from the body and is very useful in all conditions that produce a full body eruption. This was considered the sovereign treatment for all such conditions. It both calms the patient and stimulates the elimination of the disease, and there are few agitated children who are not lulled to sleep by its effects.

Chicken Pox

Chicken pox is best treated by the general treatment and by the wet sheet pack, if necessary, as described for measles.

Whooping Cough

Theoretically, whooping cough is no longer prominent as a childhood disease because of the whooping cough vaccination. For those of us, however, who are not particularly fond of having our children vaccinated, it may occur. I have found that the general treatment is usually quite effective. Chiropractic treatment is important and the use of vitamin F and ionizable calcium is successful in controlling the aftercough. This cough can continue for some time, even in the best of treated cases. If your child is exposed to or contracts whooping cough, I suggest that you call your Center physician promptly so he can guide you through this condition in such a way that there are a minimum of after problems.

Croup

Croup is a strange condition. It acts like an allergy, infection, upper respiratory condition or asthma, and yet it isn't any of these. I'm not really sure that any physician knows for sure exactly what croup is, but I've treated it enough to know that it exists and that it is a law unto itself.

It can be identified by the fact that it comes on only at night, throwing the young patient into paroxysms of coughing and asthma-like wheezing that are resistant to ordinary treatment. Having the wheezing child breathe in warm steam from a vaporizer or from a steamy shower will generally ease the attack and allow him to return to sleep. Such attacks usually abate by morning. Croup appears at sporadic intervals and doesn't seem to follow the pattern of any other familiar disorder.

In treatment, we usually recommend the basic maintenance diet. A more restricted diet is usually not necessary, although in some youngsters the elimination of starches and dairy products during the worst part of the croup may be important. A variety of homeopathic remedies are useful, but the best specific in croup is a substance called iodized lime. This is a mixture of iodine and calcium, supplied by the various homeopathic houses. If these products are used according to directions, they usually greatly aid in overcoming the nocturnal paroxysms.

Unnamed Maladies

A number of infective conditions are apparently due to viruses, but physicians have no specific names for them. They are called things like the fifth disease, the bug, the crud, what's going around and so on. They present a variety of symptoms somewhat similar to flu or upper respiratory infections, though some produce eruptions or glandular swellings.

Most of these anonymous problems respond very satisfactorily to the general treatment outlined for upper respiratory infections and/or influenza. One of the advantages of natural therapy is that it stimulates the defense and repair mechanisms of our own bodies and by doing so, the body is able to overcome these strange diseases with its own mechanisms, for it knows their nature even if we don't.

Not only is it possible to treat by natural means disorders whose natures are unknown to us, but it is also possible to treat them at the most opportune time—that is, in their very beginning— without the fear of treating incorrectly. It usually matters little to us which infective condition a patient is coming down with when we initiate treatment. As the condition progresses, we can easily modify our therapy to fit the exact disease in question, without losing any of the beneficial effects we have gained by beginning treatment early. Since most orthodox medical treatment is designed to counteract a specific named disease, it is generally necessary for them to have a definite diagnosis before therapy can begin. Thus, valuable treating time at the beginning of a disease is often lost, and sometimes the diseases are allowed to progress for some time before a diagnosis is made and therapy can be started. I must admit that our approach may not be quite so "scientific," but it is mighty satisfying.

Allergies

The most common allergies in children, I believe, are those caused by hereditary defects. The rest are probably caused by poor diet and other adverse effects of modern living.

In treating allergies by natural methods, we must check the child as we would an adult. A thorough examination is made that concentrates on metabolic tests, such as the hair test, glucose tolerance test, and tests for adrenal, thyroid, and other glandular functionings. We have recently been incorporating some of the new patient-nerve-reaction methods for diagnosing sensitivities.

With this patient work-up, it is usually possible to pinpoint the area of allergic problem and to correct it either by removing the sensitive objects, establishing a low-allergy diet, or by using specific supplementation to stabilize and balance the glandular systems. As mentioned earlier this field is the specialty of our Woodlands Medical Center.

Spinal Problems of Children

One of the most frequently overlooked problems of childhood is the group of various mechanical problems that can occur to the spine and the other articulations (joints) of the body. Hardly a youngster treated at our Centers does not have some form of mechanical problem. He will either have a sacroiliac out of place, cervical rotations, scoliosis (spinal curvature), or various vertebral subluxations in the dorsal and lumbar spine.

The most common mechanical problem of children is the same as that of their elders—subluxation of the pelvis, or sacroiliac "twist." This has been thoroughly described in Chapter III, and if you suspect this type of problem in your child, I suggest you read that chapter carefully.

The difficulty with the child's sacroiliac subluxation is that because of their resiliency, this joint can be misplaced without a great deal of discomfort. It often may slip out because of a fall or some kind of twist, feel sore for a few days, but then calm down to where it bothers them only occasionally. The parents who are probably accustomed to hearing their children complain, think little of this rather mild discomfort. In fact, when these youngsters are finally brought to our office, it is almost never with a back problem, but most frequently with symptoms such as headache, sore knees, ankle problems, or foot pains and other varieties of reflex problems from the subluxed sacroiliac. Most parents are generally surprised and chagrined when I show them what has happened. After I replace these joints, I always describe the nature of the condition to both the parent and child and implore them to come back as soon as possible if this happens again. To encourage prompt checking, we are always glad to examine patients at no charge to see if the pelvis has slipped or not. If one of these sacroiliacs is left out for a considerable period, it will cause in the child a definite spinal curvature (scoliosis), and it may take months and even years to correct such a curve of long duration.

Neck problems are encountered frequently in children. It seems that their active lives precipitate this type of difficulty. They are especially common in children susceptible to upper respiratory infections and allergies. The most common symptom of this difficulty is headache; only rarely does the child complain of a stiff neck. We find a very high percentage of children's chronic headaches are caused by vertebral misplacements of the neck.

Childhood accidents to the spine are common, and I recommend that all children be checked for such malalignments if they have any back, neck, or head problems that persist more than two days. Muscular strains usually improve in two days.

Worms

We must admit that children are susceptible to worm infections. The pinworm is the most common, and worm eggs can come from a variety of sources, but usually from the hands or fingers of one who is already infected. The pinworm is a rather small innocuous worm and doesn't do a great deal of damage, but it certainly can be irritating.

The most common way of diagnosing this condition is to put a piece of Scotch tape over the anal opening of the child as he sleeps. In the morning, the Scotch tape is pulled off and examined for the small white threadlike worms. Because the worms tend to come out of the anus at night and crawl about the skin area, they are caught on the Scotch tape and can't return.

Because these worms cause rectal itching, the child is inclined to scratch. The eggs are picked up by the fingers. If he then puts the fingers in his mouth or nose, he reinfects himself.

A variety of treatment methods are suggested for this condition, and I mention here those that I have found successful and natural. In a bad infestation, I usually give the child a colonic consisting of two quarts of warm water in which is dissolved a teaspoon of table salt. The salt seems to affect the worms the same way it does a slug: it dissolves their basic substance. Such a mixture can also be used by a mother for an ordinary enema and in most cases it effectively helps reduce the fecal irritation due to this infestation. Because worms are always in various stages of development and this treatment is only successful against adult worms, it is usually not adequate to eradicate the problem.

The use of a quarter cup of pumpkin seeds a day has cleared up many of these infections, however, especially when used in conjunction with the salt enema. Homeopathically, the remedy Cina is given. Usually in our Centers we combine the pumpkin seeds, the salt colonic and Cina for most satisfactory results.

Other worms that affect children are more serious and are best treated only under one of our Center's physicians.

Attention Deficit Disorder

The following article is by our contributor Harold E. Buttram, M.D. He has done a great deal of work with this condition of children and we are pleased to be able to include his efforts in this book:

The attention deficit hyperactive disorder (ADHD) is now epidemic in American elementary schools. Considering its long term sequelae, it is arguably one of the leading health problems of our times. Dr. Lendon Smith, well known pediatrician, has estimated that 6 to 8% of children in today's classrooms are hyperactive, whereas in the 1950s there were less than 1%. There appears to be a consensus among veteran teachers that this dramatic change came about largely during and following the 1970s.

Before addressing therapy for this disorder, we must first ask what are its causes. No one knows all of the answers to this question, but there is growing evidence that there are three major causes:

• Massive increases in neurotoxic environmental chemicals.
• Commercial food processing and adulteration with chemical additives which are rarely if ever thoroughly tested for their safety. Also there are often pesticide residues.
• Excessive use of antibiotics in treatment of childhood illnesses.

In our opinion, any treatment program which does not take measures to correct these three basic causes will not gain long term success. These and other problem areas will be reviewed in the following:

(1) Volatile Organic Compounds (VOCs)

VOCs, or solvent-type of chemicals, are basically toxic, some extremely so. Very commonly today VOCs are present at high levels in indoor air of buildings. The U.S. Environmental Protection Agency has designated this problem as the "sick building syndrome." The causes are two-fold: First, there has been a massive increase in commercial production of VOCs estimated to be over 150-fold in the past 50 or so years and, second, the energy-efficient building codes adopted following the Arabian oil embargo in the 1970s which has resulted in little or no ventilation of buildings with outdoor air. (It may be more than coincidental

211

the adoption of these building codes coincide with the dramatic changes in childhood behavior previously mentioned).

VOCs are fat or lipid-soluble, and therefore have an affinity for the lipid tissues of the body. The brain is a prime target because of its high lipid content and rich blood supply. Children are especially vulnerable to exposures, a vulnerability as much as 10 times greater than for adults.[1] Childhood exposures can and frequently do lead to learning disabilities, behavioral problems, fatigue, mood changes, poor motivation, as well as increased susceptibility to common respiratory infections.

Common sources of VOCs may include new buildings which commonly have high ambient levels in indoor air of formaldehyde, plastic vapors, glues, adhesives and paints. New wall-to-wall carpets may outgas a number of harmful chemicals. Also included are pesticides when used (pesticide sprays may remain in indoor air 21 days or more following application), tobacco smoke when not prohibited, recent renovations such as indoor painting, heavy use of disinfectants and new mattresses which may exude toxic fire-retardant fumes. Many other potential sources could be mentioned, but these are the more common ones.

Buildings high in dust and mold can bring about fatigue, mental lassitude, and adverse mood changes in susceptible individuals.

In our Centers parents or guardians are provided educational materials as to common sources of VOCs and safer alternative methods and materials. Handouts are also provided for control of dust and mold when these are a problem in the home. In a residence it is usually neither difficult nor expensive to reduce harmful VOC exposures, but there may be perplexing problems in schools when there is a lack of understanding by school officials which we have found sometimes to be the case.

(2) Toxic Heavy Metals

These include lead, cadmium, mercury and others. In our office we have used the hair test as a primary means of screening for these metals. Throughout the medical community most concern has been justifiably centered around the dangers of lead. When elevated hair lead is found, we follow it with a blood test.

Although we have not yet found a child with blood levels officially designated as toxic, it would be our policy to refer the child to a medical center for treatment. We have found a fair number with lower levels. These we treat nutritionally recommending foods high in organic sulfur (traditionally a cleanser) such as garlic, onions, beans and lentils. Supplements such as blue-green algae, deodorized garlic, and mineral nutrients including calcium, magnesium, zinc and selenium may be recommended. Parents are advised to check their home for possible sources of lead including tap water and leaded paint in older homes.

(3) Nutrition

Emphasis should be placed on plain, unprocessed foods without chemical additives and on the reduction of sugar. Sweets should be limited to special occasions and should not be an every meal indulgence.

Special emphasis is placed on the avoidance of chemical additives, especially MSG (monosodium glutamate), the artificial sweetener, aspartame, and artificial food colorings and flavorings. Numerous animal experiments in a variety of animal species have shown that MSG and aspartame are capable of causing brain and retinal damage.[2] There is no reason for believing that this does not also take place in humans. Artificial food colorings and flavorings have been shown to be a leading cause of allergic food reactions in hyperactive children.[3]

(4) The Candida Syndrome

Candida is a yeast which normally inhibits the human intestinal tract and the vagina of females. It is known that antibiotics may cause invasive overgrowth in these areas, especially with heavy or prolonged use. Dietary sugar may also promote this overgrowth, as may cortisone-type of drugs when used in sufficient quantities to depress the immune system. Symptoms may include digestive problems, vaginitis, fatigue, mental sluggishness, depression, nervous irritability, worsening of allergies and hyperactivity in children.

Few medical issues today have been more controversial that the Candida Syndrome, probably because no one fully understands its nature. It probably involves far more that just the invasive overgrowth of Candida in the digestive tract and the vagina. It may in part be caused by direct injury from antibiotics to the intestinal immune system (the secretory IgA system), sometimes referred to as "antiseptic paint" coating the intestinal lining. It may also involve overgrowth of other pathogens as well as Candida and a reduction of beneficial intestinal micro-organisms. The overall result may be an increased intestinal permeability, (the so-called "leaky gut syndrome")* leading to an increased proneness to food allergies and other sensitivities.

For diagnosis we depend on the medical history—it is always suspect when the child has been subjected to large amounts of antibiotics. We have found that laboratory tests for this condition may be unreliable, but a stool analysis is sometimes helpful. When the medical history is strongly suggestive of Candidiasis, the only option may be a therapeutic trial of medication, with a favorable response confirming the diagnosis.

---

*See protocol for this condition in Appendix C

Treatment always includes removal of sugar from the diet and elimination of chemical food additives. It may include the prescription drug nystatin, or more "natural" agents such as caprylic acid, acidophilus microorganisms to restore beneficial intestinal flora, deodorized garlic, grapefruit seed extract or other natural healing substances.

Antibiotics should be limited to more serious illnesses. Although this may sound drastic, many leading medical researchers and practitioners are coming to a similar conclusion. It is in the area of minor childhood sinus, ear and bronchial infections that "natural therapies" have a great potential in carrying the child through the illness without a need to resort to antibiotics. (See information in the earlier part of this chapter) More often than not they will be successful, although if there are indications of more serious complications, a doctor should be consulted and the decision on antibiotics left to the professional. In our office in these situations we have utilized an herbal tincture with **Echinacea, Myrrh,** and **Phytolacca** (EMP), ear drops with mullein and garlic oils, zinc lozenges or a liquid zinc preparation, vitamin C, and the appropriate homeopathic remedy. The number of potentially valuable natural agents is almost endless.

(5) The Dysfunctional Family

Unquestionably family problems frequently play a major role as underlying contributory causes of childhood behavioral problems and ADHD. In such situations family support and psychological counselling at some level may be indispensable.

(6) Food and Inhalant Allergies

Classic studies have shown that food allergies play a major role in provoking adverse behavioral changes in a large portion of ADHD children.[3,4] Common inhalant allergies (pollen, dust, mold, etc.) may also be contributory.

Identifications of food allergies include a history of dark circles under the eyes, red ears and cheeks accompanied by mood changes after eating, a history of colic during infancy, and abdominal pains and digestive disturbances in later childhood.

Identifications of food allergies may be obtained by blood tests, elimination and rechallenge diet, or by skin tests done in our office. If food allergies appear to be a problem, the doctor will help the parents decide which approach is best for their child.

Once offending foods are identified by one of these means treatment involves eliminating or reducing the problem foods and, when indicated, sublingual (under-the-tongue) food neutralization drops based on the skin tests.

214

(7) Drug Therapy Versus Nutritional Supplements

The standard medical treatment today for the hyperactive syndrome is Ritalin or other drugs, often given as a sole means of therapy. This is partly understandable. Even an hour with a hyperactive child during a rampant outburst can be exhausting to parents or teachers and these drugs usually do have a calming effect. However, they can have adverse side effects including decreased appetite and delayed growth and development. More to the point, long-term studies have shown negligible benefits in later adolescent years in terms of continued social and scholastic problems when ritalin is used as a sole therapy.[5,6]

We do not believe that, from the standpoint of the child's welfare, Ritalin is the best answer. As with antibiotics, it should probably be held in reserve for the more serious cases or when other measures have failed.

In our opinion nutritional supplements hold great promise in this area. It can be expected that critics of this approach will say it is all anecdotal; lacking in scientific proof. This may or may not be true, but when parents see their children being helped, they do not need scientific proof.

The following nutritional supplements appear to be of special value:

• **Nutrient minerals** are commonly deficient due to today's norm of diets consisting largely of refined foods. Mineral supplements may be required to support enzyme function in the body.

• **Flax seed oil supplements** provide a rich source of fatty acids necessary for growth and development of the brain, nervous system, mucous membranes and cell membranes. As with trace minerals, these are almost universally deficient in modern diets, partly due to food processing which tends to destroy the fatty acids and partly due to food choices.

• **Blue-green algae,** we believe, may prove to be of special value for the hyperactive child. Among other advantageous qualities, they contain easily assimilated amino acids which, serving as neurotransmittors, may have a steadying and calming effect on the nervous system.

• **Pycnogenol** holds promise as an alternative to Ritalin. Its primary mechanism of action appears to be that of a powerful antioxidant which scavenges harmful free-radicals generated by foreign toxic chemicals and possibly by other sources.

Additional Comments

For many families these approaches may be new, and at first glance they may appear overwhelming. If one takes one step at a time, making changes without too much haste, they are not as difficult as they may appear.

Organic foods pose a special problem. If genuine, these foods are free of chemicals, have better flavor and higher nutritive value. The problem lies in that they are not always readily available, and even when they are, they are usually more expensive and beyond the financial means of many young families. If such is the case, do the best you can with regular market foods according to the guidelines previously outlined. For most this will be sufficient. One other alterative: if you have the time and appropriate grounds, grow your own garden according to proven organic methods.

The ultimate question is, do these methods work? We should answer yes, as we have seen the results. Also it can be said that large and growing numbers of parents are seeking these approaches throughout the land, and this would not be the case if they had not witnessed or experienced favorable outcomes.

References

1. *Pesticides in Diets of Infants and Children,* sponsored by the National Research Council National Academy Press, Washington D.C., 1993. Page 3

2. *Excitotoxins, the Taste that Kills,* by Russell L. Blaylock, M.D. Health Press, P.O. Box 367, Santa Fe, New Mexico 87501, 1994.

3. Egger, J. et al, Controlled trial of oligoantigenic diet treatment in the hyperkinetic syndrome, *Lancet,* March 9, 1985. Pages 540-545.

4. Boris, M. & Mandel, F.S., Foods and additives are common causes of the attention deficit hyperactive disorder in children, *Annals of Allergy,* Vol. 72, No. 1, 1987. Pages 56-64.

5. Satterfield, J.H. et al, Therapeutic interventions to prevent delinquency in hyperactive boys, *J. Amer Acad Child Adol Psychiat,* Vol. 26, No. 1, 1987. pages 56-64.

6. Hechtam, L., Adolescent outcome of hyperactive children treated with stimulants in childhood: a review, *Psychopharmacol Bull,* Vol. 21, 1985. Page 178.

Other Diseases

There are a wide variety of other conditions for which we treat children. Most are specific difficulties and the treatment is individualized for each case. With all these conditions, the natural vitality of children helps them respond well to natural therapy. If you have a child with a problem that doesn't seem to respond to orthodox treatment, feel free to contact us and we will be glad to let you know if it is a condition that responds to natural therapy.

Congenital and Hereditary Defects

Problems that fall into these two categories constitute a large part of pediatric difficulties. Some of the congenital problems such as those due to thalidomide are beyond the help of any specific natural therapy. Some of the milder types, however, are readily helped by our methods.

Hereditary defects can also be aided where there is sufficient body vitality for a constructive therapeutic approach. It must be remembered that we all are born with hereditary defects. None of us has a body that functions 100 per cent perfectly. A child with a known hereditary defect simply has one that is visible. We all may have defects that have yet to be discovered. The man who dies early may never have had a sick day in his life, and yet he dies of a heart attack that might have been caused by a hereditary defect not yet capable of detection.

Dr. Swinburne Clymer, for whom our original Clinic was named, wrote a book entitled Prenatal Culture,* in which he describes a method by which mothers-to-be can be assured of producing children as free of congenital and hereditary defects as possible. This book, still in print, can be obtained at each of our Centers. Any of you who are interested in producing healthy children, or who have certain specific hereditary problems in your family and are afraid to bear children because you fear that they may carry forth this hereditary strain, should find this book most interesting.

A later text by Dr. Harold Buttram entitled, *For Tomorrow's Children* is also available at our Centers. This work describes what the parents-to-be need to do to prepare for the best possible conception. This work of Pre-Conception Care is one of the major thrusts and contributions of the Woodlands Medical Center in our efforts to serve humanity.

Parting Words

In concluding this chapter, I want to leave you with this thought. Although it isn't difficult to treat children by natural means, the effects of this treatment will be only short-lived if you don't faithfully follow a natural non-congestive diet after the general therapy is concluded. If the child is allowed to return to the overuse of sweets, carbohydrates, and dairy products, his problems will return, again requiring specific treatment for their correction. When parents are faithful and follow the Basic Health Maintenance Diet with even moderate determination, their children remain remarkably free of the diseases that were once such a common part of their lives. One of the easiest things to accomplish in all of natural medicine is to keep children healthy, but much of the burden rests on the shoulders of the parent.

---

*Clymer. R. Swinburne: *Prenatal Culture, How to Create the Perfect Baby* Quakertown, Pa., Philosophical Publishing House.

Chapter XIV
Specific Nutritional Therapy

Almost all our patients take vitamins, and when we give a patient a specific nutritional remedy, he automatically assumes we are giving him vitamins. This is only partially true, and it has been difficult to explain that although vitamins and minerals are useful, they make up only a small part of the nutritional elements needed and used by us in preventing and treating imbalances.

The first so-called vitamins were discovered by Casimir Funk more than fifty years ago. Since then, many other vital food factors have been discovered and isolated, and new information about the usefulness of these compounds is being disclosed constantly. There is, however, a tendency in orthodox medicine to compartmentalize these factors and to align each one with a specific symptom pattern. For example, if you have scurvy, you need vitamin C; beriberi, vitamin B.; and if you have pellagra, you need vitamin B2 and niacin. It is difficult for physicians trained in drug therapy to realize that a combination of small deficiencies of various elements may also cause problems that can't be so easily categorized. The unfortunate assumption among many of the medical profession is that if these frank deficiencies are absent, the person is nutritionally healthy and doesn't need added diet supplementation.

On the other hand, various health lecturers and self-styled nutritional experts have carried the use of vitamins and minerals to a ridiculous extreme in the opposite direction. Some of these well-meaning people saturate those who seek their aid with vitamin after vitamin and mineral after mineral in ever-spiraling amounts, until there is barely room left in their digestive tracts for food.

The wise natural healer looks with skepticism on both of these views; experience has taught him the fallacies that they both exhibit. The basic tenets on which human nutrition is based, and that are adhered to at our Healing Centers, may be stated by three simple axioms.

1. God, or Nature, if you will, desires the health and fecundity of all the world. Therefore, along with the creation of man and the other creatures were provided, in reasonably available forms, foods and other nutritional factors that would help sustain this creation in a state of optimal functioning. Every animal intuitively lives by this law, and, barring predators or natural catastrophes, usually lives its life out with a minimum of the "diseases" that affect mankind. Man doesn't live by such a natural law, however, and is able to alter the selection, amount and composition of the nutrients he takes into his body.

If one does not believe in an all-wise Creator and instead is a devotee of the Darwinian theory of evolution, the conclusions are approximately the same. In order for an organism to exist and to prosper, it must have available to it all the elements that are best adapted for its growth and functioning. If this doesn't occur, either one of two things will take place. The organism will die out or it will adapt its system to fit the elements that are supplied. Because man is an organism that has survived for some time, we must have around us all the elements necessary for our optimum health and survival. If we don't use them properly, this is our fault, not that of evolution or the all-wise Creator.

2. The complexity of the chemical processes in our body is so great and the delicacy of their balancing mechanisms so fine that it is, at least at this time in our development of science, utterly impossible for the scientist or physician to fully understand or control these processes for their own purposes. Any attempt to do so, except in emergencies, can often be fraught with severe and unpredictable consequences.

The compositions of natural foods, herbs, and other products of nature are also equally complex to meet the needs of the body's complementary complexity. These two, having developed and matured together are fit companions for one another. It is only through this complex and yet complementary structure of man and his God given food supply that a proper nutritional sustenance for man is possible.

Even our most advanced scientists have no real idea of all these complexities in both man and natural foods. If this tenet is accepted—and to me its truth is self evident—one can readily see that any attempt to add to or detract from the composition of natural foodstuffs will alter their complimentary effect on the functioning of the human body and bring about disorders and imbalances too enormous and intricate to understand. Many of us feel that man's attempt to make these changes is the major cause of many of our acute and chronic diseases.

3. The purpose of the natural healer is to preserve the normal functioning of man's body. He should in no way introduce into this body any substance that has the capability of altering this delicate balance unless he is assured he knows the full consequences of its action and the long-term effects.

If we take these three tenets and apply them to the use of vitamins and minerals, we can arrive at some interesting conclusions. From its very inception, orthodox medicine has attempted to force upon the human body, by every available route, all types of compounds that might alter body activity. Only in rare instances did the practitioner concern himself with the full consequences of what these substances might do to the highly intricate biochemical reactions taking place by the millions every second within the body.

When examined in this light, we see that vitamins can fall into the same category as that of any of the other medicinal substances. They are less toxic than most drugs, but they can alter the body's chemical reactions for the worse if not used with great care and discretion. Nutritional agents never appear alone in nature but always in complex organic structures. When we take this separate vitamin and that individual mineral, we are deviating far from nature and are entering a field that is best left to those with great knowledge and vast clinical experience.

Vitamins Versus Specific Nutritional Products

At our Healing Research Center we believe the balance of the various nutritional factors present in foods is just as important as the specific compounds themselves. This complex chemical structure in food is of such an intricacy that no scientist can now, or in the foreseeable future, construct a formula that would duplicate those of nature.

The make-up of this complex chemical structure has been investigated by many authorities. I personally believe the work of my dear friend H. C. Webber is most helpful in explaining the difference between ordinary chemical compounds and natural compounds. According to Webber's hypothesis, the plant is able to draw the various mineral elements from the soil and through chemical processes inherent in its structure is then able to combine them with other chemical substances derived from the air and soil in such a way as to form a complex chemical molecule—Webber calls it a nutritional colloid (a colloid is a large molecule, usually protein, that won't diffuse through a semipermeable membrane). This complex nutritional colloid may be likened to a miniature architectural masterpiece created out of toothpicks. It is beautiful and aesthetic but very fragile. The human digestive and metabolic systems can take these complex colloidal structures and utilize them readily in the intricate body chemical reactions.

In this way, nature has designed a process by which each kingdom in creation is necessary and helpful to every other kingdom. The plant draws from air, water and soil the necessary basic elements to produce a complex bio-matrix that is to be used by all forms of animal life for the proper maintenance and growth of their own protoplasmic substance. When the animal dies, this protoplasm is returned to the earth, where it breaks down into its basic mineral substances, from which the plant may again draw to produce the complex colloidal structure necessary for future generations of animal life. As long as this chain is unbroken, all forms of life live fairly well together, but when this pattern is altered, disease and death (Due to a breaking of natural law) are visited on all the various participants in this life cycle.

A common difficulty encountered in the proper continuance of this life cycle is based on the fact that the colloidal elements of plant structure are very fragile. Once a plant is picked, the colloids usually break down into simpler non-colloidal compounds fairly soon. Much of the wilting of a plant is brought about by this process. Webber believed that once the colloidal element begins to break down, the compounds composing it once again return to their crystal or crystalloid form. In other words, this complex structure would lose the organization that the plant had so industriously constructed.

Webber hypothesized that when this occurs, the chemical substances are still present but have been reduced to such a form that if ingested they can be the cause of many diseases heretofore unexplained. For his work, this investigator devised many methods for ascertaining whether a compound is colloidal or whether it has returned to its crystalloid state. Through these methods of testing, it was possible to discover that many of our highly regarded nutritional compounds are actually less effective than we imagine and they could with extended use prove harmful. He also found that certain processes of manufacture are able to preserve the colloid state of the basic nutritional substance so that it is possible to produce nutritional compounds that retain this most desirable chemical structure.

Webber's theories make it possible to explain many phenomena for which orthodox science has no ready answers. The work of Dr. Francis Marion Pottenger of California, for instance, is readily explained by the colloidcrystalloid theories. Pottenger, for his work with tuberculosis, wanted to do some tests on animals, and he decided to raise a great many cats for this purpose. He set up the necessary pens and other paraphernalia and purchased enough dry animal food from his local feed store to raise the cats. His cats did not proliferate, however. In addition, the kittens that were born had a variety of defects very similar to those of his human patients.

Soon this difficulty in raising cats began to stimulate the scientist's research-oriented mind more than the original project he had planned for them. After a couple of dismal generations of cats, Pottenger began to experiment with their diet. Some of the cats were given fresh liver and meat along with their dry cat food. Others were given nothing but fresh liver and meat and some were kept exclusively on the dry food.

The cats on the completely raw diet grew strong and healthy, producing offspring without congenital defects. Those on the mixed diet were almost as healthy and produced equally viable offspring. Those kept on the dry food diet, which although not raw, supposedly contained all the known food factors necessary for animal growth, continued to deteriorate until they were no longer capable of reproducing.

This new research work grew so fascinating to Pottenger that he continued with it for some time to check out various other factors. He even experimented with the waste products from the various animal groups and he found that when he fertilized soil with the excrement of the cats eating completely raw food and those eating the half raw food, seeds planted in this soil grew to healthy and luxuriant plants, whereas seeds planted in soil fertilized by excrement from the cats eating the dry food grew very meagerly and the plants were afflicted with several diseases.

From Webber's theory, we can see that animals who graze on grass containing the colloidal nutritional structure will then build a similar colloidal structure into their own body tissues. If these body tissues are in turn fed, without the destructive effects of heating, to other animals, they in turn will benefit from these nutritionally viable substances. From Pottenger's research work, we can surmise that where approximately half the food taken into the body consists of the colloidal compounds, the body is able to function nearly as well as if the diet were totally raw. On the other hand, when such colloidal intake is low, the life force rapidly withers and the body becomes subject to many diseases.

As we have seen from Pottenger's work, this colloidal structure can be broken down by heat. Light and time also break it down. If plant or flesh food is allowed to remain unused for some time, the colloidal structure will retrogress to its crystalloid structure.

Some compounds, however, are well-protected from such deterioration. Nuts have a fairly long life, and various grains, as long as their tough outer covering is not broken, retain their colloidal structure for hundreds and even thousands of years. Once this outer covering is broken, however, their colloidal structure deteriorates rapidly. For this reason, many knowledgeable authorities recommend that whole-grain flour be used within ten days of grinding.

From my own experience, I believe taste is intimately connected with the colloidal structure of food and that while a food still has its natural succulent taste, the colloidal structure is probably intact. On the other hand, when this taste is gone, it is possible that the food has lost much of its nutritional value, and its colloidal compounds have once again retrogressed to the unorganized crystalloid structure.

For the natural therapist who understands the colloidcrystalloid theory of nutrition, there is only one proper way to produce a dietary supplement. First, find a natural source high in the particular element or compound of interest. Collect this source at the height of its colloidal composition and process it in such a way that the essential colloidal compounds are concentrated to the greatest possible degree without in any way disturbing their fragile structure. The finished product then must be packaged to assure this colloidal composition through the expected life of the product.

There is great difficulty in fulfilling the requirements I have suggested. But such products can be made and are being used by natural therapists everywhere. It is to these compounds I refer when I speak of specific nutritional therapy. Most vitamin and mineral products sold in drug stores and health food stores don't conform to these requirements, and although perhaps not basically toxic, they nevertheless are unnatural compounds and have inherent in their structure the ability to imbalance the functioning of the human body. Because of these vital differences, we recommend that patients don't attempt to substitute the specific nutritional products we prescribe with similar ones from the drug or health food store. Although some of the basic ingredients might be similar, the complex colloidal structure would not be the same and the results we had hoped for wouldn't be forthcoming. To help those who insist on choosing their own supplements, I shall make some specific comments on those generally available.

Specific Nutritional Entities

Some vitamin and mineral factors are more dangerous than others. Some, while basically nontoxic, are capable of causing systemic imbalances that aren't yet completely understood.

Vitamin A

Vitamin A has recently been restricted in its dosage levels by the FDA. I believe this decision to be wise. Vitamin A can be misused and will cause, in an overdosage, an imbalance that produces symptoms almost identical to those of a deficiency. Higher dosages may be useful in treating some ailments, and as such are usually supplied from fish-liver oil or lemon grass extract. There are other sources, but these usually don't enable the high unit dosage to be produced that is favored by many physicians. Vitamin A from fish-liver oils is at least obtained from a natural source and it carries with it some of the other natural factors, such as vitamin D and vitamin F, that help control vitamin A toxicity. Whether the colloidal form is preserved depends on the processing methods used. If the lower potencies are used, little harm will come from vitamin A, although we recommend it in proper conjunction with other elements.

The lemon grass extract of vitamin A, although helpful in those without sufficient bile to properly assimilate the oil soluble form, is generally more toxic and should be used with greater care.

Beta Carotene

Beta Carotene is a precursor of Vitamin A. Many investigators find that it is better accepted in some patients than is regular Vitamin A. We have found the special liquid sublingual form to be very useful. Since it does not need to go through the liver, this form of Vitamin A can be given to patients who normally cannot accept high doses of this vitamin. We have had some very satisfying success with several cases of Sojourn's Disease (A condition producing very dry eyes) treated with sublingual Beta Carotene.

The B Complex Vitamins

Vitamin B1 (thiamine) is used both orally and by injection in high dosage for its tonic effects. Unfortunately, such dosages cause relative deficiencies of the other B vitamins, and in time the general body balance is made worse by the overuse of this vitamin.

Vitamin B2 (riboflavin) is usually not as misused as thiamine and is rapidly eliminated by the kidneys. Thus, an overdosage of riboflavin causes the urine to become a bright canary yellow.

Vitamin B3 (niacin) is used by many physicians as a drug. It produces certain physiologic effects on the body such as peripheral blood vessel dilation and a decrease in cholesterol levels. Recently, it has been shown to prevent "blood sludging." It is also used by some psychiatrists in schizophrenia. Niacin has also been called the "anti-pellagra vitamin." Some researchers believe that many of its drug effects may actually be due to its ability to correct subclinical pellagra that may have been diagnosed as other diseases. Niacin is toxic in overdosage and its use, except in moderate amounts, should be supervised by a physician acquainted with its peculiarities.

Niacinamide (the amine of niacin) is relatively nontoxic and has the same nutritional effects as niacin, but it doesn't have the drug effects.

Vitamin B6 (pyridoxine hydrochloride) is generally considered a relatively innocuous compound. However, its use for some time in amounts of 50 to 150 mg. or more a day tends to cause relative deficiencies of some other elements, particularly magnesium.

Vitamin B12 can only be produced by natural means, and it is thus nontoxic in the oral form. I don't know of any relative deficiencies caused

225

by its use. There is some evidence that the sublingual form may help in the treatment and prevention of mouth ulcers (canker sores).

Vitamin C

Vitamin C (ascorbic acid) has a relatively low toxicity and, as far as we can ascertain, doesn't upset the body chemical balances even in large amounts. Still, we at the Healing Research Center recommend a colloidal form for general supplementation, and we use the more concentrated crystalline compounds only for emergencies when heroic amounts may prove useful. For this latter use it seems to matter little whether the vitamin C is pure ascorbic acid or that extracted from rose hips or acerola berries. Many people cannot take the acid form of Vitamin C and for these we recommend the buffered form. There are many of these, some good and some not so good. Be sure to ask your Center physician for his recommendation.

Vitamin D

Vitamin D has been a nutritional football ever since it was first discovered. The most commonly used form, even in the health food field, is still the synthetic or D2 form. This is usually produced by irradiating ergosterol. Whenever a supplement lists its vitamin D as irradiated ergosterol (D2), the product is synthetic. Not only is vitamin D2 synthetic, but also it isn't the same as the natural product structurally and is therefore foreign to the body. The natural product is vitamin D3, which is generally obtained from fish-liver oils.

Vitamin D, especially D2, even in dosages just slightly above normal, can be highly toxic to some people. Having personally treated several cases of vitamin D toxicosis, I believe the FDA was not remiss in controlling the high-dosage sales.

Vitamin E

Vitamin E, next to vitamin C, is probably the most glamorous of all the food elements and one of the most controversial. If properly manufactured, it is possible to retain the colloidal structure of the vitamin E complex, but it is very easy for this structure to collapse where careful controls are not used. Vitamin E can be a variable nutritional substance but in order to obtain a good therapeutic product, not only the form of vitamin E must be considered but also the specific manufacturer.

One should always refrain from using synthetic vitamin E; these types can readily be distinguished by the name of the compound. If the name on the bottle is DL-alpha-tocopherol, the substance is synthetic. The L stands for levulo (left-turning products under polarized light) forms that don't occur in nature and are therefore foreign to the body. The natural product is always designated as D-alpha-tocopherol or dextro-alpha-tocopherol (Right turning under polarized light).

Even all D-alpha-tocopherols are not the same. Many products are advertised as a compound of mixed tocopherols, but because D-alpha-tocopherol is the only one known to be effective, you are paying for compounds of no known therapeutic value in these products.

The natural D-alpha-tocopherol can also be produced from a variety of rancid oils. The finished product is still D-alphatocopherol, or natural vitamin E, and can be sold as such, but because of changes in its colloidal nature, it won't necessarily have the same beneficial effects as another similarly labeled product from a producer of greater integrity.

Thus, great care must be exercised in purchasing vitamin E preparations. We insist that our patients purchase their Vitamin E from our Centers so that we know that they are receiving an effective and not a toxic product.

Vitamin F

Vitamin F (unsaturated fatty acids) hasn't yet been synthesized; it is extracted from various products that are high in linoleic, linolenic or arachidonic acid. If these products are produced so they retain their natural molecular structure, their vitamin F content will be effective and useful. We have two types of vitamin F compounds that we use regularly. One is in a tablet and the other is in a capsule. The tablet form is best used to help the distribution of ionizable calcium in the body while the capsule form is used to help in the treatment of benign prostatic hypertrophy.

Calcium

Calcium is supplied in two basic forms: one is of an acid reaction and is combined with phosphorus, magnesium, and other elements needed for bone building; the other is an alkaline or phosphorus-free form that acts as ionizable calcium in the blood and tissues.

Bone meal is the most common form of acid calcium. Most bone meal, however, is produced by a process using heat in one of the stages; this usually breaks down the colloidal integrity. This crystalloid calcium might be helpful for some conditions, but its lack of proper colloidal structure may in time increase arthritic deposits and perhaps the atheromatous plaques that often occur in the blood vessels with age. Bone meal entirely produced by temperatures below body heat (98.6) is available and it is the only type recommended by the Beverly Hall Corporation Healing Research Center for those who need this variety of calcium.

Alkaline calcium—calcium lactate, calcium gluconate—and calcium derived from eggshells are useful in many disorders. Leg cramps, muscle twitching, and many nervous disorders are often improved by its use. Its assimilation is helped by being taken on an empty stomach and is most effective in combination with vitamin F (see above). Used in relative moderation it seems to precipitate no adverse reactions. Dolomite a popular mixed mineral product, can't be recommended here. Being a mineral product, it is crystalloid, not colloid and it seems to increase adverse calcium buildup in the tissues.

Iron

I think there's enough iron sold in pills in a year in this country to build a battleship. Most of it is inorganic—iron sulfate being the most common form—and much of this non-colloid iron passes out through the stool in its elemental form.

Much has been written in health magazines about the fact that taking iron and vitamin E together negates the value of each. This is true in regard to inorganic iron compounds. Vitamin E helps detoxify this abnormal substance and is therefore not free for other purposes. However, natural iron and vitamin E are often found together in foods and they are well-utilized in the colloid form. Here again, as with all colloidal complexes, there is little fear that it won't be properly assimilated whenever ingested. One of the best ways to get iron is from green leafy vegetables as fresh as possible, but for those with a real problem many good forms of colloidal iron are available. We have a liquid that combines a colloidal iron with B vitamins that is well tolerated and very effective.

Iodine

Iodine is necessary for proper body function. The best way to get this mineral is in food. If sufficient seafood can't be obtained, then it may be supplemented. The most common supplements are kelp and potassium iodide.

Potassium iodide is an inorganic substance (not colloidal) and is toxic if used for an extended time. Iodized salt is usually fortified with potassium iodide and is therefore not recommended.

Kelp has become almost a ritual with some health food devotees. It is not a particularly good compound, being too high in iodine and sodium chloride (table salt) to offer the proper balance of trace minerals for which it is often suggested.

Most patients greatly overdo the use of kelp. If it is kept at a dosage wherein the daily minimum iodine ration is not exceeded by more than three or four times, there should be little danger from its use.

I recommend the use of *dulse* (another seaweed) for mineral supplementation because I believe this plant is much better balanced in minerals than kelp, although its "press" has been much poorer. Dulse can be bought in the dried form and is rather tasty if a couple of inches of it are eaten each day. Such a dose is more than adequate to take care of many of the trace mineral needs of the body.

Dr. R.S. Clymer used to recommend the food *Irish Moss* for its iodine content. It is still a good food today and most certainly carries the mineral in the colloidal form.

Magnesium

Within recent years, magnesium has become another of the glamour food elements. Dr. Clymer wrote of it extensively sixty years ago and most of what he wrote is being rehashed today. I don't deny that the mineral is important, but it is difficult to obtain as a supplement in the colloidal form. Most magnesium compounds sold on the open market contain magnesium oxide, and they are somewhat laxative (Epsom salts, the well-known cathartic, is magnesium sulfate). In a properly manufactured bone meal, magnesium should be present in balance with calcium and phosphorus. In this form, it can be given in dosages sufficient for most needs. For larger amounts, we recommend the chelated form of magnesium, because it's very similar to the natural colloidal structure and is seemingly well-accepted by the body. Since there are newer and better forms of magnesium being produced steadily, it is best to ask your Center physician for the latest word on this mineral.

Manganese

Manganese, a trace mineral, has found much use in our practice as a normalizer of ligament tone. In this capacity, we have used it particularly to strengthen the ligamentous structures around the sacroiliac (see Chapter III). We use manganese in a colloidal form that is well-accepted by the body and only rarely has had adverse effects, even in large dosages. It is combined with other synergistic agents in the form we use and if you have problems with adjustments holding please ask your Center physician to tell you about this product.

Other Trace Minerals

Many years ago, I, like other members of my profession, predicted that the '70s and the '80s would be the decades of the trace mineral. We thought that many unexplained diseases would be found to be caused, or at least aggravated, by trace mineral deficiencies. Researchers now find that

229

many symptoms can be attributed to an imbalance of these very small but vital factors. Unfortunately, the structural form of the trace mineral and its interrelated balance with its fellows are being ignored in this effort to categorize the individual specific symptomatology.

While work in this area has not proceeded as fast as we had hoped, we still believe that in time many modern diseases will be traced back to an absence or deficiency in various trace minerals.

Although specific trace minerals are used in our practice (in the chelated colloid form), I use them only in severe deficiencies, and I generally prefer a natural colloidal compound that has these elements in their normally occurring, minute, but properly balanced, form.

How Nutritional Substances are Produced

Vitamins and minerals can be produced in three ways. First, we have the synthetically produced compound. Sometimes the molecule of the synthetic product is identical to that of the natural product, such as vitamin C (ascorbic acid). Sometimes the synthetic product acts somewhat like the natural product, but it is structurally different from the natural product. Vitamin D2, which is synthetic, and vitamin D3, which is the natural product, are a case in point. The D2 prevents rickets but is not as potent as D3, and it is more toxic than the natural form.

Second, vitamins can be produced by extracting the natural crystalline form from food or other organic products in which the desired vitamin may occur. By the time the proper extraction and crystallization are done, the resulting product is quite similar to the synthetic product. In fact, the very name crystalline vitamin indicates that the substance has been reduced to a crystalloid state and that its basic colloidal structure has been lost.

Third, vitamins and nutritional products can be produced by the very careful concentration of potent food sources in such a manner that all the enzymes and compounds with colloidal structure are retained throughout the process. In this instance, the final product can truly be called "natural," and in truth it .is a living entity similar to the source found in nature. This last process is obviously the most difficult and costly. It is little used by the large manufacturers because few people are sufficiently sophisticated to appreciate its superiority. Such products are used, however, by many physicians in the natural healing arts who understand and demand what they can offer their patients.

Colloidal Nutritional Supplements

Colloidal nutritional supplements generally fall into two categories.

The first contains products to be used as nutritional support to balance out deficiencies that may be present in a patient's intake of food and drink.

The second group comprises remedies designed to correct specific imbalances in body nutrition and to aid the body in overcoming definite symptom patterns. In general, the first group can be used by anyone for supplementation of his diet; the second group should be used only on the recommendation of a natural physician for correcting conditions he has diagnosed.

The Supplemental Products

In colloidal supplemental products, an attempt is usually made to derive concentrations from a variety of sources for the nutritional grouping desired. For instance, in our Centers instead of using an ordinary B complex with arbitrarily chosen amounts of the various factors present, we use a compound in which liver, selected yeast and rice bran extracts are combined after being processed below body temperature. In such an extract, the various unknown factors that are part of the B complex should be present in sufficient amounts to be nutritionally effective. From the results achieved with such products, our theory seems to prove out in clinical practice.

The various forms of nutritional supplements can be duplicated in a similar manner. We don't attempt, however, to duplicate the high dosages so common to many crystalloid products. We believe that such high dosages are often deemed necessary because the natural-occurring synergistic products essential to the best working of some of these vitamins aren't present in the high-potency preparations; or if present, they have been reduced by the manufacturing procedures to a near inactive form. I believe this is why so many physicians feel compelled to use megavitamin therapy, in which tremendously high doses of various vitamins are used. True, at times this seems to accomplish miracles, but later follow-ups on many of these patients show that other undesirable effects are also produced by such an unbalancing procedure. I call this "unbalancing" because no one can know what this tremendous overdosing of specific nutritional elements will do to the complex body structure. It would be a miracle if one could impose such an abnormal regimen on the body without causing adverse effects.

Most physicians well-acquainted with natural therapy prefer to give nutritive supplements in a form more closely allied to that which God created. If these remedies are carefully chosen and administered, they not only prevent body imbalances, but they should also achieve therapeutic results equal or even superior to those obtained by megavitamin therapy.

Therapeutic Use of Nutrient Elements

The FDA, which is run entirely by men steeped in orthodox medicine, has always proven antagonistic to the treatment by nutritional compounds of any disease except classified deficiencies. Owing to the rules set down by the FDA, it isn't possible for me to speak of treating a disease or curing a condition by the use of nutritional supplementation. In truth, though they probably didn't mean it as such, the FDA's doctrine is accurate, for no food or supplement is capable of accomplishing this goal. What we can do by the use of specific nutritional therapy is to give to the body food factors necessary to fully carry on its work of overcoming physical and mental disturbances.

Protomorphogens or Substance Therapy

Interest in what the early naturopaths used to refer to as "substance therapy" goes back a great many years. History records that Hippocrates and Galen used this method. Brown Sequard, a great scientist known as the founder of scientific organotherapy, began the first modern interest in this subject. Henry Harrower of Glendale, California, did much to advance the concept.

Substance therapy differs from endocrinology in that the desiccated substance of the various glands and other body tissues, devoid of their hormone activity, is given to the patient in an effort to stimulate or initiate the repair mechanism naturally inherent in any body tissue. From antiquity, there were those who believed that if one wanted a strong heart he should eat the heart of an animal, if a strong liver then eat the liver of an animal and if he wanted intelligence he should eat nothing but brains. Although such a supposition was much couched in superstition, modern research in the natural field has demonstrated a certain degree of validity in the contention.

In the 1940s, Royal Lee and William Hanson wrote a book entitled *Protomorphology,** in which they attempted to prove that in the various tissue cells are compounds that they likened to blueprint substances, which could stimulate the repair mechanism of a like structure if they were diseased. For instance, if one had a weak heart muscle, one would ingest a tablet containing highly concentrated forms of this heart blueprint (protomorphogen), and this substance would aid the weakened heart to

*Lee, Royal, and Hanson, William: *Protomorphology*. Lee Foundation for Nutritional Research, Milwaukee, Wis., 1947.

repair itself. Although such a theory has never been accepted by the orthodox medical profession as a whole, there is much clinical evidence to substantiate it, and many medical men now use these substances.

Henry Harrower considered his work as endocrinology, and yet many of the substances he used, such as thymus and mammary tissue, had no detectable hormonal activity. Thus, many of the outstanding results he so carefully documents in *Practical Organotherapy* ** must have been due to the same mechanism that Lee and Hanson describe in *Protomorphology*.

Recent research by Hanson has led him to believe that the blueprint factors are actually DNA and RNA compounds present in cell nuclei. This updated approach doesn't invalidate the basic thought of the protomorphogens, however, because the DNA molecule is, in effect, a blueprint for the construction of a similar cell from this DNA structure. It is possible that all the clinical observations on organotherapy or substance therapy can now be substantiated by modern scientific thought.

Many natural healing physicians have found that certain diseases can be combatted by the careful and judicious use of these products. Such protomorphogens are particularly useful in chronic conditions because healing in such diseases is always slow and arduous. The protomorphogen factors seem to augment and direct the body healing forces toward the rebuilding of selected tissues. This effect in most of the conditions we treat isn't rapid, but because they are usually used where orthodox medicine isn't successful, there is much to recommend them.

Other Little Known Nutritional Substances

Besides the protomorphogens, other natural factors that aren't necessarily needed as daily supplements have proven useful in certain disorders. A substance we frequently use was originally called Yakatron by the Japanese physician who discovered it. Obtained from the liver, Yakatron possesses certain natural antihistamine effects. Although its effects are only moderate in some patients, others find their allergic sensitivities greatly helped by its use. Because it is a naturally occurring compound, it has no known toxicity and is free of side effects.

Thymic extract is most helpful in overcoming infections, particularly viral infections. The results are based on clinical experience, but such results have been too consistent to be doubted by any physician with an open mind.

The Lee Foundation of Milwaukee, Wisconsin, has extracted a substance from pea pods that they call E2. It isn't D-alphatocopherol, but it

---

**Harrower, Henry: *Practical Organotherapy*. Glendale, Calif. The Harrower Laboratory, 1922.

is a related substance that many natural physicians have found useful in a variety of heart afflictions.

The list of these specific nutritional factors is very long, and it wouldn't serve any useful purpose for me to discuss them all here. I desired only to present a few examples to give an idea of the little known remedies the natural physician has at his disposal.

Herbal Remedies

We consider our herbs not as drugs but as specific nutritional remedies utilized for their food like effects on specific parts of the organism. Just because a substance is obtained from a plant doesn't make it a medicinal herb in the naturalist's point of view. Digitalis, Colchicum and Belladonna all come from plants, but these, except when used homeopathically, are thought of as drugs by our profession. When I use the term drug, I refer to something that has a definite body-altering property, in contradistinction to something that offers specific organized nutrition to the body. For instance, belladonna produces much of its desired effects by actually paralyzing various nerve structures. Although at times such an effect may seem useful or advantageous, it is nevertheless produced by a drug and not a nutritional effect. Valerian also has an effect on the nervous system, but when given in naturopathic dosages, this effect is due to certain nutritional substances it provides the nervous system to aid in reducing its over sensitivity and establishing a more normal functioning. Valerian thus acts, not as a drug, but as a specific nutritional compound.

Certain herbs may be placed in either category, depending on the dose given. But this is true of many things in life, for few substances are harmless if given in excess of what the body can readily accept.

In the use of herbs for nutritional effect, we must again consider the colloidal-crystalloid concept. If an herb is so prepared so that its colloidal active principles are broken down into crystalloids, its effectiveness is greatly diminished. We generally use either powdered herbs or the homeopathic mother tinctures. I have found that homeopathic pharmacies are most painstaking in the production of their tinctures, and because of their fine therapeutic effects, I believe they have preserved a large amount of the original colloidal structure of the growing plant.

Recently we have been fortunate to have "on line" at our Centers an Herbalist who is trained in the production of his own herbal extracts. Since these are made fresh at our own facility and in the extract form are far more effective than in the simple tincture form, we are able to use them more effectively than ever before to help our patients.

Herbs in the form of teas are useful in various conditions, particularly when we desire a calming or sleep-inducing effect. In general, I prefer the tinctures to the teas, because a greater concentration of vital effective principle is present in the tinctures. The one exception to this rule is our Kidney Tea. This group of herbs is best made into a tea so that it can exert its effect on the urinary tract.

Because I hoped to present only new material in this book, I do not plan to discuss at length the various herbs used at our Centers. There are many excellent books available for this purpose. One of the most useful was written by Dr. Clymer himself, entitled *Nature's Healing Agents.** This is available from the Beverly Hall Corporation Healing Research Center.

Summary

I agree in general with the medical profession when they say that the best way to get the nutrition one needs is through the daily intake of food. If it is possible to obtain untampered, unaltered, unsprayed, naturally grown foods and to eat them in the proper balance, supplementation should generally be unnecessary. Unfortunately, few of my patients are able to obtain such a diet. For most of us, the best way to stay healthy is to do the very best we can with our food supply and to supplement this diet with specific nutritional products designed to retain, as nearly as possible, the natural colloidal structures found in fresh foods. In certain disorders and under certain periods of stress, it may be necessary to use noncolloidal substances for temporary help, but the day-to-day bulk of our supplements should be in the natural configuration.

In these days of high-powered advertising the words "natural" and "organic" have very little honest meaning when applied to a product. Legally, a product can be called organic as long as it contains some of the mineral carbon, for in scientific parlance, an organic compound is merely a compound that contains carbon and some other elements. Because all synthetic vitamins contain carbon, they can legally be called organic, though this is not at all the meaning their manufacturer hopes to give to the unsuspecting public. Remember what Macbeth said: "And be these juggling fiends no more believed that palter with us in a double sense, that keep the word of promise to our ear and break it to our hope."

Nor is the word "natural" to be believed anymore than organic; this word can also be misused in two ways. First, it is possible to extract

---

*Clymer, R. Swinburne: *Nature's Healing Agents.* Quakertown. Pa.. Philosophical Publishing House. 1965.

nutritional compounds from natural sources, but to so process them that they are little better than their synthetic counterparts. Second, some manufacturers even take the meaning of natural to mean "that which is derived from Nature," and in truth, isn't everything derived from Nature? If a product is made from coal tar, coal tar is derived from Nature and therefore a product derived from coal tar is obviously natural. Such a position could undoubtedly be defended in court. So whenever you look at labels on supplements, even those produced by highly reputable firms, remember well the statement of Macbeth.

There are available to Natural Healing Centers such as ours, many substances that, when properly used, can be most helpful in balancing the body, thereby enabling the vital force to re-establish normal function. The control of the Food and Drug Administration by the orthodox medical profession has caused an almost complete blackout of information on these products, but in spite of this opposition, they have helped a great many people to a healthier, happier life. You could be one of them.

Chapter XV
Understanding Homeopathy

Of all the methods used at the Beverly Hall Corporation Healing Research Centers, the one least understood by most patients is our use of homeopathic medication. Although homeopathy as a form of therapy is more than 200 years old and has been practiced continuously during this period, few lay people today are familiar with its fundamentals. Unlike orthodox medicine, called allopathy by the homeopath, which has an ill-defined set of assumptions about health and disease, the homeopathic practice is based on very definite conclusions about disease and its effects. For homeopathic treatment to be optimally successful, it is important for the patient to be acquainted with these basic principles and to be in agreement with the objectives the homeopath desires to obtain.

Dr. Samuel Hahnemann (1755-1843), the founder of homeopathic medicine and a brilliant scientist of his day, abhorred the completely unscientific manner in which drugs then used for healing human ailments were selected, tested, and prescribed. From his investigations and the observations of his fellow practitioners, he realized that most drugs were discovered mainly by chance, often by those not in the medical professions and they were used basically for what has become known as the "primary effect," with little regard to their actual mode of operating within the body or their secondary toxic effects.

Many years have passed since Hahnemann's original observations, yet modern-day homeopaths find that despite our current improved technology, the basic information available to orthodox medicine concerning drug functioning has advanced only meagerly since Hahnemann's time. In fact, because there has been such a tremendous proliferation of drugs since Hahnemann's time and only a moderate amount of new revelations about their use, there probably is now more accumulated ignorance about the actions of drugs currently in use than there was in Hahnemann's time.

The allopathic school takes a simplistic and almost naive view of health and disease. Allopaths consider disease as that which is represented by certain sets of symptoms that are deviations from the normal parameters of body activity. They then attempt to discover a drug or drugs that will force these symptoms to regress to a point they consider normal. Only rarely do they concern themselves with the true causes of the symptoms or with the reason that the body produces them in the first place. The general assumption is that if the various body reactions they can measure by their insensitive methods are within normal ranges, the patient is healthy. This isn't to say that allopaths don't try to find the cause of an infection, or if the ankles are swollen that they wouldn't check the heart or kidneys for malfunction. On the other hand, they probably wouldn't attempt to discover what body imbalances enable the infection to occur or what deficiencies are causing the heart or kidney malfunction.

The homeopath, on the other hand, as do all natural healing physicians, tends to consider most symptom patterns not as the disease per se, but as the body's attempt either to warn of the disease condition or to cast off the basic disease entity. If the disease were only the symptom pattern, the allopathic method would be adequate to cure all our ailments. If the homeopathic and naturalist views are correct, however, the allopathic method would all too often tend to thwart the body in its actual healing efforts, making the person less healthy than he was before the treatment.

In the late 1700s and early 1800s, Hahnemann began to develop a theory of medicine that he hoped would place the medical art on a solid foundation. He was a logical, methodical physician who did not believe in putting into the body any substance whose action he did not know as completely as possible.

He postulated that each drug used in treating the sick had a unique specific action on the body, and that before such a substance could be properly used, this unique and specific action must be thoroughly investigated to the point that the physician knew exactly what effect it would have in the human economy. In his day, there were no instruments capable of such a complete investigation, so the good doctor turned to biologic methods. After some thought, however, he rejected the much-used animal research of his allopathic contemporaries. Experience had taught him that the reactions of each species are individual and unique and one can't necessarily extrapolate information gained from one animal body system to that of another species.

Hahnemann therefore restricted all his investigation to the use of human subjects and with this he developed the method known as *proving*. In order to prove a drug, moderate physiologic doses of the compound were given to a large number of persons considered to be in good health. Young medical students were usually used because they were available and were considered to be more observant than the average lay persons. The specific drug was continued until various symptoms caused by the drug's action began to appear. These symptoms were carefully recorded by the students and the drug was continued until either the symptoms had run their gamut or until signs of toxicity appeared.

Two groups of symptoms were generally elicited. First, a prevailing group that was more or less common to almost all the drug's provers; and second, individual idiosyncratic symptoms that occurred only in one or two provers. The more consistent set of symptoms was considered the most important; although the idiosyncratic symptoms were preserved and are available in the larger homeopathic texts on materia medica. They can be useful to the homeopath in difficult cases.

From these provings, Hahnemann ascertained the specificity of each drug he tested. In other words, after an extensive set of such provings, Hahnemann had information about the specific organs and tissues affected by each drug, and he also had knowledge about the exact manner in which this drug affected these structures. While such information went well beyond what had been done previously in pharmacology, it still didn't provide him with a method of curing diseases.

At this time, the inspiration came to Hahnemann that resulted in the homeopathic school of medicine and laid the foundation for the fundamental basis of cure by all the natural therapeutic methods. Some inner wisdom brought him to see that the symptoms usually present in most diseases weren't actually the disease itself, but were in truth the body's attempts to overcome the disease and that a true healing method should encourage the body in these efforts and not discourage the body from carrying out its constructive eliminative processes.

As Hahnemann began to appreciate the true nature of health and disease, he also began to develop a method by which drugs, and the knowledge of their action, could best be used to help the sick. He hypothesized that because the symptoms produced by the body in most diseases were really an effort by the body to overcome such conditions, we should help the body in this effort in every way we can. If drugs are to be used to treat disease, the most practical way, he reasoned, was to use them to stimulate the body in its efforts to eliminate the disease.

In his provings on drugs, he discovered that individual drugs were capable of stimulating specific tissues in the body in the same manner that the different disease processes could. "If the drugs and disease cause similar effects, what would happen," he asked himself, "to a patient, who has a certain set of symptoms which the body is creating to overcome a disease, if I gave a drug which in a healthy person would cause that identical set of symptoms? Would this drug stimulate the body in its efforts to overcome the disease more rapidly than it could without this help?" Such reasoning put into practice was the beginning of homeopathic medicine.

When this new method was put to the test, Hahnemann was over-joyed to discover that it was more successful than even he had hoped. He found that when the specific drug that caused a certain set of symptoms in a healthy person was given to a diseased patient with a similar set of symptoms, a speedy and apparently complete recovery ensued. For example, belladonna, when given in large doses to a healthy person produces a hot, dry, very red, sore throat. When such a throat is encountered as a disease entity, it usually is rapidly cured if small amounts of belladonna are given. Thus, although the allopath and the homeopath both use this drug in their treatment programs, the conditions and principles behind the administration of the drug are entirely different.

Let's use the sore throat again to show the difference between these schools. The allopath holds that if he can destroy the bacteria, the disease is cured and the body will be healthy once again. Hahnemann and the homeopaths would look on this matter from an entirely different viewpoint. They know our body is always inhabited by bacteria; in fact, almost all the known pathogenic bacteria can be cultured from the healthy human throat. The homeopath would therefore consider the sore throat an attempt by the body through an inflammatory process to eliminate a morbid or unhealthy condition that may have been building up in the body, rather than consider it a disease per se. The homeopath would consider bacteria as the agents by which this morbid matter is destroyed and not necessarily as detrimental agents. This would be particularly true of recurring sore throats that are controlled but not cured by the usual antibiotic therapy.

The disease process then is actually this morbid or toxic matter that has accumulated within the body. The throat inflammation is the body's attempt to overcome and cast off this disease material. The homeopath gives the patient a remedy that will help the body in its efforts to eliminate this matter. When this is done, the bacteria, their job finished, disappear and the throat returns to normal.

Antibiotics, as used by the allopath, prevent bacterial growth and suppress the acute inflammation, thereby leaving the body with the disease still fulminating within its depths. Homeopathic treatment helps the body to cast off the disease so that when the symptoms subside by the use of homeopathic remedies, not only is the patient pain-free, but also the morbid disease matter itself is eliminated. In other words, the patient usually becomes healthier after the proper treatment of conditions by homeopathic methods, whereas all too often he may become less healthy when treated by allopathic methods.

Over the years, there have been many explanations about why

homeopathic medicine works. One theory is that because the remedy and the disease are nearly identical in their effects, there is created within the body a neutralization somewhat like that caused when two out-of-phase sound waves of identical frequency cancel one another.

Hahnemann's original explanation, however, was not quite so complicated. He merely said that the drug has a stimulating effect on the specific cells affected by the disease and that this reaction greatly hastens the body's attempt to cast off the ailment. In chronic diseases, he believed that the body's attempts to overcome the disease were unfortunately quite feeble, thus enabling such chronic ailments to persist. Here he particularly thought the homeopathic stimulative method to be very important to properly direct and activate the vital force in its efforts to overcome such conditions.

The Minimal Dose

The foregoing discussion explains the choices of the homeopathic remedy, but there is another unique factor in homeopathic medication that has always been an obstacle to the general public's acceptance of this method. This reticence has to do with what is known as the "diminutive dose." The homeopath uses dosages of medicine that are so small by standard physiologic measurement that in the higher dilutions it is utterly impossible to detect by chemical or other analytic means any of the drug within the carrier material. It seems that only a very minute part of the drug is needed to produce the stimulative activity.

Perhaps this feature of homeopathy, more than any other, has held it up to constant ridicule by the allopath. Hahnemann, nevertheless, developed this technique only after long experience and experimentation, and he used it only because it proved to be the most satisfactory method of treating with drugs in his estimation.

In his early prescribing, Hahnemann used fairly large physiologic doses of his remedies. He soon found that although he would cure the disease for which he prescribed his drug, he often left the patient with other problems because of certain toxicities inherent in the remedy. In order to offset these toxicities, he began to diminish the size of the drug dose given. Although he'expected less success with his cures, he believed this was best for the long-term health of the patient.

To his amazement, he soon found that his patients got well faster and the cure seemed more permanent than it did with larger dosages. Once he had observed this phenomenon, his fertile brain wouldn't rest until he'd found just exactly to what extent the dose reduction could be carried out with continued beneficial results. From extensive investiga-

241

tion, he found that many remedies became more effective for certain types of cases as they were further divided, especially when this division was done in specific steps with certain measures taken to ensure adequate dispersal of the original drug.

This process, called trituration, is still used by all authentic homeopathic manufacturers. In this procedure, a specific amount of the pure drug is taken and mixed with ten equal parts of a dilutant; either milk sugar or alcohol is usually used. This first dilution is then shaken a certain specific number of times. This remedy is then called a 1x or first trituration. For the 2x or second trituration, a specific amount of the 1x mixture is taken, again mixed with ten parts of dilutant, and shaken for proper mixture and division. For a 3x, a portion of the 2x is taken, mixed again with ten parts of dilutant, and this procedure repeated for the other dilutions.

Thus, the method is one of geometric progression. The first trituration is a 1 to 10 dilution, the second a 1 to 100 dilution, the third a 1 to 1000 dilution and so on. Because the homeopath commonly uses remedies of 30x and 200x, these triturations contain almost an infinitesimal amount of the crude drug. In some of the highest triturations, it is possible, owing to the size of the molecules, that there may be none of the original crude substance at all in the dose.

This being true, one can see why allopaths ridicule homeopathy. For if there is none of the crude drug left in the higher triturations, how can they possibly be effective? Strange to say, according to homeopathic theory and practice, the more a drug is divided, the greater its strength or ability to heal becomes, especially in chronic ailments. In fact, the homeopath believes these higher potencies have such a powerful effect that they must only be given with great care and when one is very sure of the specific symptom pattern.

Hahnemann taught that each drug has a specific character that causes its basic effects on the body. This character, although due to the physico-chemical structure of its molecule, is independent of this molecule, once such a character is established, in the same way that the Soul inhabits the body and yet doesn't directly depend on the body for its existence. It is this "soul of the drug" that does most of the healing in homeopathy, and it is this nebulous entity that is released for its most complete action by the process of trituration and shaking (succussion) to which these drugs are subjected.

Near the end of his life, Hahnemann took to curing his patients in some instances by merely having them smell a vial containing the proper remedy for their condition. Although such a procedure was a natural outgrowth of his investigations, the technique hasn't been continued by modern practitioners, perhaps from a fear that their patients may consider them even more unusual and less scientific than they seem to be anyway.

Long experience has shown that the lower homeopathic potencies (those up to 6x) are most useful in acute or short term diseases, whereas higher potencies (12x, 30x, 200x, or higher) are best adapted as long-term, deep-working remedies in chronic ailments.

Many remedies, by their very nature, are short-working and therefore best adapted to acute conditions. Aconite is a good example. This drug is used by the homeopath in the first stage of infective and feverish conditions, but its usefulness wanes as the fever lowers. On the other hand, certain other remedies, such as sulfur, calcarea carb, tuberculium and silicia, are usually used as constitutional remedies, for they are very deep-working remedies that can be used for months and even years with continued good effect and will root out many well-seated chronic diseases. We frequently treat a patient's chronic condition with a deep acting constitutional remedy while also addressing intercurrent acute problems with separate "acute" remedies. Furthermore, since most of our patients have more than one constitutional layer that must be treated in succession with the appropriately indicated remedies, this process of overcoming deep constitutional problems may take several years to complete. It is the art of the master homeopath to effectively address both the acute and chronic needs of his patient while he strips away layer after layer of constitutional disease.

How to Best Use Homeopathic Remedies

In using homeopathic remedies, certain important precautions should be taken so that their optimum effect may be realized.

They should be taken dry under the tongue, whether the liquid or the more common trituration tablet is used. If they are swallowed with water, as are most medications, their effectiveness is negated. When placed under the tongue, their medicinal power is rapidly absorbed into the blood in the same manner that nitroglycerin is absorbed.

Because the homeopathic remedy is so subtle, it should not be taken just before or just after having eaten or drunk. At least fifteen minutes should pass after a meal before a homeopathic remedy is taken, and a longer time is preferred.

For a homeopathic remedy to function correctly, the use of allopathic drugs should be restricted because their use tends to counteract the full effectiveness of most homeopathic remedies. I don't find this as true with the low homeopathic potencies as it is in the high potencies.

For this purpose, commonly used compounds such as tea, coffee, Coca Cola, and cigarettes, must be considered drugs, because they contain substances that have pharmacologic effects on the body. Although patients who have these habits can be helped by the homeopathic method, the cure is much more rapid if the patient attempts to live a life without the use of physiologic stimulants or inhibitors during the treatment.

There is an old saying, "You have to get worse before you get better." In general this is a lot of nonsense and it is used by many physicians to cover their inability to help their patients. With homeopathic remedies, however, this maxim may well be true. We attempt with homeopathic remedies to further stimulate the specific organs that are producing the symptoms. At first this stimulation may result in a short-term intensification of these symptoms, but this soon passes as the vital energy of the body responds to this stimulus and rapidly overcomes the disease. The homeopath is encouraged if his patient worsens slightly soon after taking the remedy, because this positively indicates that he has selected the correct remedy and it is having its desired effect. If the remedy is ill-chosen, it doesn't affect the proper tissues and no symptom intensification will result.

The Homeopathic Laws of Cure

In treating acute disorders, the homeopathic method frequently works rapidly with good success. To the unknowing patient it seems to work much in the same fashion as do allopathic medications. Thus, the patient will present himself to the physician with a certain set of symptoms. He is given the indicated homeopathic remedy, and although there may be slight temporary symptom intensification, this is followed by a rapid cure of the condition and the patient is returned once again to his normal activities. From the patient's viewpoint, the allopathic cure and the homeopathic cure of acute ailments are similar. Of course, this similarity is only on the surface and the long-range results of the two methods can be very different as described before.

The outer differences between the allopathic and homeopathic schools are very distinct in the treatment of chronic diseases. To the homeopath, these chronic diseases can best be eliminated by stimulating the repair mechanism of the body, which he likes to call the *Vital Force*, with the properly chosen homeopathic medication. It may take many different remedies to correct most chronic conditions because these diseases are usually due to multiple causes and a different drug or group of drugs is needed for each cause.

The homeopathic and natural healing physician look on chronic disease as the consequence of improper nutrition, emotional tension, improper treatment with allopathic medication and an over abundance of stress from which the body is not able to recover. The symptoms or the final manifestations that occur are merely an end result of these accumulated body assaults. While allopathy attempts to battle these manifestations when they become objectionable, the true natural healing physician directs his efforts to overcoming the underlying causes, thereby resulting in a patient who is disease-free, not one who is just symptom free.

Herring's Laws

In the treating of chronic diseases, the homeopaths have discovered that the elimination of these conditions proceeds in a certain specific order and rules have been laid down outlining this healing procedure. These rules are known as Herring's Laws in honor of Constantine Herring (1800-1880), who is considered the father of American Homeopathy.

Herring's three laws may be expressed simply as follows:

1. Symptoms of a chronic disease disappear in a definite order when the patient is properly treated in accordance with homeopathic recommendations. The symptoms usually disappear in the reverse order of their appearance—the most recent symptom disappears first; then an earlier symptom remanifests only to abate when the proper remedy is given. This process continues until all the unresolved disease conditions are eliminated, even though some may go back to early childhood. This procedure is called the *reverse progression of symptoms*. This procedure of symptom regression isn't restricted to homeopathy alone, but is to be expected when most natural methods of therapy are used to overcome chronic ailments.

2. Herring's second law states that the symptoms tend to move from the more vital organs to the less vital organs and from the interior of the body toward the periphery or skin. This law functions because of the body's attempt to preserve itself. If a disease that produces morbid matter can't be eliminated, the body tries to deposit the residues of this condition in as harmless an area as possible. The skin is one of the safest, but the various connective tissues and joints are also frequently used by the body for this purpose.

Only when the disease process is overpowering does the body allow it to invade the vital organs, and even then the body makes every possible attempt to keep the disease processes out of the heart and brain. When a patient comes to us with disorders of the vital organs, we know the vital force is weak or these areas wouldn't be affected and therefore the cure will be prolonged. Under treatment, the symptoms will subside and recede from the more vital areas to the less vital areas, and the symptoms may even end with a healing reaction on the best eliminator of all—the skin.

3. Herring's third rule states that the symptoms move from the top of the body downward, disappearing first from the head, then from the thigh to the knee, ankle, and foot. We frequently encounter this last pattern, wherein the pain will go from the abdomen into the hip, then thigh, then knee and then in and out the foot. These patients often comment: "You know, Doctor, I'm sure when it gets down to the foot, it will just go out the toes and be gone." They usually are correct.

The functioning of the third law is based on a principle similar to the second. Because the more vital areas are found in the head and upper portion of the body and those of less importance are encountered toward the extremities, the third law is a symptomatic extension of the second law. Its nature is important to the physician but not particularly to the patient.

From these laws, a patient may realize that under proper homeopathic treatment he could re-manifest symptom patterns from an earlier stage of his life, only if these conditions weren't fully corrected originally. If he had so lived that the body didn't have residual disease material, it wouldn't be necessary to go through this retracing regimen.

I have always found this concept for the cure of chronic diseases one of the most fascinating aspects of natural therapy. Such a concept is completely rejected by all but a few allopaths. This rejection is to be expected, of course, for if they accept it, they would also have to accept the fact that most of their methods of therapy are injurious to the patient in the long run. Although there are many fine men in the medical field who have for years been harboring grave doubts about basic allopathic practice, I fear it will be many more years before they are able to accept the homeopathic and naturalistic view of chronic ailments.

The Nature of Homeopathic Cure

Over the years, the homeopath has accumulated provings for thousands of homeopathic remedies. Although in common practice only a few hundred are used, this great number of provings enable the matching of symptoms to almost any encountered disorder. The prudent homeopath doesn't, however, attempt to use homeopathic remedies to cure all ailments. One of the basic principles of Hahnemann was to find the cause of the disease and correct it. If this could be done best by means other than the use of a remedy, then this would be the most practical way to treat the patient.

Dr. George Royal, the famous homeopath, relates the story of a patient who once came to him with a pain in his mid-back, which gradually increased during the day, but which soon disappeared after he left his job. Royal tried one or two remedies, but the pain did not change. One day the patient appeared at Royal's office with a large button in his hand. "Dr. Royal," he said, "this is the cause of my trouble." The button was used on his suspenders where they crossed in the back, and it was applying a constant pressure on a vertebral nerve as the patient sat in his chair at work. Once the man discovered this and removed the button, his ailment was corrected, and no further homeopathic medication was needed.

The modern homeopath, therefore, is fully acquainted with advanced nutrition and specific nutritional substances. He is also familiar with many of the therapeutic modalities used in the natural field, while still being knowledgeable about orthodox allopathic surgery and drugs.

The homeopath knows that, at times, emergency measures must be taken and physiologic drugs may be required, but most of the exasperating conditions of mankind and especially those that respond poorly to orthodox medicine will respond well to homeopathic methods.

Homeopathy—Advantages and Disadvantages

Most of the disorders described in this book can be helped by homeopathic treatment. In our Centers, we almost invariably use this type of therapy along with the other forms of natural medicine. Homeopathy does have, however, one great advantage over every other form of therapy. Because its indicated remedy is chosen only by the symptom pattern of the patient, a remedy can be found for every possible condition, irrespective of whether a definitive medical diagnosis can be established or not. In allopathy, even with the finest modern methods of examination, the causes of many disorders are not readily found and, not finding a cause, the allopath is unable to offer adequate treatment. Such a deficiency can't occur with homeopathy. Because a remedy choice is made exclusively on the symptom pattern, one can always be found for every patient, because even an undiagnosable disease will have symptoms. If this remedy is wisely chosen, an improvement in the patient's condition is almost sure to follow, assuming the problem is among those susceptible to homeopathic treatment.

Another advantage of homeopathy is that it is truly safe. The remedies are prepared in such dilution that they are absolutely harmless and without any adverse side effects, even to the most delicate constitution or frailest infant.

Still other advantages are that the remedies are easily given and readily acceptable, even to children at ages when it is almost impossible to get them to accept other tablets or compounds. Also the remedies are inexpensive; the most potent of the homeopathic remedies cost the patient no more than a few dollars.

The disadvantages of homeopathy are few for the patient, but somewhat greater for the physician. This method takes time and dedication on the part of the physician. It isn't easy to find the proper remedy from among the thousands available. It takes great skill and much time in complicated cases for the physician to properly prescribe for and treat each patient. It generally isn't possible for him to command fees commensurate with the time involved, and homeopathy thus hasn't become popular.

This last disadvantage is now being relieved by the computer. At our Centers we now have special computer programs that help us to find the proper remedy in a few seconds instead of the hours and even days that it has taken in the past. If you are given a homeopathic remedy, ask your physician to show you how this program works, it is most fascinating.

In chronic disorders, considerable time is necessary to effect a proper cure. In these disorders, however, the allopath has little to offer in the way of a cure. With a combination of homeopathic and other natural methods, a cure can be effected as rapidly as the body will allow.

One other disadvantage of homeopathy is that it is psychologically weak. The practice of giving little sugar pills under the tongue to cure very severe disorders doesn't seem adequate to most patients. If they have a disorder that to them is serious they want something big and complicated done to correct it. For this reason, besides others of course, surgery is popular even though many medical reports show that a good fifty per cent of surgery is completely unnecessary. Most patients like a show, and homeopathy doesn't put on a good show, except in the fabulous cures it produces. Most homeopaths I have known are quiet, dedicated and unassuming men who are not likely to seek the limelight, so even their best cures are little heard of. In truth homeopathy has had very poor public relations. I hope by this chapter to correct some of this anonymity.

In ending this chapter, I want to quote the preface to the first edition of Hahnemann's *Organon of Medicine.** This edition first appeared in 1810:

"According to the testimony of all ages, no occupation is more unanimously declared to be a conjectural art than medicine; consequently none has less right to refuse a searching enquiry as to whether it is well founded than it, on which man's health, his most precious possession on earth, depends."

---

*Hahnemann, Samuel: *Organon of Medicine*. Philadelphia. Pa.. Boeriche and Tafel, 1901.

Postscript: Recently, a great aid to the Homeopath has been introduced in the form of a comprehensive computer database of nearly all the important Homeopathic literature of the last two-hundred years. With this program, the Homeopath can make a search for the proper remedy in a matter of seconds, rather than the days, or even weeks, that it might have taken in the past. We are pleased to let you know that our Healing Centers now have this revolutionary program on line and are able to use it for all your Homeopathic needs.

Chapter XIV
Prostatic Problems

Disorders of the prostate are among the most troublesome conditions that beset the middle-aged man. The three most common difficulties are inflammation of the gland (prostatitis), benign prostatic hypertrophy (simple enlargement) and prostatic carcinoma (cancer).

Prostatitis

Prostatitis may occur at any adult age, but it is most common between twenty-five and forty. It is usually caused by some infective agent that comes from another part of the urinary tract. Orthodox treatment consists of antibiotics, although these aren't universally successful, and the prostatitis tends to return after the initial treatment is finished. Some clinics have treated this condition by direct injections of antibiotics into the prostate. They reported a good rate of cure, but I haven't investigated these claims and therefore can't substantiate or deny the efficacy of this method.

In our Clinic, we have traditionally treated prostatitis with the electrical magnetic waves of diathermy, microwave and **Magnatherm**, and a variety of specific nutritional compounds to help stimulate the reticuloendothelial system. These treatments are usually effective in overcoming acute prostatitis. The **Depolar Ray** is especially helpful in this condition though to be effective the treatment must extend from one-half to one hour each visit. The new **Low Level Laser** has also shown good promise of being effective in this condition. Most certainly this condition would fall into this reported field of efficacy.

Prostatic Cancer

The prostate is a relatively common site of cancer. Fortunately, the prostate is usually palpable and the hard, irregular masses of cancer tissue can usually be discovered early. We recommend the middle-aged man to have this examination with the same regularity that his wife has a Pap smear. If such examinations are done regularly, there is no reason for prostatic cancer to develop beyond the stage where it can be successfully treated surgically. Although we aren't surgically inclined, if a very high rate of cure can be obtained through surgery and only tentative help by other means, we aren't afraid to recommend surgery. When the cancer is found in its early stages, surgery is usually quite successful. Therefore we generally recommend it, unless the patient is vehemently opposed.

Nowadays we also have the PSA blood test to check to see if there might be some cancerous activity in this organ. We have found that where the PSA begins to rise, we can often stop this rise and even lower it in many patients by the use of the same basic treatment that we use for benign hypertrophy.

The above paragraph was written some twenty years ago and during the interim there have been several interesting studies concerning prostatic cancer. The first of these tended to show that this cancer is often very slow growing and that the survival rate of those who had it operated on and those who did not was almost the same.

Later, with the bringing to light of several famous people who died of this cancer and others who were saved from this fate (just in the nick of time) by immediate surgery, there seemed to be a big push to remove all such tumors, regardless of the earlier studies.

Since cancer is not my specialty, I cannot really comment on the paradoxical nature of these two finds except to wonder if the earlier finding might not have been thought of as threatening to the surgical community and so they initiated a campaign to counteract it. This much in the same way that the orthopaedic surgeons are now waging a campaign to nullify the Government report of acute low back conditions which favored manipulation over surgery.

Benign Hypertrophy

By far the most common prostatic involvement is the benign enlargement (hypertrophy) that comes with middle or old age. Some physicians consider this condition a natural physiologic change that occurs in the aging male. We, at Beverly Hall Corporation Healing Research Center do not agree. Although this condition is common and we make it a general practice to examine every male over the age of forty for this type of enlargement, we find relatively normal prostates in many of our older patients who have attempted to follow the natural life style we recommend.

Much research has been done in a search for the cause of this disorder. The results of this work have given us many clues as to its cure. Most of the early research seemed to show that this condition was caused by an apparent deficiency of one of the various fatty acids—which at that time was called Vitamin F. These acids—linoleic, linolenic and arachidonic—when given to the patient with prostatic enlargement, help in alleviating the symptoms and in even causing a decrease in the prostatic size.

Further investigation demonstrated that trace minerals in various

252

combinations might help. Zinc in particular has been singled out as a possible vital factor and some authorities have recommended eating pumpkin seeds to supply zinc, thereby alleviating the disorder.

Still later work has shown that the specific amino acids— glutamic acid, alanine, and aminoacetic acid—when supplied in a raw assimilable form and in a specific proportion are very beneficial in correcting the general symptom pattern of benign prostatic hypertrophy. A compound of these amino acids has so proven its value that it is the only product I am aware of that is allowed by the FDA to state on labels that it is helpful for the symptomatic relief of benign prostatic hypertrophy.

There is an interesting story behind that labeling, by the way. The original product had been on the market for some time and had gradually gained acceptance by physicians of all persuasions. Then one day, a member of the FDA decided that this should not be; a nutritional product couldn't help this disorder and so it was ordered off the market. Usually, when such an action is taken, the company, not having the vast sums needed for a battle that are available to a federal agency, takes down its tents and steals off into the night. Fortunately for the middle aged men of America, the heads of this company weren't about to give in so readily and they took the government to court to prove the value of their product. During this trial, renowned urologists from all parts of the country took the stand to tell of their successful experiences with this compound. And in the end, not only did the government lose its case, but the company also won the right to label their product as being useful for the symptomatic relief of benign prostatic hypertrophy.

Another useful agent in the treatment of benign hypertrophy is the herb *Saw Palmetto*. This classic (and classy) herb has been used for this purpose for centuries and is as beneficial today as it was when it was discovered. At our Healing Research Center we treat this condition with remedies that contain all these salubrious compounds and others not so well known.

In general, I believe that prostatic enlargement results from nutritional deficiencies that become manifest in men as they reach middle age. Treatment therefore should not only be directed toward supplying the nutrients already discussed, but also in making certain that the patient's whole basic nutrition is as balanced as possible.

Sexual Activity

Because the prostate is an integral part of the sexual apparatus, I think that its integrity can be affected by conditions that influence sexual function. The obvious purpose of the prostate gland is to supply a thickened medium to make up the bulk of the seminal fluid, which carries the sperm into the vagina during ejaculation. Many authorities have conjectured that the prostate is also a hormone-producing gland. Some of these authors have thought that certain hormones produced in the prostate are absorbed by the vaginal mucosa, having a beneficial effect on the general female economy and a stabilizing effect on her nervous system. (See Chapter 26)

If the prostate functions as most other glands do, and we have no reason to expect it to work differently, the more it is used, excluding obvious excesses, the better it should work. If, on the other hand, it is inactive for long periods or is otherwise abused, it may become congested, something that could play a part in producing hypertrophy. If sexual intercourse is engaged in by a married couple every few days, the prostate, barring rather severe deficiencies, should have every opportunity to retain its normal structure. Assuming, however, that sexual relations are sporadic, occurring maybe once or twice a month, the circulation of the formed prostatic fluid is definitely inhibited and it is possible that this gland may eventually become hypertrophic owing to the stagnant condition of its secretions. It does seem that as some men grow older the prostate slows down the production of its excretion and so congestion may not occur as rapidly as in a younger man or one whose hormone structure is such that his prostatic fluid production does not diminish with age. For these men, the release of the prostatic fluid is still beneficial but it may not be necessary (or possible) to have intercourse as frequently as in the younger or more virile man.

This theory of prostatic stagnation is definitely not accepted by most medical practitioners. These same practitioners, however, do not have any more satisfactory explanation for this problem and until they can either adequately disprove my theory or come up with a superior one of their own, I shall continue to suggest to my male patients that they make every attempt to continue normal sexual relations at reasonable intervals as late in life as possible. It is usually possible for me to tell the exact status of a middle-aged man's sexual activity by palpating his prostate gland. Only rarely has such an examination failed to give me truthful information.

Treatment

The treatment of this condition in our Clinic is broken down into three parts—first, that which must be done by the patient himself; second, that which can be helped by nutritional supplementation; and last, treatments that must be carried out under the supervision of the treating physician.

From the foregoing discussion on sexual activity and prostatic stagnation, one may correctly surmise that we first apprise a patient of the nature of his prostate gland, its normal purpose, and what he can do through the proper regulation of this sexual activity to aid his physician in correcting his disorder.

In unmarried patients, or those who are at an age when sexual activity is no longer practical or possible, we suggest a regimen of breathing exercises designed to absorb the prostatic secretions back into the general body circulation. The more sophisticated of my readers may find such suggestions naive, but clinical experience has proven the usefulness of this method.

Clinical experience has also shown that promiscuous activities by men not only do not help, but actually tend to aggravate prostatic difficulties. My own theory is that the vaginal secretions of different women are almost as dissimilar as their faces, and although it is possible for a man to adapt and actually thrive from the effects of a single vaginal secretion bathing his sexual organs, a mixture of secretions produces a result that is somewhat chaotic to his sensitive sexual structures. I find, therefore, that prostatic difficulties often accompany promiscuity as readily as they do habitual masturbation and married continence.

My experience has shown that a harmonious life with one woman, including sexual activity at a consistent regular rhythm late into life, is the best possible external environment to assure a healthy prostate gland.

Nutritional Supplementation

Most of the nutritional products used to help prostate difficulties have already been discussed. Vitamin F can be obtained from a number of sources. The original product used for this purpose was vitamin F perles from the Royal Lee Foundation. I like to support originators by using their products until I am sure that a competing product is definitely superior; if this occurs, I then use the more effective compound. In our Center, we still use the original vitamin F perles. Although one of several cold-processed oils— safflower, soy, and sunflower—might be effective if used for a long time, we find the concentrated F perles more effective.

In using zinc and other trace minerals, we recommend the chelated form, or the colloidal form. I often recommend a complete spectrum of trace minerals for my prostate patients. There are several products that contain the amino acids found to be most useful to help this condition. Here again I like to stick with one of the old classical formulas since it seems to work consistently better than the others.

Saw Palmetto can be added in many forms. We are now beginning to use a form distilled fresh by our own in-house herbalist. You just can not beat freshness in herbal compounds.

Office Treatment

Office treatment has proven an invaluable part of prostatic therapy. Once the gland is considerably enlarged, the correction of deficiencies and poor sexual habits don't relieve the swelling without proper local treatment.

The first procedure we use is a good prostatic massage. To carry out this procedure, the patient is asked to assume a knee-chest position and the doctor slowly inserts a cotted, well-lubricated index finger into the patient's anus. Both sides of the prostate are carefully and thoroughly examined, and the prostate is then massaged in such a way as to lift the gland off the urethra (urinary tube), to break up any mild adhesions and loosen the gelatinous-like substance present in the enlarged gland. At first we treat these cases as often as once a week, although as soon as good improvement is made, the patient is reduced to bimonthly and later to monthly office visits.

In our Centers, we use either diathermy or **Magnatherm** before the prostatic massage is given. This treatment helps prepare the body tissues so they can more readily respond to massage.

The **Depolar Ray** is helpful in all cases and is never omitted from our prostate therapy. This little known therapeutic device generates an alternating magnetic energy that seems to stabilize some of the unknown factors that may play a role in prostatic hypertrophy. Although the **Depolar Ray** is not a cure-all for prostatic disorders, it has nevertheless proven itself to be invaluable in the treatment of prostatic hypertrophy for the last forty years.

Prognosis

It hasn't been necessary, to my knowledge, for any of our prostatic hypertrophy patients to require later surgery. In our experience this ailment responds well to natural therapy. Obviously, the earlier we start therapy, the better and more rapid are the results. Even with advanced cases, however, we usually can relieve the symptoms, enabling them to live a relatively normal life.

The two common types of surgery performed for this enlargement are not without their own attendant difficulties. In transurethral resection, a cutting edge is passed up the urethra and a section of the prostate is removed from the inside. This is useful in some patients, but usually it requires another operation ten to fifteen years after the first one, unless natural therapy is instituted.

The more radical total removal of the prostate offers permanent cure, but it tends (as can the transurethral resection) to definitely alter the patient's sexual life. Most surgeons are loath to mention these sexual difficulties before surgery, but it is rare for a patient not to have sexual weaknesses after either operation.

Prostatic operations are currently very popular among physicians. It's not necessarily their fault, however, that such operations must be performed. Most men have an inherent dislike and fear of medical treatment, and therefore usually won't seek attention for a prostate disorder until it is well advanced. If we could treat these men at an earlier state, much surgery could be avoided.

By constant publicity, we have convinced the women of our country to get their Pap tests and to examine their breasts, and from these simple procedures many disastrous problems have been prevented. Unfortunately, no such efforts have been made to have prostates checked on a similar basis. For this, I make a plea here and now. If you are forty or older, please go to a physician knowledgeable in these methods and have your prostate examined. If he finds it enlarged, let us help you follow the recommendations in this chapter. Prostate disorders strike right at the very seat of your manhood, and there is no reason you should be robbed of the many pleasures that should be yours in middle and later life.

Chapter XVII
Fasting—Pros And Cons

Of all the methods used by the natural physician, no method is as powerful nor as controversial as the fast. More disorders of the human economy can be overcome by the fast and its variations than by any other single therapy. Yet the fast is but rarely used by most practitioners because so few are trained in the proper technique and procedures needed to obtain the best results.

Types of Fasts

We use three basic types of fasts at our Centers. The first is the relatively short fast, which is recommended during most acute conditions. This is used during influenza, childhood diseases, colds, and other acute conditions, particularly when the body temperature is elevated. In these acute disorders, we usually recommend a modified fast in which fruit juices diluted one to one with un-fluoridated and un-chlorinated water are prescribed.

The second, and most common, type of true fast is the short complete fast, which is used to overcome a large variety of chronic disorders. This type of fast, which usually lasts five days to two weeks, is often repeated every few months until the results desired in a specific disease are obtained.

Last, at times nothing but the extended fast, lasting three weeks to three months, will serve our needs. This is the most powerful of all the fasts, but it is most difficult to undergo and must be handled with great care, even by the most accomplished physician .

The Rationale Behind Fasting

One of the reasons fasting, particularly in chronic diseases, has never found much favor with orthodox physicians is that it depends on an intelligence in the body that most of them are not prepared to accept. This intelligence, which homeopaths and naturopaths call the *vital force* and which has been called *innate* by chiropractors, must be accepted as fact for an adequate understanding of fasting. The true naturalist reasons in this fashion. There is, he says, within the body a force at work, constantly striving to preserve and strengthen our being. This force attempts to control the various mechanisms and chemical reactions of the body in such a way that life is perpetuated and the organism functions in the most efficient manner under the circumstances it finds itself in.

If one believes in a just and loving God, such an assumption is easily accepted, for surely if God is as wise and as benevolent as He must be, He would devise an organism that has the ability to constantly work for its own betterment. The natural healer, therefore, accepts, as a basic premise of his method of treatment, that within the body there is a force sufficiently potent to correct the infirmities and diseases that may affect it. When this inner vital force does not heal, the natural physician reasons that it must be impeded by adverse circumstances and it is the physician's duty to discover the reasons for this failure and to correct them so that the vital force can continue its healing ways.

From long investigation, the naturalist believes there are only a few reasons why the vital force may become so inhibited. First, it can't perform properly if it doesn't have the necessary nutrients with which to carry out its duties. Second, its action will be sluggish if it is heavily encumbered with congesting matter clogging its functioning life lines. Third, it can't fulfill its duties if it is being poisoned by harmful emotional pressures that can produce a nearly constant drain on its already strained abilities. Last, and particularly germane to this subject, it can't do its job in some instances unless it is given a free hand and unobstructed opportunity to proceed to a salubrious conclusion.

To fulfill these four specific needs of the vital force, the natural physician first attempts to discover any deficiencies that may exist within the patient's system. Then, by the selection and administration of proper foods, and if necessary, specific nutritional substances, he supplies the body with the needed materials the vital force requires to establish normal functioning and overcome the ailment.

In selecting a diet for his patient, the natural physician carefully restricts the menus to foods that don't congest and that will therefore enable the various body eliminative channels to be as free as possible under the circumstances of the basic disorder. Concurrently, the natural physician also uses whatever therapeutic methods he thinks best to aid the body in its decongesting attempts.

If necessary, he counsels the patient on proper mental attitude to be fostered during the cure, so that the patient's own thought and emotional processes won't impede the vital force in its work.

The three foregoing methods of aiding the vital force are in themselves adequate to cure many chronic ailments. Some, however, are too stubborn to give way to this simple, but basic, schedule and they may require the fourth to be implemented. The fourth, as you remember, is a proper opportunity and environment in which to work.

If some severe chronic conditions are to be cured by the vital force, it must have nearly unimpeded control of the body— that is, it must have the ability to adjust to the various mechanical, chemical and electronic mechanisms of the body with the least possible interference from the outside. With our present degree of understanding, this is best accomplished by the fast.

If we look at the fast in this light, we are in effect saying to the vital force, "Here, vital force, I give you back your body. I shall sustain it only with water, which is neutral and necessary to keep the cells from dehydration. I won't put into the body any drugs that you will have to fight, nor will I give it any food that you may or may not need at this time. I will therefore not force you to use your energies to digest substances that I have chosen but that you may not desire. So here, dear instrument of God, take this body, use all your strength and energies to make it whole. I won't interfere until you, through the various signals that you may give me, indicate that you once again want me to give the body food and other substances that you may require."

I realize that such an approach must seem naive to those unaccustomed to natural methods. However, such a view is based on sound scientific fact. In the body, millions of chemical and electronic changes occur every second. To say that man is able to understand and control all these reactions is impudence in the extreme. The vital force of the body alone is capable of the intricate integrations of actions needed to re-balance the system to overcome many chronic diseases. Man's attempts to control body function in these ailments have nearly always met with long-term disaster.

In the much less complicated world of animal and plant ecology, man has recently discovered that in almost every instance where he has attempted to use his intelligence to control Nature, he has done far more harm than good. Many hardheaded scientists now agree that only when man works in harmony with Nature is the greatest benefit for him and his environment to be realized. Now that we have finally realized such a truth in the external world, it is to be hoped that we realize that this knowledge is even more applicable to the internal world of our own bodies.

The character of most chronic diseases is entirely unknown to even the greatest of physicians, including those in the natural field. The ignorance of physicians about the fundamental cause and nature of chronic ailments is profound. After reading many thousands of medical articles over the years, I find the authors all too often end their detailed description of the disease with an apologetic statement something like this: "The actual cause and fundamental mechanisms of this disease are entirely unknown, however, and it is hoped that future research will better clarify this rather embarrassing situation." Although these exact words may not be used, this spirit of their thought is repeated time after time in medical textbooks. These are not the books given to the lay public. Any physician with an honest heart readily admits the extent of our ignorance about the true cause and cure of chronic diseases.

Our knowledge of acute diseases isn't that sure and unshakable either. We are told that various bacteria and viruses cause disease, yet all we really know is that these bacteria are present in these diseases. If we inject these bacteria into healthy people, some will become sick and some will not. Is the disease really caused by the bacteria, or are bacteria scavengers that, according to many naturalist physicians, are simply the agents used by the body to cure the real disease? If the system is weak enough, a disease may take hold by the installation of an infective agent and yet in many persons it does not.

Why then does one man get a disease and another not? No physician knows for sure. If we took out of this body the vital healing force and left the full care and healing of our diseases to our physicians, I'm sure the human race would have perished thousands of years ago. Ben Franklin once said, "God cures the disease, but the doctor takes the fee." Although this may not be entirely true, it is not entirely facetious.

The true nature of practically all ailments, acute or chronic, is known only to God and the inherent healing power in man. The only diseases that man can be entirely sure of are the ones that he has created himself by poisoning his food, water, air and the medications he takes. Therefore, if this healing force alone has a full understanding of the disease, isn't it only rational that in the attempt to overcome this disease, we give this all-knowing healing force every opportunity to function and exercise to its fullest ability? This we do by the fast.

Here and here alone do we free this vital force from all outside interference and let it do with the multitude of body functions as it will. During the fast, the wise and dedicated physician sits at the feet of this great internal power and watches its working with awe and admiration. He is a willing servant, ever ready to help this force if it gives the slightest hint of such need. Being a good and dutiful servant, however, the physician knows all too well not to interfere in his Master's affairs until commanded.

The Procedure of the Fast at Our Healing Centers

The first type of fast, the semi-fast, carried out in acute conditions, is simple. We place the patient with a fever on a diet of half water and half fruit juice mixed. The patient is allowed as much of this solution as he desires and this routine is continued until his temperature returns to normal, at which time the patient is placed on a general eliminative diet of fruits and vegetables, a little lean meat or fish and perhaps some cottage cheese or yogurt, until full strength returns. Then he can return once again to the Basic Maintenance Diet. In children with extended fevers, it is sometimes necessary to add food of an eliminative type once the fever has dropped below 100°. In most cases, though, the fruit-and-water solution is all that is necessary until the temperature returns to normal.

The General Fast

The short fast for chronic conditions is the most common of the general fasts; the extended fast is handled exactly as is the short fast, except that additional laboratory measures must be taken as precautions by the physician.

In conducting the general fast, one must always have in mind the objectives. The purpose of this fast is not to lose weight, to increase spiritual enlightenment or to feel better immediately, for those who fast often feel worse at various periods during it. The purpose of the healing fast is to balance the body chemistry, to cleanse the body from abnormal and deleterious congestions and to cure certain physical infirmities and diseases that may be present in the body. Every thought of the physician during the fast should be directed toward these purposes by helping the vital force in every conceivable way. To this end, he must not forget the four fundamental needs of the vital force. These four needs must be met before and during the fast or his success will be incomplete.

In our Centers we never start patients on a fast without a previous period of preparation. Patients about to fast are first given a thorough general physical and laboratory examination. Where time allows, we also request a hair test, vitamin and mineral analyses, and other specific methods of analysis (see Chapter I).

If we find the patient is a good candidate for the fast and is in need of it, we place him on a high-nutrient diet supplemented with colloidal nutritional elements, in an effort to saturate his body with all the materials that the vital force may need later in its healing and repair. While this nutritional build-up is being accomplished, we attempt to decongest and cleanse the body through a variety of natural methods. Tissue de-sludging massage, herbal colonic therapy, body manipulation and a variety of special hydrotherapy methods all may be used to produce a system as decongested and as circulatorily efficient as we can obtain.

During this time, the patient is also counseled on the basic purposes of the procedure he is about to undergo. The nature and purpose of the fast are explained to the patient as I have explained them here. They are also taught of the temporary adverse feelings and emotions that may come with the proper functioning of this internal vital force. During the fast itself, we provide these patients with reading material to help put their mind in the proper constructive attitude so as to make the greatest possible constructive use of this method.

After the patient has been adequately prepared—which may take anywhere from a week to a month, depending on the condition to be overcome and the original status of the patient—the fast is begun.

Although most authorities agree that the most effective fasts are carried out with only water to drink, there is much debate about the type and amount of water that should be used. Some authorities believe in forcing fluids; others believe in restricting the amount taken to an absolute minimum. Some physicians opt for distilled water, others suggest spring water and still others make no recommendation at all.

In our Centers, we have used each of these methods successfully depending on the specific patient. In general, we invariably follow a course of moderation. Forcing fluids seems useful only during acute conditions and only rarely is such a method necessary or even useful in fasting for chronic ailments. Some physicians believe that the fast is more productive if fluids are restricted to a bare minimum. They believe that in this way the body is able to wring out the various toxic substances from the body. There may be some truth in this, but on the other hand, when fluids are restricted it is difficult for the kidneys and bowels to carry on their proper elimination processes.

In fasts with restricted water intake, it is possible that permanent damage may be done to the kidneys. I therefore restrict this method to highly selected patients and then only for a very short period. To force or restrict fluids is an attempt to control the vital force and this is counter to our basic purpose. I therefore conduct most fasts by allowing the patient to take water as directed by the vital force through the agency of thirst. If the body needs more or less water for a better healing, I let it tell us.

Much more debate centers around the type of water given than the amount. Some physicians believe that unless a fast is conducted with the use of distilled water, no real improvement is to be expected. These proponents seem to forget that the fast has been used as a treatment from the beginning of mankind. It is in fact one of the instinctive healing procedures of all animal life. It worked for early man and animals and as far as I know none of these ever used distilled water.

Although certain types of conditions may benefit from distilled water intake during the fast, I generally recommend that high quality spring water be used. I make this suggestion partially from clinical observation and partially from a philosophic viewpoint. Clinically, I have used distilled, spring, and well water, and results from spring or well water have always equaled, if not excelled, those from distilled water.

Philosophically, I believe that by offering the body an unnatural product—distilled water—we are in a sense again attempting to influence the vital force in a negative manner, by introducing substances into the body that may cause the vital force to make adjustments not to the best benefit of its objectives. By using distilled water, which tends to disturb the mineral balance of the body, we take away from the vital force things it may need, thereby destroying the balance the vital force is attempting to establish and preserve.

Effects That Occur During Fasts

It takes at least three days for body functioning to come to a standstill and accept the fact that the patient is giving the vital forces full control of its own organism. Although a certain amount of cleansing and decongesting takes place in the first three days, no real healing of chronic ailments is ever accomplished this early. During these first three days, the patient usually has some problem with hunger, or rather I should say, with appetite. Having built up a habit pattern of eating two or three times a day, the body doesn't easily adjust to a changed pattern. Once the third day is past, an entirely new phase is entered and hunger usually ceases to be a problem. The body becomes almost self-sufficient and from the fourth day on the patient usually feels as if he could continue the fast forever.

Weight loss during a general fast is evident, but it is much less than one might anticipate, because the body makes every effort to economize its necessary functions and there is very little wasted energy.

During the fast, we usually have our patients rest a great deal. We want to conserve as much body energy as possible for the vital force to use as healing power. If there is much activity, this deducts from the healing ability of the body.

Some authorities recommend total bed rest during the fast. We find this unnecessary and actually detrimental to the patient's economy. Certain body functions, particularly those of the kidneys in calcium metabolism, are upset by a continuous reclining position. The patient is allowed, however, as much rest as he desires during a fast. There may even be periods, for a day or two, when the patient desires complete bed rest. This is allowed, as the vital force may at certain times during the fast withdraw practically all the body energy to the internal environment to overcome a particularly difficult problem.

Patients vary greatly in their feelings and the symptoms displayed during the fast. Some of our patients state happily that they have never felt as well in their lives as during their fast. Others may display a variety of unpleasant symptoms. It isn't unusual for a variety of skin eruptions to develop during the healing fast, because this is one of the best ways the body has of casting off toxic substances. Any disagreeable reaction associated with such eruptions is rapidly controlled by the use of one of the other physical therapeutic methods available at our Centers.

High blood pressure usually drops during a fast, whereas low blood pressure often increases to normal levels. The blood pressures of all patients are watched carefully during fasting. If the level drops too low, the fast is broken.

Urine examinations are made daily, and blood samples are taken whenever the need arises. Most patients tend to show acid bodies in the urine (ketosis) after a few days of fasting. If this is kept within moderate levels by the vital force and if the patient is in good physical and emotional shape, we usually don't become overly concerned. On the other hand, if the ketone levels begin to rise above the allowable range, or if the patient begins to feel overly tired or ill, we add very small amounts of pure cranberry juice to his water. In almost all instances, this slight amount of juice—as little as ¼ of a cup a day—corrects the ketosis and gives the patient a feeling of well-being. By following this method, it is possible to extend fasts in some patients far beyond what might have otherwise been advisable.

I realize that by adding cranberry juice, even in this very small amount, we break the philosophic rules I laid down for fasting. Experience has shown, however, that the results of the fast seem unaffected by the use of cranberry juice. Without this juice, it would be necessary to stop some fasts far sooner. The benefits of the longer fast far outweigh any slight inhibiting effect the cranberry juice might have.

Most of our general fasts last anywhere from five days to two weeks. If the condition, though chronic, is of fairly recent origin, a single fast of this duration may be sufficient for its eradication. For more deep-seated conditions, however, it may be necessary to use several of these short fasts to accomplish our full purpose. We usually allow a month to two months between fasts and generally each ensuing fast is made longer than the last. With each healing fast, the patient's health improves and he becomes all the more an advocate of this ancient, but unique, method of cure.

The extended fast, that is a fast extending from three weeks to three months, is occasionally used. It requires a very specific type of person—

one who is heart and soul sold on fasting—to undergo the rigors of this procedure. We, at our Centers recommend it only rarely. I believe that most who use the extended fast could produce the same results from a series of short fasts. It must be admitted, however, that a few specific conditions seem to respond only to the extended fast. This treatment must be carefully handled, and is one of the most intricate and arduous tasks a patient and physician can undertake.

The Breaking of the Fast

Every physician, who has his patients fast, has his own favorite method of breaking the fast. At our Centers, we are rather conservative and use some of the more ancient techniques.

When the patient has fasted sufficiently, I suggest that he begin the breaking period by taking diluted fruit juices with his water on the first day. On the second day, he may take the juices straight if he so desires and small amounts of solid fruit or vegetables are added. If he responds well to this food, yogurt, cottage cheese and a small amount of raw almonds or sunflower seeds are allowed on the third day. On the fourth day, the patient is allowed fresh fish, vegetables, nuts, and fruits. On the fifth day, he is returned to the Basic Maintenance Diet, unless there is a reason for keeping him on a semi-eliminative regimen.

The breaking of the fast is usually handled adequately by the foregoing regimen. For some of more delicate constitution, it may be necessary to extend this period or to use a variety of specific substances to aid the body in preparing itself for food once again. These special cases must be individually controlled by the physician.

Some Parting Thoughts on Fasting

Short fasts of three to four days can be carried out by almost any patient at home without any complicated repercussions. Such fasts are useful and often exhilarating and they can help overcome certain uncomplicated congestions and minor disorders. They are not adequate to eliminate serious or longterm chronic ailments, however.

Fasts longer than three to four days should be done only under the supervision of a physician trained in this therapy. Once one passes into the fourth day of a fast, it is possible for the body to produce a wide variety of eliminative reactions that must be handled by someone knowledgeable in their nature, otherwise adverse effects could result from the patients misunderstanding of these reactions .

Some early authors on fasting thought that the fast should continue until the breath becomes sweet, the tongue clean, and the mind clear. In some chronic disorders, the patient would die before this objective is reached in a single fast. There is no sure guide for knowing exactly when a fast should be broken. This is another reason why any fast more than three or four days should be attempted only under proper supervision.

A question often asked me is: "If a fast is so useful and powerful to eliminate disease, why doesn't every doctor use it?" The answer is disarmingly simple. The fast is little used by most physicians because they are not taught about it, they have had no experience with it in their practice or in hospitals and, of course, since it requires no medication, no drug company is going to sponsor research into its effectiveness.

Few doctors without such outside influence are oriented in this age of medical complexity to fathom the powerful influence of the fasting method. Even if they had the inclination or knowledge to conduct a fast, few physicians have the physical plant available to carry it out satisfactorily. The medical profession has generally restricted healing to two establishments—the crowded office and the hospital. The fasting patient needs daily observation and a quiet serene environment in which this technique can be carried out. This certainly can't be done in a physician's office and few hospitals would accept such cases because they believe their beds can be put to much better use for the severely ill. The medical establishment is not geared emotionally or physically to use fasting in any form.

Years of private practice have taught me that many patients are not properly served by the office and hospital practice of orthodox medicine. Many patients can't be adequately treated in the office or home, but they don't require or benefit from the antiseptic, sterile, extremely costly hospital environment. This is one of the main reasons we have built our Healing Sanctuary. We have here on fifty country acres a facility where patients can stay in nice homey rooms that resemble a luxury motel more than a hospital or sanitarium. These rooms are directly connected with a vast treatment center so that the patients can be checked readily each day by their physicians, but with seclusion and privacy an integral part of their environment. In this atmosphere, the true fasting method can be carried out with ease and safety, and perhaps this is one reason our fasting treatments prove so successful.

An old friend of mine and a great physician, John B. Bastyr, of Seattle, once told to me, "Fasting will cure every disease of mankind if only the patient lives long enough." The purpose of the physician is to see that the patient not only lives through the fast, but also that the fast is conducted so that its deep penetrating healing is best directed.

Chapter XVIII
Sight Without Glasses

Many methods have been suggested over the years to treat vision and to correct refractory errors without the use of glasses. Undoubtedly the most extensive and well known work in this field was that done by the ophthalmologist W. H. Bates. In 1920, Dr. Bates published *The Cure of Imperfect Sight by Treatment Without Glasses,** a text now extremely rare. Many other more easily obtainable texts using his methods have been written and can be recommended, but the whole extent of his work can't be adequately understood without some knowledge of his original theories as delineated in his original book.

The difference between orthodox ophthalmic theory and the Bates theory is shown in Figure 13. Orthodox theory holds that accommodation (focusing) of the eye is accomplished only by relaxation of the ciliary muscle, which enables the lens to assume a variety of shapes and focal lengths, thereby focusing on objects both far and near. In the Bates theory, the lens remains fairly constant in shape, but the eyeball changes its position, owing to action of the various extrinsic muscles of the eyeball.

In developing his theories, Bates was not a closet scientist; he had a full active practice and had examined tens of thousands of eyes during his career. In his book, he details the results of hundreds of thousands of experiments he made, first in an effort to prove the orthodox accepted theory of eye accommodation, which he could not prove, and then to show validation of his own theory.

Bates' methods of photographing the eyes were unique with him and he was doing work seventy-five years ago that hasn't yet been adequately duplicated by modern scientific investigators. Those interested in the scientific explanation of these methods are recommended to obtain his book, though it is long out of print; it possibly could be obtained in some of the larger used book stores.

Bates taught that the cause of practically all refractory eye problems—those corrected by the fitting of eyeglasses—was due to eyestrain. This was particularly true in younger persons, and he also taught that the best treatment of these errors was by relaxation and the elimination of strain rather than by merely placing a positive or negative lens in front of the eye so that the patient could see more clearly despite his strain.

---

*Bates, NV. H.: *The Cure of Imperfect Sight by Treatment Without Glasses.* New York. Central Fixation Publishing Co.. 1920.

Personally, I believe that both the orthodox and Bates theories of accommodation may function simultaneously in ocular disorders. I see no contradiction in the conclusion that certain amounts of accommodation may be accomplished by a change in the convexity of the lens, whose elasticity decreases as the individual grows older, helping account for the hyperopic eye of the elderly, while strain that alters the shape of the eyeball could account for many refractory defects, especially in younger individuals, that can be successfully corrected by the Bates method.

The Bates method of treatment is very effective in many cases, a fact that I can attest to personally. All during high school, I needed and wore eyeglasses for myopia. During the end of my senior year, I read my first book by a disciple of Bates, and following the methods suggested, I soon was able to rid myself of eyeglasses. For almost thirty years I had no need for glasses. By my mid forties the typical hardening of the lens began and so now I need glasses for reading but my far vision which was corrected by the Bates method is still good. Whether the Bates theory is completely accurate, I can't say with certainty. But his treatment methods are effective, and I believe much good would be accomplished if his methods of eye care could be taught in hygiene classes in every high school in our nation.

The Bates Theory

Not only did Bates hold views contradictory to those of orthodox ophthalmology about the process of accommodation, many of his other findings are in direct opposition to their recommendations. Bates believed (and my own experience has verified it) that the refractive ability of the eye varies from day to day. Thus, one day, a person may see very well, whereas the next day his eye is less able to accommodate.

If we try to fit glasses on such a person, we can fit them only to the eye state at the time of the fitting. When the eye changes, the glasses can't and they are thus inappropriate. The eye must therefore adjust to the lens; when it must do so, it is not free to operate as a natural agent and is weakened to that extent.

Bates has this to say on the subject: "As refractive abnormalities are constantly changing, not only from day to day and from hour to hour, but from minute to minute, even under the influence of dilating drugs, the accurate fitting of glasses is of course impossible. In some cases, these fluctuations are so extreme or the patient so unresponsive to mental suggestion, that no relief whatever is obtained from correcting lenses, which necessarily become under such circumstances, an added discomfort. At their best, it cannot be maintained that glasses are anything more than a very unsatisfactory substitute for normal vision."

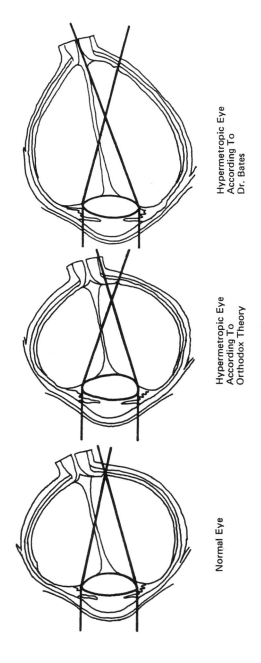

Hypermetropic Eye
According To
Dr. Bates

Hypermetropic Eye
According To
Orthodox Theory

Normal Eye

Figure 13

271

I don't want to imply that we ask our patients to throw away their glasses. I want only to show that corrective glasses aren't necessarily the ideal way of correcting all refractory problems and that another method may often prove quite effective. Even the patient who isn't able to completely eliminate his glasses usually is able to use progressively weaker lenses, whereas each change of lens previously had required a stronger prescription, signifying a weaker eye mechanism.

Bates surmised that most refractory eye problems are caused by the strain to see. He believed that the relaxed eye made proper accommodation quite readily, but that under the various strains put on civilized man, the eye is one of the first organs to react adversely to these pressures and that this is the major cause of our refractory problems.

He also stated that the eyes aren't necessarily rested by sleep—that during sleep one could even stare with the eyes closed and that relaxation must be taught. He also believed that eyes aren't necessarily tired by use but by the strain that often accompanies such use. One of his fundamental theories was that the act of seeing is a passive act—that is, to see requires no active participation on our part. In fact, he felt any attempt to see produces eyestrain automatically. This strain may take many forms, resulting in many abnormal conditions. Circulation to the eyes is disturbed by this strain, and normal circulation can only be restored by proper mental control of this eyestrain. He was certain that eyestrain could not only produce errors of refraction, but also, through abnormal inhibition of the proper circulation, other disorders such as cataracts and glaucoma. (We have no knowledge of any evidence he presented to prove this connection, however.)

In complete contradiction to most authorities, Bates taught that the usual do's and don'ts of eye care aren't based on observed fact. He didn't think that bright lights are necessarily harmful to the eye; rather he believed that the eye had the necessary methods of accommodation to correct for these and that light is to a degree the life blood of the eye. In fact, as a part of his treatment, he used to suggest a certain amount of sun gazing, in which the patient would sway back and forth looking at the sun with his eyes closed, and then occasionally open the eyes for a fraction of a second to allow the full light of the sun to penetrate to the retina. Admittedly, this must be done only momentarily or the retina can be damaged, but when used in moderation it has helped improve eyesight in many.

Bates held that darkness is the biggest danger to the eyes, though he did think that sudden contrasts of light—a change from light to dark or from dark to light—are in themselves beneficial. In fact, Bates recommended that his patients go to the movies in the early days of the so-called "flickers," for he believed the flickering image on the screen was actually an exercise for the eye and. if properly observed, following the methods I describe on central fixation, would prove of great benefit. If Bates were alive today it would be interesting to know what he would have to say about television and computer screens. I would not be surprised to find that he might not feel that they are beneficial for long periods of viewing.

Another accepted orthodox dictum not upheld by Bates' investigations was the theory that fine print and dim light are bad for the eyes. In his book, Bates says, "On the contrary, the reading of fine print, when it can be done without discomfort has invariably proven to be beneficial and the dimmer the light in which it can be read and closer to the eyes that it can be held, the greater the benefit. By this means severe pain in the eyes has been relieved in a few minutes and even instantly. The reason is that fine print cannot be read in a dim light and close to the eyes unless the eyes are relaxed, whereas large print can be read in good light and at ordinary reading distance although the eyes may be under strain. When fine print can be read under adverse conditions, the reading of ordinary print under ordinary conditions is vastly improved."

To lay at rest another accepted theory, he had this to say about reading in moving vehicles: "Persons who wish to preserve their eyesight are equally warned not to read in moving vehicles, but since under modern conditions of life, many persons have to spend a large part of their time in moving vehicles and many of them have no other time to read, it is useless to expect that they will ever discontinue the practice. Fortunately the theory of its injuriousness is not borne out by the facts. If the object regarded is moved more or less rapidly, strain and lowered vision are at first always produced, but this is always temporary and ultimately the vision is improved by the practice."

To finish his list of do's where other people have listed don'ts, Bates has this to say about reading in bed: "There is probably no visual habit against which we have been more persistently warned than that of reading in a recumbent position. Many plausible reasons have been deduced for its supposed injuriousness, but so delightful is the practice that probably few have ever been deterred from it by fear of the consequences. It is gratifying to be able to state therefore that I have found these consequences to be beneficial rather than injurious. As in the case of the use of the eye under other difficult conditions, it is a good thing to be able to read lying down, the ability to do it improves with practice. In an upright position with good light coming over the left shoulder, one can read with eyes under a considerable degree of strain, but in a recumbent position with the light and the angle of the page to the eye unfavorable, one cannot read unless one relaxes. Anyone who can read lying down without discomfort is not likely to have any difficulty in reading under ordinary conditions."

At the end of his chapter on reading, Bates presents in summary his theories about reading under difficult conditions, and I think we can do no better than to again quote the original: "The fact is, that vision under difficult conditions is good mental training. The mind may be disturbed at first by the unfavorable environment, but after it has become accustomed to such environment, the mental control and consequently the eyesight are improved. To advise against using the eyes under unfavorable conditions is like telling a person who has been in bed for a few weeks and finds it difficult to walk to refrain from such exercise. Of course discretion must be used in both cases. The convalescent must not at once try to run the marathon, nor must the person with defective vision attempt, without some preparation, to outstare the sun at noonday. But just as the invalid may gradually increase his strength until the marathon has no terrors for him, so may the eye with defective sight be educated until all the rules with which we have too long allowed ourselves to be harassed, in the name of eye hygiene, may be disregarded. Not only with safety, but with benefit."

The purpose of this chapter is not to present the methods of the Bates eye treatment in a form capable of being used for complete correction of eye difficulties, but merely to acquaint the reader with the basic method and some of the lesser known theories of Bates. If you are interested in helping yourself to improved vision, I can highly recommend that you speak to one of our healing center physicians about your desire.

There are a few cornerstones of Bates' work, however, with which you should be familiar and that can help every one to better eye health and functioning.

Fundamentals of Bates Technique—Central Fixation

The basic fundamental of all Bates treatment is to get rid of mental strain, which affects the eyes. This first effort to accomplish this should be directed toward understanding and applying central fixation.

Bates taught that the eye sees accurately only with a very small amount of the retina. This part, known as the macular area, is a small depression in the retina in which large numbers of eye elements are compacted. This area is located on the central axis of the lens and it is at this point only that we see in perfect focus. We have vision from the rest of the retina, but this vision is out of focus and if we try to focus on objects with the periphery of the retina, strain is automatically produced and our vision is adversely affected. Bates stated that proper vision is produced by rapidly moving this macular area to investigate any object we wish to see. Because accurate vision is only possible at this small macular area, by moving the eyeball this spot can be made to fall over the various parts of the object we are investigating. In summing up central fixation, Bates said, "The staring eye is a straining eye. The normal eye is almost never at rest, but is constantly moving and shifting in its effort to properly visualize whatever we wish to see."

Palming

As an aid to relaxation, Bates recommended palming (Fig. 14). The idea was to exclude as much light as possible from the eyes without them being shut. Palming was suggested whenever the patient felt pain or discomfort from the eyes or whenever eyestrain could be sensed. As a part of the palming technique, Bates also recommended that the patient try to visualize black. He believed that by using the memory to envision the color black in front of the eyes, relaxation was produced. He documented many cases in which long-term eye difficulties were corrected almost instantly when the patient was finally able to visualize black.

Shifting

Bates considered rapid eye movement such a natural part of eye health that he designed the technique known as shifting to keep the eye in motion even when reading. During reading you should keep the eye moving from word to word and make no attempt to visualize the entire sentence or paragraph in one gulp[. Normal shifting is almost completely inconspicuous, because it is incredibly rapid and the inability to shift properly produces staring— according to Bates, the first step on the road to refractory problems.

The Long Swing

One of his most satisfactory therapeutic exercises for the eyes is known as the universal or long, swing. It is also sometimes called the elephant swing (Fig. 15). One places the feet about eighteen inches apart and the hands are dropped loosely to the sides. The body is turned at the waist as far to one side as it will go and then slowly back to the other side as far as it will go. The arms are allowed to swing freely during this rotation.

The eyes are at first shut, then gradually opened as the exercise progresses. No effort should be made to see any object. Every attempt

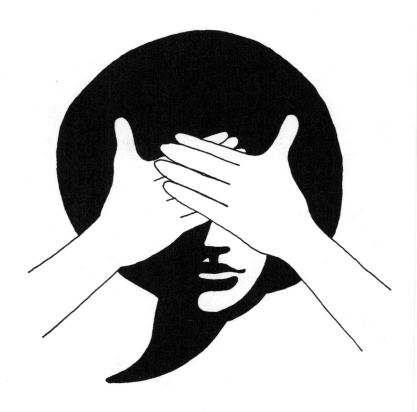

Figure 14

276

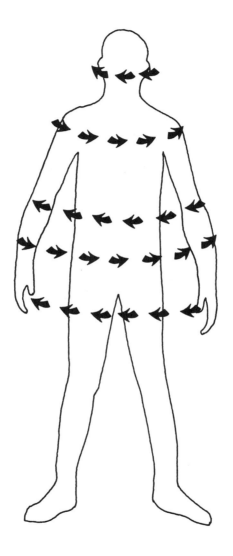

Figure 15

should be made to relax the eyes and facial muscles during the long swing. As this procedure is continued, you will become so relaxed that you feel like sleeping for days. If you can't obtain this degree of relaxation at first, continue the practice until such a state is obtained.

Many other treatment specifics are used in the Bates method, but if your chosen text includes the foregoing, it is undoubtedly authentic.

Maintenance Therapy

One of the difficulties with the Bates method, as with so many other natural treatments, is that it takes time and patient cooperation for best results. Fortunately, such improvement, once obtained, can be fairly easily maintained if the patient trains himself to follow certain simple procedures.

As the patient perseveres with the Bates therapy, he will reach a point at which he can readily detect strain occurring within his ocular apparatus. He must train himself, as he senses this strain, to immediately produce an automatic counter-relaxing action that will correct this build-up.

Although I did my own personal Bates therapy nearly fifty years ago and have not repeated it since, by following this tactic I've been able to keep my eyes free of the myopia I had at that time. In talking to people, there may be times when for a second or two I close my eyes to relax them. I have trained my own protective apparatus in such a way that whenever my eyes feel dry from staring, or strain, they automatically shut and remain shut until this strain passes. This period rarely lasts longer than a few seconds. It has now become so automatic that I am unaware of its action unless it is brought to my attention. After a patient finishes the Bates therapy at our Centers, we take great pains to teach him this type of relaxation. If he learns this method well, his condition will remain stable with little additional effort.

To achieve this relaxation, it isn't sufficient alone to close the eyes, for one can continue to stare after the eyes are closed. All the muscles surrounding the eyes must relax. In our Centers, we teach the patient to relax practically all his face muscles, including those of the lower jaw. Where this is done, not only are the eyes rested, but also many headaches are prevented because tension of the face and neck muscles may cause many of these ailments.

Parting Words

If the Bates method is as useful and practical as I have led you to believe, why isn't it in more general use? Why don't many of the good and honest ophthalmologists investigate and use it if it's of value?

Although I can't speak for others, I can give a small insight into the working of medical authority. To this end, I submit the last two paragraphs of Bates' book, which I think is self-explanatory:

"Between 1886 and 1891 I was a lecturer at the postgraduate hospital and medical school. The head of the institution was Dr. D. B. St. John Rusa. He was the author of many books and was honored and respected by the whole medical profession. At the school they had got the habit of putting glasses on the nearsighted doctors and I had got the habit of curing them without glasses. It was naturally annoying to a man who had put glasses on a student to have him appear at lectures without them and say that Dr. Bates had cured him. Dr. Rusa found it particularly annoying and the trouble reached a climax one evening at the annual banquet of the faculty when in the presence of 150 doctors, he suddenly poured out the viles of his wrath upon my head.

"He said that I was injuring the reputation of the postgraduate by claiming to cure myopia. Everyone knew that Donders said it was incurable. And I had no right to claim that I knew more than Donders. I reminded him that some of the men I had cured had been fitted with glasses by himself. He replied that if he had said they had myopia, he had made a mistake. I suggested further investigation. 'Fit some more doctors with glasses for myopia,' I said, 'And I will cure them. 'It is easy for you to examine them afterward and see if the cure is genuine.' This method did not appeal to him, however, he repeated that it was impossible to cure myopia and to prove that it was impossible, he expelled me from the postgraduate, even the privilege of resignation being denied me.

"The fact is that except in rare cases, man is not a reasoning being. He is dominated by authority and when facts are not in accord with the view imposed by authority, so much the worse for the facts. They may and indeed must win in the long run, but in the meantime the world gropes needlessly in the darkness and endures much suffering that might have been avoided."

Postscript: Of late a new eye operation called *Radial Keratotomy* is gaining some prominence. In this operation, that is designed to correct myopia, incisions are made in the lens of the eye and this is supposed to allow the eye to then focus properly on the retina. Since I have not treated any patients who have had this operation I cannot comment on its effectiveness, though I'm certain that the good Dr. Bates would turn over in his grave if he knew that they were attempting to use surgery to correct something that he was curing one-hundred years ago with some simple non-invasive methods.

Chapter XIX
The Heart and Natural Therapy

When I first started my professional career, I assumed that it would be easy to cure every patient that presented himself at my office door. Perhaps in youth if we didn't have such confidence, we would never begin anything, for surely we don't have the experience yet to really be assured of the success we desire.

Although all patients didn't respond to my natural remedies as well as I had hoped, I did have excellent success with one group to whom the natural remedies seemed particularly well adapted. With the ensuing years, I have greatly refined and expanded my techniques; yet the methods I used with my early patients are practically the same as I use today with only minor variations. This group of patients are those with heart conditions, which respond extremely well to the herbal and nutritional remedies that are a basic part of the armamentaria of our profession.

Of the large variety of heart (cardiac) disorders, many are of such a nature, either because of organic changes or because of the severity of their disorder, that even the best natural remedies have only a minimal effect. Long experience has taught me, however, that most early heart conditions (excluding severe congenital problems) respond well to natural remedies, used either by themselves or in combination with the more orthodox prescribed drugs.

Types of Heart Conditions

Heart conditions can be divided into several specific groups. In youth, the most common of these are the disorders caused by bacterial or viral infections such as those due to scarlet fever, rheumatic fever, diphtheria, and other infectious diseases of childhood that can adversely affect the heart structure. Bacterial endocarditis is an infection of the lining of the heart that stems from a variety of systemic bacterial infections.

Many of these conditions can be kept from injuring the heart if the original infection is treated early by natural means. However, if the infection is bacterial rather than viral, and seems to be overwhelming, it is probably best to use the indicated antibiotic to prevent the spread of the infection. This is one instance in which antibiotics have proven extremely useful, and it is better, I believe, to accept the possible adverse effects of antibiotic therapy than to risk permanent damage to the heart.

When heart damage has occurred, the heart valves are frequently left with little nodules called Vegetations, which may in time calcify.

Though it isn't generally considered possible to remove these vegetations, it is possible with natural herbs to support the muscular structures of the heart so that the general movement of blood is aided and the patients' symptoms are often greatly improved. The degree of such improvement depends on the extent of damage, but I have found that it is a rare patient, indeed, who is not aided by these therapeutic methods.

With the development of blood chelation methods, it is now possible to dissolve some of the calcium crustations on the heart valves that follow these infections. This new treatment can now offer nonsurgical help to patients for whom the outlook was very bleak just a few years ago. (See Chapter 22 on Chelation.)

Muscular Weakness·

One of the most common types of heart disorders—simple muscular weakness—is often missed in its early stages by orthodox medical diagnostic techniques. Most orthodox heart diagnosis has been tailored to detect the character and quality of the more severe disorders and toward this end they have developed many fine sensitive instruments. I have little quarrel with the great advances in this field. However, I find that many patients with mild heart weakness are often ignored or misdiagnosed by general practitioners. There seem to be two reasons for this: first, their methods of detection aren't designed to detect these early muscular disturbances; and second, if they do discover them, the drugs they use are so strong that they must think twice before using them for such a heart problem.

On the other hand, in the natural field we have devoted much time and effort toward discovering chronic ailments in the very earliest stages and then treating them with natural remedies whose actions are mild but thorough, and therefore well adapted to these heart conditions.

Through the use of certain instruments (particularly a phonocardiograph known as the Endocardiograph) and methods, these muscular weaknesses can be detected when the only symptoms are general tiredness and the tendency to become easily exhausted. These symptoms are often attributed to anemia, low blood sugar, or just plain laziness, when in fact the cause may be a mild degree of cardiac muscular insufficiency.

Coronary Problems

When most people think of heart problems, they think of the heart attack, or possibly of the heart pain called angina pectoris. Heart attacks and angina pectoris are related in that they are caused by a disorder of the coronary arteries. The coronary artery is a small artery that branches off the aorta (the large artery emerging from the heart) and supplies the heart muscle itself with blood. Despite what many persons believe, the heart muscle is not able to absorb any of the blood that passes through it. It, like every other organ in the body, must have its own specific blood supply and these small coronary arteries—one on the left and one on the right—supply individual sections of the heart muscle. If these tiny arteries become clogged with cholesterol or perhaps a small blood clot, the blood supply to a section of the heart muscle is stopped, producing a heart attack or coronary occlusion. In angina pectoris, an artery is not completely closed off but is narrowed so that the muscle is able to get some blood but not as much as it needs. If a patient with angina pectoris is under physical or emotional stress, in which the heart needs more oxygen, the artery isn't able to supply it and the heart muscle develops a cramp because of oxygen deficiency. This cramp produces the pain we call angina pectoris. If the patient takes nitroglycerine or another vasodilator, the coronary artery is temporarily dilated, enabling more blood to pass through, thus bringing more oxygen to the heart muscle. The cramp is then overcome and the pain will subside.

Many physicians believe that a narrowing of the coronary artery is not always necessary for angina pains to occur. They hypothesize that in certain persons the artery can be thrown into a nervous spasm that causes the artery to narrow, producing a pain similar as that in angina. This spasm is also relieved by nitroglycerine or similar drugs. These patients are often given tranquilizers and sedatives such as phenobarbital to prevent the spasm from recurring.

Many natural remedies have an effect similar to that of nitroglycerine in helping to dilate the coronary arteries. Their effect, however, is usually slower, though nontoxic, and often more prolonged. In general, such remedies are given to the angina patient to be taken daily. The patient is advised, however, if an attack does occur, to use his nitroglycerine to prevent serious consequences.

The spastic angina symptoms can usually be helped greatly by natural methods, which are aimed at overcoming the overly sensitive nervous system and also by psychologic methods designed to help the patient achieve a more stable nervous system.

Physicians who use the blood chelation method believe that is what will revolutionize the treatment of these patients. They believe the deposits in the coronary arteries can be dissolved by this therapy. Our work has proven to us that this is correct, and many patients now can be saved from an early grave by this treatment.

Nervous Disorders of the Heart

The heart is supplied with a nerve system to control its regular activity. This system is fairly complicated, but it is supplied with various fail-safe mechanisms prepared to take over if the first-line system breaks down. Even so, several nervous problems can affect the heart.

Tachycardia

Tachycardia (rapid heartbeat) can be due to several conditions. General systemic toxicity from infection or from other toxic influences can cause the heart to beat quite rapidly, especially in infections accompanied by a fever.

Tachycardia can also be caused by weakened muscle structure. In this instance, because a smaller amount of blood is ejected from the heart with each beat, the heart must beat more rapidly to keep the necessary volume of blood flowing. Tachycardia may also occur from a variety of mineral imbalances, particularly potassium deficiency.

Tachycardia can also be caused by emotional or psychologic disorders. A condition known as paroxysmal tachycardia is temporary and may be caused by a variety of emotional reactions.

Bradycardia

Most people have experienced spells of rapid heart beat. Slow heartbeat (bradycardia) is less well-known. In bradycardia, the nerve conduction to the heart is such that the heart beats much less than its normal seventy-two a minute. In severe cases, it may beat as slow as thirty-six times a minute. This latter condition occurs in heart block. If the beat is a constant thirty-six a minute, it is usually referred to as complete heart block. Beat rates between forty and fifty-five are found in partial heart block.

In the well-trained athlete, the heart may beat between fifty and sixty times a minute. In the athlete, the heart muscle has been strengthened to such a degree that it is capable of putting out sufficient blood volume at this lower rate. On the other hand, if the average patient has a heartbeat much below sixty beats a minute, there probably is some difficulty with his nerve conduction system.

In the heart is a nerve structure known as the pacemaker, whose job is to send the normal seventy-two-beat-a-minute impulse throughout the heart musculature. If something happens to the pacemaker so that it becomes incapable of sending its signals to the heart, the heart doesn't stop because the good Lord has put into it a separate selfcontained regulating system. This self-contained system, which will continue the heartbeat as long as is necessary without outside nervous influence, causes the heart to beat at approximately half the normal rate—about thirty-six to forty beats a minute. Although such a basal beat is adequate to maintain life, it isn't necessarily to the best interest of the patient to allow such a basal rate to continue long without outside regulation.

Natural remedies have proven successful in initiating adequate nerve irritability in many of these patients so that the heartbeat rate can be increased to near normal. However, in true complete heart block, in which the pacemaker is beyond regeneration, it is perhaps advisable to have one of the new electronic pacemakers installed so that a more normal heartbeat and its attendant normal volume of blood flow can be re-instituted. If this is necessary however, the patient needs to be alerted to the fact that many unscrupulous vendors have been shown to be offering used and otherwise undesirable electronic pacemakers to physicians so feel free to discuss this matter with our surgeon before you agree to such a placement.

Arrhythmias—Heart Irregularities

Heart palpitations usually are imaginary in that only the patient becomes conscious of the heartbeat, for when the heart is examined by a physician, its rhythm is normal and regular. Such instances are quite common during menopause and in the emotional person with a highly sensitive nervous system. Such palpitations, in themselves, are generally innocuous; treatment should be directed to overcoming the underlying physical or psychologic difficulty.

True arrhythmias (heartbeat irregularities) may consist of a regular irregular beat or an irregular irregular beat. Confusing as it may seem, this is exactly what happens. In a regular irregularity the heart may skip every third or fourth beat, actually producing a regular irregular beat. Some hearts, on the other hand, because of the nature of the nerve conductivity, have a completely irregular pattern—the spacing between beats has no discernible rhythm.

Many arrhythmias respond dramatically to natural methods. Some of the more chronic ones may not seem to change rhythm, but the patient usually feels much improved under natural therapy. It seems that while the arrhythmia may not be demonstrably helped, the cardiac musculature is improved and the circulating blood volume per minute is increased, with an increased sense of well-being felt by the patient.

Other heart disorders may occur, but most of them fall into the aforementioned four categories. For instance, the rather common disorder known as congestive heart disease, with its attendant cardiac edema, either of the lungs or the legs, is really nothing more than an advanced form of muscular weakness; this can be helped by the methods that help other muscular weaknesses. In severe congestive heart disease, strong drugs may be required but many times even these can be greatly increased in efficiency by the simultaneous use of natural methods.

The Treatment of Heart Conditions By Natural Therapy

Heart conditions that may be caused by infective agents are usually best treated before the heart is affected. If the recommendations already made about the natural treatment of the various childhood diseases are carried out, one will seldom be distressed with the later aftereffects of heart disease.

Rheumatic Fever

In juvenile rheumatic fever, much care must be taken in handling the young patient and such a condition should never be treated without the aid of a competent physician. Even the mildest case of rheumatic fever can leave a damaged heart if it isn't promptly and properly cared for. The old medical saw that "rheumatic fever licks at the joints but bites the heart," isn't without foundation. In my experience, the most common cause of cardiac muscular weakness has been a mild and sometimes unrecognized rheumatic fever that occurred during the patient's childhood.

The orthodox medical care of rheumatic fever consists of rest and the extended use of antibiotics to keep the infection under control. We have found this method to be generally effective, although it does expose the patient to all the known dangers of long-term antibiotic therapy. These antibiotics can also be augmented with the indicated specific nutritional supplements and herbal therapy. In the patients we have treated, the results have proven very satisfactory.

In caring for the rheumatic child, the physician shouldn't be afraid to demand from the parents adequate rest and the proper dietary regimen for his patient. With even the best of therapies, the heart may be damaged if the diet isn't all it should be or if proper rest is not given at specific vital times in the course of the disease.

When heart damage has occurred, either from untreated or unsatisfactorily treated rheumatic fever, the usual remedies given for general muscular weakness of the heart have proven vital.

Muscular Weakness.

Most of the heart is made up of muscle tissue that, unlike the other muscles of the body, must work constantly from before birth until death.

It is allowed to rest during this period only a small fraction of a second between each beat. Thus, the occurrence of cardiac muscle weakness is easy to understand. Although the vital force of the body will do everything in its power to keep any injury to the heart muscle to a minimum, many toxic substances do injure this muscle and such weakness, especially the mild variety, is common.

Digitalis and its various derivatives are the most common drugs used by the medical profession in treating cardiac muscular weakness. Although digitalis is powerful and has certain toxic and cumulative effects, it is effective and particularly useful in severe cardiac weaknesses.

Owing to digitalis's toxic effects, however, most physicians don't use it in mild cases of cardiac weakness and it is here that the nontoxic heart herbs have a vital place in treatment.

When the heart muscle is weakened and isn't able to exert sufficient pressure to adequately circulate the blood, edema (fluid in tissues) may occur in the feet and legs. This fluid may also accumulate in the lungs owing to a weakness of the right side of the heart, producing cardiac asthma. Edema is usually treated with diuretics (products that stimulate the excretion of urine, thereby eliminating water from the system).

Most of these congestive heart disease patients are treated medically with digitalis (in one form or another), and if needed, diuretics. Digitalis has a mild diuretic effect and in some instances this alone is sufficient. In severe cases, diuretics are also almost always used.

When these disorders are treated naturally, we attempt to substitute a combination of the herbs Cactus Grandiflorus and Crataegus Oxyeantha in place of digitalis. The cactuscrataegus combination is the sovereign heart remedy of the natural physician. It isn't as strong or as rapid as digitalis and won't help in emergencies, but used by itself in mild muscular weaknesses it will do all that digitalis does without the cumulative effect or toxic side effects. Also, cactus-crataegus may be used for an extended period without fear of any possible difficulties. In fact, this combination seems to overcome certain organic difficulties with continued and regular use.

In severe cases of heart muscle weakness in which digitalis and/or diuretics are being used, cactus-crataegus can also be used. Even in these cases, considerable improvement is usually experienced when cactus-crataegus is used in addition to the orthodox therapy. I have never experienced any conflicts from these remedies used together.

From long experience, I believe that the cactus-crataegus combination is not simply a harmless digitalis. Even though it can do the work of digitalis in milder cases, it also has many specific actions entirely of its own that are deep in their workings and far more curative than any of the known orthodox therapies. Of all the herbal medications used in our office, with the possible exception of our EMP, the cactuscrataegus combination is used more than any other. I have never known it to fail to produce improvement in cardiac muscular weakness. It is truly one of the great sovereign remedies of natural healing.

Although the cactus-crataegus combination is the bulwark of our work on heart muscle disorders, other natural herbal remedies and nutritional remedies have proven their effectiveness. Convallaria (lily of the valley) is one of these. The action of convallaria, however, is somewhat different from that of cactus-crataegus. Convallaria increases coronary circulation, promotes more vigorous and regular heart action, corrects dyspnea (difficulty in breathing), and increases urinary activity. Convallaria is indicated in extension of the heart ventricles, in palpitations, in dyspnea due to cardiac asthma, and is helpful in irregular heartbeat. It is a heart tonic. It is of much value too as a diuretic and combines well with other diuretics just as digitalis does. Unlike digitalis, convallaria isn't toxic. It is used, along with cactus-crataegus, where cardiac edema occurs along with the general cardiac muscular weakness.

Other herbs such as pheasants eye (Adonis), Strophanthus, Capsicum and Lobelia, are also used in this type of a heart condition, however, these must be used with great care and only by a physician who is well-trained in the individual characteristics of each of these herbs and in the characteristics they exhibit when combined with our other remedies.

In Chapter 14, we discussed protomorphogens. Theoretically it should be possible to extract a protomorphogen of heart muscle to assist in the strengthening of this organ and such a protomorphogen is produced by several of the manufacturers who supply the natural physician. This protomorphogen is used for almost all our patients with cardiac weakness, and when used in addition to the herbal substances, it helps greatly to speed up cardiac improvement. The heart protomophogen is not a short term option. It must be used for six months to two years to obtain the proper degree of muscle improvement. Any attempt to use it for a shorter period usually results in disappointment both for the patient and the physician.

Our medical division, Woodlands Medical Center, has found that a combination of various natural minerals infused into the blood can have a very beneficial effect in these heart muscle problems. These methods work very well in concert with the natural program outlined above.

288

Angina-like Problems

The usual medical treatment for these disorders, other than some of the newer surgical methods (By-Pass), is nitroglycerine, amyl nitrite and other vasodilating drugs. Although most of these drugs don't have particularly lasting side effects, they are likely to cause headaches and other disorders precipitated by the rather violent blood vessel dilation.

The natural remedies for this condition are milder, more extended in their action and usually successful in all but the most severe disorders. A fraction of the vitamin E compound extracted from pea pods and called vitamin E2 has shown promise in the milder forms of angina.

We usually suggest the use of vitamin E2 immediately at the beginning of any cardiac pain. If the cardiac pain does not diminish rapidly, the patient is requested to use his usual dose of nitroglycerine or other prescribed vasodilator. With this regimen, we make no attempt to deprive the patient of the useful effects of orthodox medicine; rather, we try to help the patient so that such medication becomes less and less necessary by improving his basic condition through natural means.

One remedy we have also found useful in this condition is Pangamic Acid (vitamin B15). Pangamic acid was originally discovered and isolated by Hans A. Krebs, the famous discoverer of the biochemical cycle known as the Krebs cycle. Unfortunately Krebs wasn't very well appreciated by those in authority, and his product, though admittedly harmless and natural, was banned from production by the FDA for some time.

Some years after this action, Russian investigators also produced pangamic acid and hailed it as one of the great discoveries of the century and, in stories issuing from that country, some of their top scientists stated that this boon to aging humanity should be put on every dining room table and should be used as freely as salt or sugar. There were at that time and for all I know, still are, clinics in Russia in which the only therapy used was pangamic acid and very dramatic results were reported in disorders of the aged. (Whether these are now active in the capitalistic Russia is unknown.)

For a while after the Russian disclosures were made, Krebs was allowed to produce this substance for sale in the United States. This was during the period following Sputnik, when we didn't want Russia to outdo us in any scientific endeavor. As soon as the furor over the Russian discoveries subsided, however, the FDA again lowered the boom on the production of pangamic acid. Recently, however, the Russian formula has become available in the U.S. and we are now back to using the remedy in our heart cases. It is not known as B15 however.

Of course, one of the best and at times most dramatic treatments for this condition is intravenous Chelation. While this method is still debated in the medical community our physicians at the Woodlands Medical Center have helped thousands of these patients to better health.

Heart Irregularities

For the various arrhythmias that beset the nerve conduction apparatus of the heart, the most commonly used medical drug is quinidine, a derivative of quinine. Although its action is not entirely understood, as is true of many allopathic drugs, quinidine is useful in stabilizing cardiac arrhythmias. This isn't always true, however; in my own experience, some arrhythmias have been aggravated by this and other quinine derivatives.

At the present time newer and more effective drugs have been developed. The so called Beta Blockers are being used to settle some of these arrhythmias.

In the natural field, we generally treat arrhythmias with the cardiac herbs already mentioned and through the use of specific extracts and combinations of the B complex vitamins. Some functional arrhythmias seem to be due to specific B complex vitamin deficiencies. In fact, cardiac arrhythmias are an integral part of beriberi (B. deficiency) and other frank B complex deficiency diseases.

Mineral Imbalance

Attention to the electrolyte structures of the body (the fluid compounds of the body, containing such minerals as calcium, sodium, magnesium, and potassium) may be important in overcoming functional cardiac arrhythmias. In persistent arrhythmias for which no pathologic condition can be found, we recommend that a blood test and a hair test be done to check the body mineral balance. Most of these patients can be helped once the physician is aware of the specific balance of the minerals in the body.

Severe pathologic arrhythmias are often helped by general cardiac treatment through natural means. The combination of cactus-crataegus, convallaria, heart protomorphagens, vitamin E, vitamin B complex, vitamin C, and other factors has been known to help even the most severe organic arrhythmias, although we never promise a complete cure to these patients. Nor do we suggest that the patient discontinue his orthodox therapy unless through careful investigation and testing, we are sure that such therapy has nothing to offer him at the time.

Diuretics

In treating congestive heart disease, diuretics are often necessary to keep fluid from collecting in the various dependent parts of the body. Such fluid, which collects because of the inability of the heart to keep the blood properly circulating, causes additional strain on the vascular system, further weakening the heart if the fluid isn't removed.

To accomplish this, diuretics are given. Since the drugs used for this purpose are essential in many cases, they usually have toxic side effects so, wherever possible, we try to substitute natural non-toxic remedies.

Since the effect of the fluid build-up in the body is usually far more dangerous than the toxic effects of the diuretic, the physician of natural therapy is justified in taking a patient off diuretics only if he is absolutely sure that his natural methods will produce an equal or superior degree of fluid removal. If this can't be done, he must never remove the medical diuretic.

Some natural diuretics often prove more useful in specific instances than the drug diuretics. In general, however, the natural compounds are much milder and may not be as vigorous as the situation demands. A combination of a small dose of a drug diuretic combined with a natural diuretic is often as good as or better than a larger dose of the drug diuretic alone and this combination results in less toxicity and fewer side effects than the drug alone. If you are on diuretics or feel that you may need one, feel free to discuss this matter with your Center physician. You can be certain that he will guide you to the best combination for your needs.

The Pros and Cons of Vitamin E

I am fully aware of the work of the Shute brothers of Canada regarding vitamin E and heart diseases. Even though I use vitamin E on almost all my heart cases, I believe that although this vitamin is helpful, it is nowhere near as specific as the herbal remedies. I have never noticed sufficient success with vitamin E alone to use it as a single therapy for heart conditions. This is not meant to dissuade heart patients from the use of vitamin E. I suggest, however, that this vitamin should not be expected to correct heart disorders that are better treated with other natural remedies. Vitamin E must be used with caution in those with high blood pressure because it will raise some pressures.

Office Treatment of Cardiac Conditions

In general, the various office therapies so useful in many acute and chronic conditions have not proven of great value in cardiac disorders. Over the years we have used various forms of diathermies, diapulses, Magnatherms and others modalities for anginas and muscular weak-

291

nesses. Although I find them useful in specific cases, there have also been just as many cases in which the condition seemed to become aggravated by the use of these therapies. Therefore, such office methods are used by us with great care and discretion in all cardiac disorders.

In counter distinction to these various modalities, we have found that massage, chiropractic, and nerve-relaxing manipulative therapies are useful in the cardiac disorders. However, our treatment of these patients is usually much milder than for the general run of patients.

Homeopathy

The homeopathic method is useful in almost all cardiac disorders. I have found these remedies most helpful in treating the residual symptoms that may occur after the basic problems are controlled by the herbal and nutritional approach. This is particularly true now that we have instituted our new computerized search for the most effective Homeopathic remedy.

Early Diagnosis of Cardiac Conditions

Because heart disorders respond best to natural therapeutic methods in their earliest stages, the physician who practices this method should diagnose the disorder as soon as possible. To this end, the natural therapist has made extensive use of two instruments whose principles are accepted by the orthodox profession but are little used in medical practice. These are the Phonocardiograph (generally known by the trade name Endocardiograph) and the Cameron Heartometer, which records on a circular graph a tracing of the pulse beat from the brachial or femoral arteries.

The phonocardiograph charts the heart sounds by the use of a small sensitive microphone placed over the four cardiac valve areas that are usually listened to by physicians with their stethoscopes. The sounds produced at these areas give us much information about the rhythm and the muscular integrity of the heart. Unfortunately, the human ear has limited sensitivity, and it isn't possible for small minute changes in duration or rhythm to be readily picked up during normal stethoscopic examination. When the phonocardiograph is used, however, these heart sounds are graphed by a stylus on a piece of rapidly moving waxed ribbon, and the cardiac sounds are thus indelibly recorded so they can be carefully examined at the physician's leisure.

With the use of the Heartometer, the various arrhythmic or muscular disorders can be detected because of the graph alterations of the pulse wave (by the pulse wave we mean the variation in the pressure produced in the artery by the muscular contraction, or beat, of the heart).

[This information on the **Cameron Heartometer** has been left in this edition of *It's Only Natural* for historic reasons only. This company is no longer in business and so the needed supplies for this instrument are not now available.]

It is possible to detect muscular and arrhythmic difficulties in very early stages of development with both these instruments.

The electrocardiograph, which is generally used by the orthodox practitioner and which is also used in conjunction with the foregoing instruments by natural physicians, operates by graphing changes in the electrical potential or nervous supply to the heart. Such an instrument is of inestimable value in arrhythmias and after specific cardiac disorders, particularly cardiac arrest (heart attack).

In early muscular weakness, however, often no alterations in the electrocardiographic pattern appear, and if one of these hearts is tested in the orthodox manner, no problem or disease may be found. Thus, the wise natural physician uses all three instruments. For the very earliest discovery of muscular weakness, the phonocardiograph is probably the most effective.

By the use of these cardiac instruments, it is possible for the natural physician to begin therapy of heart disorders long before his orthodox compatriot will be able to offer help. Not only are we able to detect disorders earlier by these means, but also because of the basic nontoxic nature of our remedies, we are able to prescribe the indicated therapy at a time when the stronger allopathic medicines would be entirely inappropriate. Digitalis, for instance, would be far too toxic to prescribe in very early myocardial weakness and most orthodox physicians, even if they were able to detect this weakness, probably wouldn't prescribe digitalis because its adverse effects would outweigh any benefit gained. On the other hand, the cactus-crataegus combination may be used from the earliest stages of cardiac muscle weakness and we find that nothing but benefit can be derived from such prompt administration.

In some patients, even an early diagnosis by the phonocardiograph is difficult. These patients may present many of the symptoms of cardiac muscular weakness even though such a condition can't be demonstrated by any diagnostic procedure developed at this time. In these instances, I usually prescribe cactus-crataegus therapy for one month. If the patient's symptoms are caused by a mild cardiac problem, they will usually experience great improvement in this trial period; if such improvement occurs, the herbal remedy can be continued as long as deemed necessary.

293

However, if during this period the patient experiences no improvement, either subjectively or objectively, the herbal medication is discontinued and other causes for the symptoms are sought.

Parting Words

In summarizing this chapter, I want to emphasize that natural therapeutic methods are well-adapted to many cardiac problems. In fact, there is almost no type of cardiac condition that can't be helped in some degree by properly selected natural remedies. The relatively mild disorders can usually be completely controlled by the use of these agents. The severe disorders may require the concomitant use of orthodox drugs, but their improvement can still be hastened by the natural remedies. Even terminal disorders have often been staid, at least temporarily, by these natural methods.

Chapter XX
Hyperlipidemia:
You and Your Blood Vessels

The word Hyperlipidemia may be new to many of my readers. Almost everyone, however, has heard of cholesterol and its relationship to heart disease, hardening of the arteries, and a variety of other chronic diseases.

Investigation has shown that not only cholesterol, but also another group of fatty substances—the triglycerides—play an important part in these ailments. Hyperlipidemia may be an elevation of cholesterol, triglycerides or both, and it manifests itself in one of five types of primary lipid metabolic disorders, caused either by an overproduction or deficient removal of cholesterol and/or triglycerides. (These types are no longer used as much as they were twenty years ago when this was first written, but the basic principles are still the same.)

We now realize that what we thought was originally one condition is actually one of five different primary conditions. As if this were not enough, it is also possible that the elevation of the blood fats (hyperlipidemia) may also be a secondary manifestation of some other disease, the clinical findings of which may be subtle or even absent. This could occur with such diseases as diabetes, hypothyroidism, nephrosis, biliary obstruction, glycogen storage disease, dysproteinemia and acute pancreatitis, and it may even be associated with other metabolic dysfunctions such as impaired glucose tolerance, hyperinsulinemia and hyperuricemia.

Thus, the condition that was previously treated by simply putting a patient on a low-cholesterol diet has now proved to be very complicated, but it is one that can be diagnosed and properly treated by modern scientific methods. Hyperlipidemia has been called the most endemic disease in America today, and it is undoubtedly the number one cause of death in this country.

Unlike most of the other treatments discussed in this book, this information on hyperlipidemia is in no way unique to our Healing Centers, but it is included here for two reasons. First, we consider such information vitally important to a large percentage of our patients. Second, simple clarified information on hyperlipidemia hasn't yet been made generally available to the public.

To determine if a patient is hyperlipidemic, we make it routine to run cholesterol and triglyceride tests and electrophoretic phenotyping on all patients in whom we suspect some form of fatty metabolic disorder. We also run these tests on all patients over forty who present themselves for a general physical examination, because it is impossible to determine by symptoms alone which patients are hyperlipidemic. Time and again, I have run such tests on husband and wife because he wouldn't have it unless she did, only to find that the presumably healthy wife had hyperlipidemia, whereas the great concern for her husband was unfounded.

Owing to the growing interest in this condition among physicians generally, the costs of such tests have come down considerably in the last year and can now be given to almost every patient at moderate expense.

If the patient has elevated blood cholesterol or triglyceride levels, but isn't one of the five primary phenotypes of hyperlipidemia, the physician must search for possible primary diseases that may be causing secondary hyperlipidemia. When any one of these primary diseases is found, its proper treatment should correct the blood lipid levels.

It is interesting to note in this connection that impairment of the glucose tolerance level is often present in phenotypes 3, 4, and 5, and some authorities suggest that a standard oral glucose tolerance test should be done in every subject with hyperlipidemia, regardless of the type suspected. Often hyperinsulinemia (overproduction of insulin) may be present with decreased glucose tolerance. When hyperinsulinemia is present, the physician must be careful to avoid drugs that adversely affect glucose metabolism. Prime examples of these drugs are thiazide diuretics.

Many authorities recommend that thiazide diuretics be avoided in the patient with elevated blood lipids. Unfortunately, many patients with elevated blood lipids also have high blood pressure and one of the most common groups of prescribed drugs for high blood pressure is the thiazide diuretics. Many authorities have noted that blood uric acid levels are often elevated in patients with elevated triglyceride levels and so a uric acid test should be run on each patient with hyperlipidemia. Interestingly, thiazide diuretics also tend to increase the uric acid level and therefore in another instance may again increase the problems of hyperlipidemia.

Although a relation between gallstones and hyperlipidemia hasn't been established, many authorities suggest there is a high frequency of these two conditions occurring concomitantly, therefore making it advisable to check patients who have elevated blood lipid levels for gallstones.

The treatments of most of the primary hyperlipidemias are centered around dietary restrictions. Some drugs are available, but most are toxic and are prescribed even by the most conservative physicians only after dietary restrictions have obviously failed.

The specific dietary recommendations for each of the five different primary types of hyperlipidemia differ from each of the others. Therefore, any form of dietary suggestion can only be given after a patient has been thoroughly examined and the proper electrophoretic tests given. Any attempt to treat hyperlipidemia without full and complete diagnostic measures is useless.

With the recent knowledge of fat metabolism and its effects on the body, it is now theoretically possible to stem the rising incidence of cardiovascular deaths. Our main objective now is one of testing as many of our patients as possible so we can detect the specific type of lipid disorder and take corrective measures early in disease to prevent disastrous future events.

The above was written over twenty years ago and while many new ideas about this condition have come and gone most of what we wrote then is still germane today.

However, to bring this subject up-to-date, we also include here the following paper prepared on this subject by Dr. William Kracht, D.O. one of our most dedicated and knowledgable physicians.

Diet, Life-style, and Nutritional Supplements For Your Heart and Blood Vessels

The cause of atherosclerosis, or plaque formation on the blood vessel walls, is not limited to just one factor. Genetics indeed play a role, but this inheritance factor can be modified by our diet, lifestyle and behavior. Heavy metal accumulation in the body's tissues (iron, lead, mercury and cadmium) can promote this plaque formation. Food allergies can damage the lining of the artery wall. Chlorine and fluoride may also play a role in this process. Low levels of antioxidants in the body combined with elevated "free radical" molecules can change the cholesterol and fats in the body to "more aggressive floggers." Partially hydrogenated fats found in processed foods and oils are not metabolized in the body and thus become stuck in our cell walls and act to block normal cellular metabolism. High sugar, high fat and low fiber in our typical American diets are known to accelerate this plaque formation. Lastly, tobacco use, alcohol consumption combined with a sedentary lifestyle and the stresses of modern life promote the development of heart and blood vessel disease seen today. The following is a brief outline covering diet, lifestyle and nutritional supplements important in preventing and treating heart and vascular disease.

Diet

The best diet to lower your blood cholesterol and fats and help protect the heart and blood vessels from "clogging" is a high complex carbohydrate, high fiber, low fat diet with the addition of vegetables for trace minerals and certain other beneficial foods and supplements. Cholesterol actually plays a small part in this big picture. The amount of cholesterol in our food accounts for only 10%-20% of the body's total cholesterol. The remaining 80-90% is manufactured by the liver and intestines from fats, proteins and certain forms of carbohydrates (starch) in your diet. Thus, the goal is to decrease the "bad" fats, sugars and proteins that lead to cholesterol synthesis and substitute better foods for your heart and blood vessels. The following guidelines are given as an addition and emphasis to the Basic Maintenance Diet (see Appendix B)

High Complex Carbohydrates

Eat no simple sugars. Avoid foods and beverages that have sugar listed as one of the first three ingredients. These include cakes, candies, ice cream, certain cereals, Jell-O, ketchup, etc. Remember all excess sugar is converted into fat. Sugar may play a larger role in heart and blood vessel blockage than cholesterol.

Use no white flour or products that contain white flour.

Raw unfiltered honey, unsulphured black strap molasses, pure maple syrup and date sugar may be used in small amounts as acceptable sweeteners.

Follow the recommendations on high complex carbohydrates in the Basic Health Maintenance Diet.

High Fiber

Oats (oatmeal, oat bran) and legumes (dried beans, peas and lentils) are the best whole food fiber foods to lower cholesterol.

Flax fiber and psyllium are good fiber sources. The least expensive method is to buy whole flax seeds (store them in the freezer) and grind two tablespoons in a blender for 15-30 seconds and then use the powder to your desire. You also gain the benefit of the good oils (essential fatty acids) from the flax seed in addition to its fiber benefit. If psyllium is used, one teaspoon three times per day (One tablespoon per day total) of the pure powder is recommended.

Oat bran, 3-4 tablespoons per day may be supplemented to the diet to give 15-20 grams of nutritional dietary fiber. It can be stirred into juice, water or added to cereal or baked into baked goods.

Low Saturated Fat

Pay particular attention to the section of "Fats" in the Basic Maintenance Diet. Avoid fried food as the devil avoids holy water.

Olive oil is the best oil for lowering cholesterol. If you like sardines or tuna, try to obtain these packed in olive oil. Make your own salad dressing with olive oil. Buy extra virgin.

No hydrogenated vegetable oils. This includes margarine. Again, a little butter may be better than margarine but try to use olive oil any time you want to use butter or margarine.

Keep fatty meats to a minimum, instead substitute cold water fish that have the "good" fish fats: haddock, salmon, sardines, mackerel, herring, flounder. Fish with lowest levels of mercury include pollack, salmon, bass, sole, cod, haddock, flounder and shellfish

Cholesterol

The most important aspect of cholesterol in foods to understand is the fact that cholesterol is changed when exposed to high temperatures (it becomes oxidized) making it even more likely to cause "clogging" of the blood vessels, thus adding fuel to the fire. When it comes to honestly viewing cholesterol, it is the oxidized form that really causes problems. The best way to understand oxidation is to look at rust. Rust results from metal that has become oxidized. The same process happens to our body's tissues when internal oxidation occurs. Again, avoiding fried foods is one of the best ways to prevent this internal oxidation.

Eggs in moderation are all right occasionally providing you are following the rest of this diet. You may poach, softboil, or lightly scramble (low heat) but don't hard-boil or fry (again, this causes oxidation). Egg Beaters are not recommended as they have partially hydrogenated fatty oils and a higher content of oxidized cholesterol!

Beverages

Avoid tap water that contains chlorine and fluoride. Chlorine may cause blood vessel wall damage and fluoride is toxic to nervous tissue. Use bottled spring water preferably in glass.

Avoid coffee, black tea and cola. If you choose decaffeinated coffee, be sure to obtain water processed and not chemical processed decaffeinated brands (Sanka and Brim). Herbal teas (especially ginger) are preferable as are coffee substitutes such as Postum and Pero.

Avoid alcohol. It is high in sugar and increases the risk of heart disease. The only exception may be small amounts (One glass or less per day) of red wine. However, wine contains sulfites and pesticide residues and this should be taken into consideration. Try naturally sparkling spring water with lemon or lime as your social drink

Miscellaneous Foods to Help Lower Your Risk of Heart Disease

Use ginger, garlic and onions liberally. These foods can help lower cholesterol levels and decrease the stickiness of platelets thus decreasing the possibility of blood clots. Garlic can also raise HDL levels. Garlic and onion have the additional benefit of helping the liver's detoxification ability.

Grapefruit has been shown to be very effective in lowering blood cholesterol levels, probably from its fiber content.

Soybeans (topic) and other vegetable protein in place of meats and dairy products. Soy has very low fat and has been found to lower cholesterol levels.

Alfalfa sprouts—Have been shown to regress blood vessel plaques in monkeys. Make liberal use of sprouts.

Cultured milk products—yogurt, kefir, buttermilk

Pineapple, chickpeas (humus), eggplant are all able to help lower blood cholesterol levels.

Use ginger and cayenne pepper as spices instead of salt.

Lifestyle and Behavior Modifications

Discontinue all uses of Tobacco products. Tobacco products are probably the number one cause of heart disease and blood vessel clogging. Statistical evidence reveals a mean increase of about 70% in the death rate and a 3-5 fold increase in the risk of heart artery disease in smokers compared to non smokers. No program can be assured of success while continuing the use of tobacco products. If you are undergoing chelation, tobacco products are capable of completely defeating the action of EDTA due to the release of killer free radicals. Tobacco is admittedly one of the most addictive substances commonly used. If discontinuing tobacco products is difficult for you, please let us know so that we may help establish a cessation program for you.

Exercise

Exercise is protective against heart disease. Exercise is also one of the few tools we have for raising the good HDL cholesterol in the blood. A carefully graded, progressive, aerobic exercise program is a necessity.

The best program to start is simply walking. Start slowly if you have not been exercising and slowly increase the amount of time to 30 to 60 minutes 3-5 days per week. If possible, try to reach a pace of 15 minutes per mile. Although not really aerobic exercise, Tai Chi can also be added for muscle stretching and motion. If you are over 50 or have known heart or vascular disease, do not start an exercise program before talking to your Center doctor.

Stress Management Techniques

Stress Management Techniques are an integral part of a heart and blood vessel program. Dr. Dean Ornish found it to be of utmost importance to his success in treating heart disease but also the most difficult for his patients to follow. Autogenic training is the word we like to use to describe stress management techniques. The stress response in the body has been shown to raise cholesterol levels, raise blood pressure, and cause spasm of the blood vessels in the heart. This is quite evident as more heart attacks occur Monday mornings than any other day of the week. At our Healing Centers, we have available autogenic training tapes and other self biofeedback exercises that can be done in the comfort and privacy of your own home. These tapes and stress management techniques are inexpensive and essential in preventing the progression of many types of medical conditions, and moreover, are essential in helping to reverse them.

Supplements

The following briefly discusses some of the more common nutritional and herbal substances that may be beneficial in heart and vascular diseases. Your Center doctor will outline a program to meet your individual needs.

Vitamin C—Helps to prevent the accumulation of cholesterol plaques on the blood vessel walls. It also helps repair tiny "cracks" in the blood vessel walls that act as a nidus for blood clot formation. It also functions as one of the body's chief antioxidants. Recommended doses range from 1000-6000 mg. Per day.

Vitamin E—Another antioxidant—prevents platelet stickiness and may increase good HDL levels. Recommended doses range from 200-1200 IU/day.

Antioxidant Formula—A balanced antioxidant formula that combines both vitamins, minerals and plant substances that act as potent antioxidants and free radical scavengers is recommended.

Magnesium—is probably the most important mineral in heart and blood vessel disease. It is nature's "calcium channel blocker" and helps relax tense vessels and muscles and promotes proper function of the heart and blood vessel cells. Recommended doses range from 300-1000 mg. a day. The glycinate, malate and citrate forms appear to be the best absorbed and utilized.

Calcium, Zinc, Copper, Chromium and Selenium—are all other trace minerals essential to help lower blood fat levels and promote normal functioning of the heart and blood vessel cells. A balanced high potency trace mineral supplement in recommended.

Vitamin B6 and Folic Acid—are important if the homocysteine levels in the blood or urine are elevated. Elevated homocysteine levels have been demonstrated as a risk factor for vascular disease.

Niacin—in the form of "inositol hexaniacinate" is a very effective cholesterol lowering nutrient. It also elevates good HDL and also lowers triglycerides. Dosages range from 300-1,800 mg. a day.

Carnitine (or Acetyl L-Carnitine)—is a type of molecule that is synthesized from the amino acid lysine and functions to helps the heart muscles to utilize oxygen from the blood. Doses up to one gram a day may be used.

Lecithin granules (from soybean)—Helps lower cholesterol and free fats (triglycerides) and may increase HDL levels. Doses of 1-2 tablespoons per day are recommended.

Pantethine—is especially helpful for elevated cholesterol levels and angina symptoms. Doses range from 300-1200 mg. a day.

Essential Fatty Acids—At this time we recommend flax seed oil for your essential fatty acid supplementation. Doses range from 1-2 tablespoons per day. Keep the bottle in the refrigerator and use it within one month's time from opening. One may also use fish oil capsules but there is a recent concern over their mercury content. Doses for the fish oil capsules (Max EPA) are 1-2 pills three times per day with meals or one may use Cod liver oil, one tablespoon per day; it is cheaper than fish oil capsules. You may want to alternate the flaxseed oil and cod liver oils every other day.

Be sure to buy small bottles, add 800 IU of Vitamin E oil (it acts as a preservative) and keep them in the refrigerator.

Gugulipid—is the extract from the mukul myrrh tree native to India and demonstrates significant cholesterol and triglyceride lowering effects and without side effects.

Ginkgo Biloba—is an extract from the ginkgo tree leaves and has been shown to promote blood flow, especially in the brain. It is also a very potent antioxidant.

Coenzyme Q-10—is a substance demonstrated to promote normal heart function and may be helpful in heart failure and angina.

Crataegus and Cactus—are other plant remedies that demonstrate favorable effects upon the heart and blood vessels.

Thus we have for you some of the most up-to-date information to help you prevent a build up in the blood vessels of placque, America's most serious killer. Let me implore you however to not attempt to treat yourself for this problem. The information is constantly changing and it is the responsibility of our Center physician to keep abreast of all that is new. Let him (or her) guide you in this field especially, since the path to cleaner blood vessels is fraught with many unseen dangers.

Summary

Of all the chapters in this book, this could be one of the most important to your own life. I want to emphasize one simple message: If you are in middle life, and have not had a complete lipid profile you may be in danger. Let your Center physician know that you want this test.

Chapter XXI
Arthritis—Fact And Fancy

By far the most common chronic disease in America is arthritis. It seems that every few weeks someone publishes a book guaranteeing to eliminate this scourge of middle and old age, but unfortunately we have more arthritis with us than ever before. Thus, either no one reads or follows the advice given in these books or the methods recommended don't work. My money is on the latter.

There are at least three common (and many not so well known ones) disorders called arthritis and each is a separate and distinct disease entity in and of itself. These are osteo arthritis (hypertrophic arthritis), rheumatoid arthritis, and gouty arthritis.

When the single word arthritis is used by most lay people, hypertrophic arthritis is usually being referred to. This type of arthritis generally afflicts those from middle age on and is characterized by a build-up of calcium deposits in and around the bony surfaces within a joint. In its most extreme form, osteoarthritis may be called crippling arthritis, although this name is not really appropriate and tends to cause more fear than elucidation in the mind of the patient.

Osteoarthritis

Osteoarthritis is a cold, stiff condition. The joints are difficult to move, but they usually aren't hot or inflammatory. Osteoarthritic joints usually improve by movement but stiffen with rest.

Rheumatoid Arthritis

In many ways, rheumatoid arthritis is the exact opposite of osteoarthritis. Rheumatoid arthritis generally attacks people in their 30 s or early 40's, though it sometimes waits until the 50's before it rears its ugly head. This type of arthritis is inflammatory—that is, the joints are usually swollen, reddened, hot and very painful if any attempt is made to move them. The pain and swelling usually appear in attacks or spells. Certain joints may appear fairly normal for some time, only to suddenly swell and become very sore and inflamed. This may last for some time and then the inflammation dies down. The joint, though never quite normal again, at least becomes usable for a while.

The underlying basic nature of rheumatoid arthritis is not fully understood and although the anti-inflammatory sterols such as prednisone are able to relieve the attacks, they are not curative. In time their use precipitates more degeneration than if the patient had remained untreated with them. Rheumatoid arthritis does respond moderately to salicylates; thus the most knowledgeable and conscientious physicians usually recommend aspirin or aspirin-like compounds rather than the sterols if the patient can be controlled by these nonsterol compounds.

In general, the inflamed joint of rheumatoid arthritis should be rested; any attempt to exercise the joint when it is swollen usually results in further aggravation of the problem. Such a reaction is directly counter to that of osteoarthritis. In rheumatoid arthritis, usually only a small amount of calcium is deposited in the joint, the basic lesion being one of degeneration or deterioration of the joint material. The calcium deposition is probably due to an attempt by the body at repair.

Rheumatoid arthritis is so entirely different from osteoarthritis that an entirely different name should be found for it. Even though the physician understands the character of these two conditions, arthritis is arthritis to a lay person, and very few are able to readily distinguish between osteo and rheumatoid. Because there is probably no chronic condition in which self-treatment is so prevalent as arthritis, and because the therapy for rheumatoid arthritis is considerably different from that for osteoarthritis, we feel the medical community should attempt either to rename rheumatoid arthritis or to make sure that the distinction between it and osteoarthritis is completely understood by each patient and the general public as well.

Gouty Arthritis

Gouty arthritis is the least frequent of the three, but it seems to be on the increase in recent years. In the early days of my career, I assumed that gout was confined to the aristocracy of the Middle Ages and, like the plague, died with this feudal time. The truth is that gout is more prevalent today than at any other time in history.

We have all seen pictures of the captain in the Katzenjammer Kids sitting with his foot swathed in bandages, as he endures his gouty attack. As I remember, my hero, Benjamin Franklin was also, occasionally, laid up with this malady. Although the joint of the great toe is one of the most common areas for gout to manifest, it is possible for this rather ambiguous condition to cause distress in almost any joint. It is an axiom in our Centers to suspect "hidden gout" whenever any painful condition of the bony frame does not respond to treatment within a reasonable time.

Gout can usually be diagnosed from elevations in the blood uric acid levels, although only a slight elevation of the uric acid may cause widespread problems in selected individuals. Some patients present all the symptoms of gout but do not show an elevated blood uric acid. We usually place these patients on temporary gout therapy. If improvement takes place, we consider it to be an instance of occult (hidden) gout.

In former days, kings and other royalty became gouty from an over-use of red meats, wines, liquors and an insufficient supply of fresh leafy vegetables. The poor of those times couldn't afford such a lavish diet and were thus inadvertently spared by their poverty from this painful affliction. In our day, almost everyone can afford a fare that often causes gout in susceptible persons. Gout has now become most democratic and is ready and willing to afflict even the most humble. It is undoubtedly because of our affluence that gout has become so common—a disorder that every doctor must consider in a person who complains of skeletal aches and pains.

Treatment of Osteoarthritis

Most books for the public on arthritis discuss osteoarthritis, which can be easily treated in mild cases, but which becomes almost impossible to help in severe cases. Its symptoms may range from mild stiffness of the fingers, occurring in the morning, to crippling so severe that the patient is practically incapable of moving. Osteoarthritis can be responsible for both of these extremes and anything in between.

I dislike using the word arthritis for the milder forms of this disease. If one of my patients at some time has encountered a person with severe osteoarthritis, the term would be enough to strike fear into his heart, which could only worsen the condition. Thus, we usually refer to mild osteoarthritis as minor calcium deposits or simple joint stiffness, which in truth is what it is.

In its milder forms, this disorder is usually easily treated, particularly when it is restricted to a few peripheral joints. The patient is placed on a special diet and ultrasound is used through the affected areas. When the areas to be treated are small, like the hand or foot, we usually sound under water; otherwise we use a cream between the sound head and the patient's skin. Three to ten treatments are usually necessary to bring this type of arthritis under control; only rarely is more energetic treatment needed.

Recently we have added the Low Level Laser Therapy to all our arthritic therapy with mind blowing effect in some patients. Frequently, almost immediate pain relief is experienced by some patients. In many instances the pain of the arthritis is relieved before the end of the three to four minute treatment. While the pain may return, we have seen many cases where just one treatment has lasted for many weeks.

When the osteoarthritis is more general, it is necessary for a whole-body-regeneration plan to be instituted. The patient is first placed on a collagen disease diet. Manipulative therapy diathermy and **Magnatherm** treatment are given as thought appropriate. Ultrasound treatments are given to the worst offending joints. Nutritional supplementation is used after thorough testing for nutritional deficiencies has been completed. Water and fruit juice fasts are used in selected cases. And now of course the **MicroLight 830 LLLT** is added to this therapy and the results are much better than ever before.

In general, our treatment of osteoarthritis is effective but undramatic. We don't use a magic wand to overcome this extensive condition, but with the best natural therapeutic methods we can bring great relief to most of our patients.

This last paragraph was written many years before the LLLT. I left it in this edition because of the words "magic wand." If there ever was a magic wand the LLLT is it. (It even looks like a magic wand.) This little wonder is revolutionizing the way we treat arthritis. We can only view with great anticipation what will come now as others attempt to better the work of the Danish firm that developed this therapy.

Vinegar and Honey

A popular folk remedy for osteoarthritis is apple-cider vinegar and honey. Dr. D.C. Jarvis, who popularized this treatment, stated that it supplies potassium in a form that is usable by the body. In his experience, this potassium tends to correct the chemical imbalances causing, or at least aggravating, this type of arthritis.

Many of our patients have insisted that their condition has been improved by using cider vinegar and honey. I can't deny these assertions, though I don't think the acetic acid present in the vinegar is beneficial on a long-term basis.

I believe that much of the benefit attributed to this combination results from the acidity produced by the cider vinegar in some of the body tissues. It can be shown that calcium won't be deposited in an acid medium. Because the joints are normally acid in reaction, calcium should not be deposited there. Many authors have thus postulated that calcium can be deposited in arthritic joints because for some reason or other these joints have become alkaline in reaction. Therefore the improvements reported by those who use the vinegar-and-honey method may result from acidification of the articular areas by this combination.

We use another acid called orthophosphoric acid, which is extracted from wheat bran for this purpose. The advantage of orthophosphoric acid is that it is a food factor, natural to the body, and therefore is less toxic than cider vinegar.

Calcium and Arthritis

Most of my patients are completely confused about the relationship between calcium and osteoarthritis. Some authors insist that because osteoarthritis is a condition in which calcium is deposited in the joints, the patient has too much calcium and should avoid all foods containing it. Other authorities suggest that it is the mishandling of calcium by the body that causes the problem and that the osteoarthritic needs more calcium. These authorities recommend large amounts of bone meal to help the arthritic condition. There is some validity in both opinions, though the dogmatic and unknowledgeable following of either could lead to disastrous results.

Paradoxically, in osteoarthritis, the bones lose calcium at the same time it is being deposited in the joints, apparently because of an imbalance in the hormonal and enzymatic systems. Unless the management of these are taken into account, calcium can be injurious to osteo arthritis patients.

I don't recommend that people older than forty take bone meal, except when provided in a form that supplies the various enzyme factors necessary for its proper metabolism and assimilation. For most of these patients we suggest one of the alkaline calciums such as calcium lactate, calcium gluconate, or egg-shell compounds. If a bone-type calcium is desired, and often one with adequate enzymes can be useful in treating some cases of osteoarthritis, we suggest those that contain the necessary enzymes needed for calcium metabolism.

Diet and Arthritis

Many diets have been suggested over the years for osteoarthritis. In my experience the collagen diet given in the appendix of this book has proven the most useful for our patients. It isn't as restricted as most, but it does take a certain amount of diligence and resignation on the part of the patient to follow it correctly. If the patient is faithful, results are sure to follow, and it is a rare patient whose arthritis doesn't improve while on this diet.

If one of our patients does not fare well on the regular arthritis diet we may try to eliminate the night shade plants (peppers, tomatoes, egg plant and potatoes). This will often make dramatic improvement in those arthritic patients who are sensitive to these foods.

Diet and Fasting

One of the most successful forms of therapy used in our Centers for osteoarthritis is the water fast. Almost no other condition responds so well to the fast as does osteoarthritis, particularly if the patient happens to be one of those full fleshed persons so commonly afflicted with this disease. The loss of weight resulting from the fast usually proves most advantageous to their general health.

Emotional Attitude and Arthritis

Some authors believe the emotional attitude or nature of a person has a great deal to do with his arthritis. Although I have noticed such a relationship in some of my patients, I can't agree that it is a common cause of osteoarthritis. However, I make every effort to encourage my patients to establish as positive and happy an emotional outlook as conceivable under their circumstances. Because such attention to emotional integrity is an integral part of our therapy, little additional help is needed for the arthritic patient. My experience has been that once you are able to reduce the patient's pain level (For instance with the LLLT), their emotional attitude improves dramatically.

Physical Therapy and Arthritis

Most of the physical therapeutic methods used in treating osteoarthritis have already been described. We generally use ultrasound, diathermy, **Magnatherm**, sine wave and/or galvanic therapy with our patients. (And now the LLLT) These methods are old standbys and like all old friends are more or less taken for granted, even by patients. It is only when the patient is not able to have this type of treatment for a while that he realizes how much benefit is derived from its use. It is not uncommon for pain to return with a vengeance when the patient is unable to take advantage of his regular physical therapy.

Homeopathy and Arthritis

The first chronic patients that Hahnemann treated were those with osteoarthritis. Although the homeopath doesn't prescribe according to disease (as does the allopath), some remedies are more suited to this type of problem than others. The two most commonly used homeopathic remedies for osteoarthritis are Bryonia alba, and Rhus tox. While these aren't a cure for the crippling stage of this disorder, they nevertheless can offer much harmless pain relief in patients responsive to their action.

The true homeopath, of course, always chooses the remedy according to the totality of the patient's symptoms. Where well chosen, such remedies can prove of inestimable value in this condition.

Chelation

By the use of certain agents (see also Chapter 22) placed into the circulating blood by the intravenous slow drip method, it is now possible to dissolve some of the calcium deposits formed in hypertrophic arthritis. We have been investigating this method for many years and it has shown great promise in selected patients.

The Treatment of Rheumatoid Arthritis

In our Clinic we consider rheumatoid arthritis to be more a condition of glandular imbalance than of a general degenerative nature. Rheumatoid arthritis is treated by us much in the same way that we treat adrenal exhaustion (see Chapter II). That is not to say that patients with adrenal exhaustion will develop rheumatoid arthritis. They won't unless other factors necessary to precipitate this disorder are present. Perhaps the stress of rheumatoid arthritis brings about adrenal insufficiency.

The emotions, as in all adrenal insufficiency type patients, are an important factor in treating rheumatoid arthritis. Each rheumatoid patient is evaluated regarding the nature of his emotional stability. Where needed, private counseling sessions are made an integral part of his therapy, although in some patients such measures are happily unnecessary. In most patients, the basic improvements produced by our treatment seem to be sufficient to raise the lowered spirits usually encountered in this disorder, thereby bringing them to a more positive frame of mind.

Specific diets don't seem as remedial for the rheumatoid arthritis patient as they are in osteoarthritis. It is important, however, that the patient refrain from all forms of refined foods and those with chemical additives, and toward this end we insist that he follow our Basic Health Maintenance Diet as carefully as possible. Several specific dietary deficiencies have been indicted as being factors in this disease, but none of these have been adequately proven.

Specific Nutritional Therapy

In the specific nutritional therapy of rheumatoid arthritis, we usually concentrate on supporting the adrenal glands and in correcting the trace mineral balance in the body. If we think the patient is unable to get sufficient high biologic protein in his diet, we may supplement with concentrated protein compounds.

Pangamic acid (DMG) is considered by some a near specific for rheumatoid arthritis. Our experience is not so optimistic, but many rheumatoid arthritic patients do respond to DMG with various degrees of benefit.

311

Physical Therapy

The physical therapy used in rheumatoid arthritis is much different from that used in osteoarthritis. In osteoarthritis, rather heroic measures are often required to help the affected parts; in rheumatoid arthritis, one must use all forms of physical therapy with care and discretion. Very mild forms of massage, ultrasound and Magnatherm have been used in our rheumatoid arthritis patients with good success, but the treating physician must feel out the sensitivities of the patient with discernment and carefully tailor his treatments to fit the patient's specific state at the time of the treatment.

If the patient is in a state of inflammatory swelling, only very mild and gentle therapeutic measures can be used. If the patient is over treated at this time, his pain will be increased and the disorder aggravated. As the patient improves, the physical therapeutic methods can become more vigorous, but at no time do we use the vigorous methods used in osteoarthritis.

The major exception to this rule is the use of LLLT. The rheumatoid arthritic patient seems to respond well to this "magic wand" and as yet we have had no adverse effects even in those patients who were treated very thoroughly.

Chelation

According to various authorities on blood chelation, both rheumatoid arthritis and osteoarthritis are benefitted by this therapy. The complete rationale behind this result is not well understood. Some attribute it to the general detoxifying effect that results from systemic chelation.

The Treatment of Gouty Arthritis

Gouty arthritis is generally considered more easily treated and less severe than extreme forms of osteoarthritis or rheumatoid arthritis, but it is nevertheless aggravating enough if one happens to be the victim. In general, gouty arthritis is believed to be caused by an improper metabolizing of purines in the body. A breakdown of these substances can cause uric acid to build up in the blood. This acid may then unite with alkali to form salts such as sodium urate and ammonium urate, which are slightly more soluble than the acid itself. Because of this feeble solubility, the urates are often deposited in joints, resulting in the severe pain of gouty arthritis. The uric acid is derived chiefly from nucleoproteins, which are found in nearly all foods of animal origin except eggs and milk, but these proteins are more common in the glandular organs such as sweetbreads, kidneys, and liver. Legumes, peas, beans and asparagus also contain significant amounts of nucleoproteins.

In gouty arthritis, an apparently hereditary imbalance makes it difficult for the body to properly break down the nucleoproteins. Where such a situation exists, it is necessary to place the patient on a diet that is relatively free from these offending substances. No other form of therapy is entirely successful in treating this disease.

Orthodoxly, a variety of drugs are used to help eliminate the excessive uric acid from the system. At our Healing Centers, we find that a gouty diet, certain nutritional compounds and homeopathic remedies may well control a case of gout without the use of such drugs as long as the patient is cooperative.

The suggested diet for gouty arthritis appears in the appendix of this book. Such a diet is imperative if attacks are to be prevented—important because every time an attack occurs owing to dietary indiscretions, a certain amount of joint tissue is injured. Even though the attack may pass, the injured tissue can't be regenerated. Although through natural means a patient can be helped to weather an attack, it is a much more practical goal of therapy to prevent such attacks. Each attack weakens the structure of the affected bones, and a state can be reached eventually in which almost no therapy is wholly satisfactory in preventing distress from the gouty deposits.

Cherry Juice—A Real Remedy

Many years ago, the literature from the Lee Foundation of Milwaukee recommended the use of cherry juice in controlling the symptoms of gouty arthritis. More recently an article appeared in *Prevention Magazine* on the advantages of the same remedy. To the best of my knowledge, it is not known what substance in cherries has a beneficial effect in gout, but cherries have proven very helpful in many patients with this painful complaint.

The suggested dosage is half a pound of cherries a day or its equivalent of cherry juice concentrate. We have found these concentrates fully as effective as any other form of cherries.

The use of cherries in gouty arthritis has proven so successful that we have begun to recommend it in other forms of arthritis and have been pleased with the results. It isn't known exactly whether some of these patients had a small amount of gouty arthritis complicating their other problems, or whether the cherry juice has a wider effect than its use in gout. Whatever the case, we find it a delightful, effective, and inexpensive remedy that even the Food and Drug Administration can't prevent us from using, making it a true rarity in the natural armamentarium.

Specific Nutritional Compounds

Although we use specific nutritional substances in each gout patient, they must be individually optimized for each patient and there is therefore no specific grouping to be recommended.

In acute attacks, owing to the irritative effects of the sodium urates, potassium bicarbonate has been recommended to counteract and neutralize this sodium salt. Potassium bicarbonate is somewhat difficult to obtain, although you might ask your local pharmacist to see if he can obtain the food-grade potassium bicarbonate for you. Half a teaspoonful taken in a glass of water often helps mitigate an acute gout attack. If your druggist cannot obtain the potassium bicarbonate for you, ask your Center physician. He will be able to help you find a supply.

Physical Therapy

Physical therapy is useful in gout, but it must be handled somewhat similarly to that used in rheumatoid arthritis. When the patient is experiencing gouty inflammation of the joint, one must use great discretion in using any physical therapy over this area, for it is possible to aggravate the condition. Once dietary and remedial measures have brought the inflammation under control, physical therapy can be used with good benefit as long as the work is done within the tolerance of the patient. Treatments should be so regulated that they are never painful. This is just the opposite of osteoarthritis, in which the most adequate treatments are usually mildly painful and the improvement is felt later.

While at the time of this writing we have had very little use of the LLLT with gouty arthritis, there is no reason to feel that it is not beneficial here as well as with the other forms of this disease.

Parting Words

Many books have promised cures for the arthritides, and I'm sure a great many more will be written, offering the same optimistic promises. Few of these books, however, will bring arthritis victims the help they desire.

The arthritides can be helped and in many instances actually cured. Such results, however, require a willing patient, a conscientious, devoted physician with a knowledge of body metabolism and natural therapeutics, and time and perseverance on both their parts. In severe cases, such a cure doesn't take place in a week, a month or even a year, but it can be done where there is true desire and effort on the part of physician and patient.

Arthritis is at one and the same time one of the most disappointing and yet one of the most rewarding disorders to treat by natural means. It is disappointing in that only rarely are rapid results obtained (written before the LLLT); it is rewarding in that when with time, work and patience, good results are obtained, something has been accomplished for which both patient and physician can be very proud.

Postscript: Several years ago we discovered the most dramatic remedy ever for all forms of arthritic pain. It was a Chinese proprietary product called **Tung Shueh**. This item was a combination of eighteen Chinese herbs and was without a doubt the world's finest non-toxic controller of arthritic pain (and most other types of bone-muscle-fibrous tissue pain) ever discovered.

This remedy was so good that we could not believe it did not contain some unlabeled powerful drug, even though none of us knew of any known drug that relieved pain so well without any other discernable side effects. We had this remedy tested by a variety of very competent laboratories and none of them could discern any such drugs in the "little round black pills."

This **Tung Sheuh** was so good that we soon discovered many seemingly identical copies of it available in health food stores and other similar sources. We checked as many of these as possible but none that we tested had any of the therapeutic effects of the original remedy.

Finally, about a year ago, we were told that the plant that made this marvelous remedy had been closed by the powers that be. It would seem that the motto of the giant drug cartels, "If you can't beat them, destroy them" had triumphed once again. The world would once again be left with only two choices—buy from the drug cartels or suffer.

We mention Tung Shueh for two reasons:

One, if you find such a remedy in a store or advertised it is probably not the real thing. Not surprisingly, there seems to be little effort to stop the sale and importation of the fake **Tung Shuehs**. Since they don't work they are no threat to the Drug Cartels.

Two, someday it may be possible to again obtain the authentic original **Tung Shueh**. If this happens we want you to know of the real wonders that these little round black balls can perform.

Chapter XXII
The Wonders of Chelation

There's a new therapy on the horizon that may prove a boon to many patients with disorders that heretofore have resisted some of our best efforts. This therapy is known as blood chelation. Chelation is a process in which a metal ion—such as lead, mercury, zinc, and calcium—becomes bound or chelated with a protein molecule to form a separate substance.

In medicine this process has been used in two ways: First, it is an excellent manner in which to combine certain mineral ions for use in nutritional supplementation. It is believed by many physicians experienced in this field to be one of the most satisfactory ways to prescribe supplemental minerals. Second, specific chelating agents can be injected into the veins to combine with mineral substances present in the blood with subsequent elimination by the kidneys. By this process the bloodstream and other tissues of the body can be freed of toxic or injurious substances. This second type of chelation is discussed here.

Because this procedure consists of introducing into the venous blood supply a substance not inherently natural to the body, although it is nontoxic, this method wouldn't normally come under the heading of natural treatment. Also, because chelation requires venous injection, it can only be done legally in this country by a medical or an osteopathic physician. We added it to the therapies available at the original Clymer Health Clinic over twenty five years ago because there is no more practical nor harmless way of accomplishing the results it offers. A great amount of evidence supports the claim that EDTA chelation not only can remove heavy metals from the blood, but also can help in increasing blood supply through arteries diseased by arteriosclerosis .

Despite such glowing claims, we were not fanatical about chelation at the original Clymer Health Clinic nor are we so at Woodlands Medical Center ;where this treatment is now an important part of the therapeutic arsenal. We use it only when we are sure that other less expensive and more natural treatments have been ineffective. Chelation by itself is rarely a complete answer to the patient's problem under any circumstances, because even though it may remove the immediate causes of his difficulties, unless he changes the habits that produced these difficulties originally, the condition will return again. Chelation aids the naturaltreatment of the patient, but it is not a substitute for the usual methods and techniques used at our Centers.

317

History

Chelation—this "new" method of therapy—has been used in medicine for more than twenty years, and it has been put to a wide range of applications in many medical centers throughout the world. The most universally used substance for this type of chelation is a compound called EDTA. EDTA was first used in 1948 to chelate lead from persons with lead poisoning, and it is still used for this purpose today. It has proven of particular use in children who have been poisoned by eating lead-base paints. Chelation has also been used in such conditions as mercury poisoning, radioactive metal toxicity, scleroderma, snake bite, and in calcinosis. Only somewhat recently have physicians begun to use chelation for vascular atheromatous disease.

Concurrent with the investigation of this agent in the common vascular disorders, biochemists and biophysicists are becoming intrigued with the wide range of physiologic metal chelation that occurs at the micro-cellular level of enzymatic reactions in the body—particularly in regard to such metals as potassium, magnesium, manganese, molybdenum, calcium, zinc, and copper. Most basic chemical functions within our body are brought about through the operation of various enzymes and enzyme-like substances. Most enzymes are able to function properly because of certain specific amounts of various trace minerals that are a part of their integral substance.

If the trace mineral balance can be altered by various toxic substances in our body and the toxic substances can be removed through chelation, much of the future in medicine may well center on chelation. This work could open large vistas into a wide range of disorders for which both the cause and possible treatment have heretofore been vague or undetermined. Such conditions as the psychotic disorders, the so-called collagenous diseases, and many disorders of metabolism and enzyme deficiencies may be helped by chelation.

All physicians know that their offices are filled with patients with vague and unexplainable ills. Most of these patients are treated as neurotics and given various tranquilizers or are encouraged to undergo psychotherapy. Is it not possible that what these patients really have is a disorder of the enzymatic balance of their body, probably owing to the intake of the many toxic substances that now pervade our environment? If chelation can help to reestablish normal enzymatic function, think of what a boon it could be to a large percentage of our population. At present, however, the most immediately encouraging results of chelation are in the various so-called degenerative diseases, for which there have been very few successful therapies.

Disorders that Chelation Can Help

Following is a list of conditions successfully treated by chelation that has been assembled by physicians who did much of the early research work. Many of these problems are common and are generally considered incurable: scleroderma; digitalis intoxication; heavy-metal poisoning (especially acute plumbism); calcinosis (pipestem calcinosis of the vessels, prostatic calcinosis); vascular atheromatous disorders including atherosclerosis, atheromatous deposits, arteriosclerosis obliterans, peripheral vascular insufficiency with intermittent claudication, and acute brain syndrome secondary to cerebral ischemia secondary to calcific atherosclerosis; myocardial or coronary insufficiency; collagenosis; arteriosclerosis including cerebrovascular arteriosclerosis; arthritis including hypertrophic and rheumatoid; calcific tendinosis; calculi; diabetic retinopathy; multiple sclerosis; macular degeneration of the retina; cataracts; Parkinsonism; emphysema; poisonous snake and insect bites; calcified necrotic ulcers; heart valve calcification; hemochromatosis; calcific bursitis; calcified granulomas; and hypertension.

This list was made up for physicians, and many of the names may be so much Greek to you. I will try, however, to single out some of the more important conditions and describe them in simple terms.

Scleroderma

Scleroderma is little known, and yet it is a disease that most physicians will encounter in their regular practice. It often accompanies the vascular condition known as Raynaud's disease. In scleroderma, the skin of the fingertips becomes very hard, and can feel almost like bone. The EDTA chelation treatment for this condition is so successful that Medicare will pay for it. Medicare will also pay for chelation therapy in digitalis poisoning, which can occur when a heart patient has had large doses of digitalis for too long a time.

Lead Poisoning

Chelation is almost specific for lead poisoning (plumbism) and insurances under the banner of IND will pay for chelation when used for an overabundance of lead in the blood.

I have recently read propaganda put out by various oil companies attempting to convince us that we are worrying unnecessarily about the use of lead in automotive fuels. They say that the small amount of lead that these fuels put into the air isn't going to hurt us in any way, shape, or form. Not long ago the Philadelphia Zoo was having considerable trouble with illnesses of many of their animals. When blood tests were taken of the animals, high lead levels were found. This zoo is located near several large highways, and the zoo officials stated that they were definitely positive that the only way these animals could have obtained such high lead levels was from breathing the fumes produced by vehicles on these highways. If this can occur in zoo animals, it can surely occur in man. Toxicities with lead, mercury, and other heavy metals are today not just a possibility but are a definite endemic problem.

Arteriosclerosis

Pipestem calcinosis is merely one form of arteriosclerosis in which heavy deposits of calcium have been laid down in blood vessel walls to such a degree that the blood vessel feels like a pipestem when palpated. This problem is related to other vascular atheromatous disorders, including arteriosclerosis, atheromatous deposits, arteriosclerosis obliterans, and peripheral vascular insufficiency with intermittent claudication. All these conditions are related to fatty and mineral deposition on the blood vessel walls. These deposits diminish blood flow and raise the blood pressure. Depending on the vessels affected, we are presented with a variety of symptoms.

If the clogging is in the legs, it can cause intermittent claudication, in which the legs cramp after walking a short distance owing to lack of oxygen in the muscles. If the coronary arteries of the heart become narrowed, the condition is called angina pectoris. If they close off entirely, a heart attack or cardiac arrest results. If the affected vessels are in the brain, the clogging could cause a stroke; if it is just general diffuse narrowing, a loss of balance, forgetfulness, and the vague psychotic symptoms of the general senile syndrome may result. The symptoms are many but the condition is basically the same, and one that more and more physicians believe can respond advantageously to the chelation therapy.

Arthritis

What is here called hypertrophic arthritis is also known as osteoarthritis. According to many authorities, both this and rheumatoid arthritis respond well to chelation. Because in rheumatoid arthritis very little calcification occurs, such response must be related to the detoxifying effects of chelation and perhaps to its normalization of enzyme function. At present, its mode of operation is not certain, but physicians who have used it are convinced that it is beneficial in rheumatoid arthritis.

Eye Disorders

Diabetic retinopathy, macular degeneration of the retina, and cataracts seem to be due to deterioration of the blood vessels of the eye and the resultant poor circulation to the eye tissues. Wherever the disease is caused by impaired circulation, chelation will be of help.

Multiple Sclerosis, Parkinson's Disease, and Emphysema

Chelation has also been suggested for treating multiple sclerosis, Parkinson's disease, and emphysema. If these conditions have been treated successfully by chelation, as some authorities relate, such success is probably due to the correction of enzyme imbalances .

How Chelation Works

Chelation is a most interesting therapy, and it is of particular interest to the natural physician in that, like his remedies but unlike those of the allopath, most of its side effects have proven useful and not harmful. For instance many of the conditions such as emphysema and Parkinsonism, that have been helped by chelation were originally helped as side effects—the chelation had been given for some other problem, but in the process the emphysema and Parkinsonism were also helped.

If I may be allowed to theorize a bit, it seems that chelation could be called a natural therapy. Evidence shows it isn't the chelating agent alone that produces so much of the benefit, but rather that the chelating agent simply removes certain congesting and inhibiting substances that have held the vital healing force of the body in bondage. Once these bonds are loosened by EDTA, the vital force can go about its job once again to heal and stabilize the body.

Most physicians who use chelation have been surprised to find that their patients continue to report progress and improvement for several months after the original chelation therapy is finished. From their knowledge of the agent, these physicians know that there is no effect from the chelating agent itself over this period because ninety-eight per cent of the EDTA is eliminated within forty-eight hours. I believe only the liberating of the natural healing force of the body can account for these excellent prolonged effects.

When properly handled, chelation has proven entirely safe. However, it must only be carried out by those well versed in its requirements. The patients must be given a very thorough examination before chelation can be used. Those with healed tubercular lesions of the lungs and/or severe renal disease are generally not accepted for therapy. In the first instance, chelation might break down the calcium around the healed tubercular lesions, releasing the tubercular bacillus. In the second, because the chelated compound must be eliminated by the kidneys, a certain degree of kidney function must be assured or the toxic compounds released can't be eliminated and the kidneys are further damaged. If the condition is a matter of life and death, the physician may take a chance and use chelation with poor kidney function. There are many reports of this being done with great benefit to the patient.

Some practitioners give chelation therapy only in the hospital; such cautious care is not generally required. It is necessary, however, for each patient to be watched carefully during the chelation, and most physicians usually don't have the facilities for carrying this out. At Woodlands Medical Center, we are fortunate in having sufficient room and personnel for carrying out chelation safely and effectively without the cost and regimentation of hospitalization. A portion of our staff devotes its entire time and energies to caring for chelation patients. In this way, we believe we can give the most effective, safe, and inexpensive service.

Chelation treatments can be given as often as every day, or we can take our time and spread out the treatments to give the body time for its healing work. Patients who stay at our Centers are usually given five treatments a week; local patients may be treated by the more leisurely method. After the initial series is over, the patients are checked in three to six months; if necessary, another series of five treatments is then given. Many mild enzyme imbalance disorders can be helped with a simple series of five treatments. Almost all the conditions in which there is an overabundance of calcium require a full series of fifteen to twenty treatments.

At our Centers, we can house out-of-town patients in comfortable air-conditioned rooms while they undergo their chelation treatments. Those who come for this therapy can undergo other forms of treatment at the same time, so that complete body regeneration therapy can be attempted. Our live-in patients are provided with natural organic foods selected for each individual patient. In this way, we make every attempt to give the inner vital force the greatest possible help to establish health within its being.

Parting Words

In the years to come, you will hear more about chelation. It isn't a perfect cure, but it offers more help for certain heretofore untreatable disorders than any other form of therapy at present. By itself, chelation therapy can be very useful, but when combined with other forms of natural therapy it can be a godsend to those with certain afflictions. I hope that none of my readers ever need chelation therapy, but if the need should arise you can rejoice that such a method is available.

322

The foregoing on Chelation was written many years ago for the first edition of *It's Only Natural* While many changes in this treatment have evolved, we felt that you would like to still have our original commentary on this subject. That which follows is a recent update on Chelation written by Dr. William G. Kracht one of the physicians now administering this therapy at Woodlands Medical Center.

Chelation for the Twenty First Century

Chelation (pronounced "Key-lay-shun") is a painless, non invasive treatment administered in a physician's office. It is composed of a molecule called EDTA (ethylene diamine tetracidic acid) that binds to metals such as lead, cadmium, aluminum, iron, copper and calcium so they then can be eliminated through the kidneys. Thus chelation removes toxic build up of metals and minerals from the body. It also acts as an "antioxidant" (similar to Vitamin E) further protecting the arteries and other tissues from the damaging effects of "free radicals". EDTA also appears to restore the natural calcium/magnesium balance that is necessary for proper relaxation of the blood vessel wall muscles. Finally EDTA appears to restore normal enzyme functions of the cells. EDTA appears to have several additive beneficial functions and effects upon the body, which enable it to be a key therapy in many conditions.

These and probably other ways all combine to make chelation treatments beneficial for a variety of conditions to include, but not limited to, impaired circulation and/or blockage in any blood vessels of the body, heart disease, high blood pressure, prevention of heart attacks and strokes, and to relieve angina. In addition, chelation patients have reported that the therapy has improved sexual function, increased vision, increased memory and concentration, and reduced symptoms of other medical problems such as arthritis, multiple sclerosis, Parkinson's disease, macular degeneration, glaucoma, scleroderma, and psoriasis. There is also evidence that it may help prevent Alzheimer's disease and there is even one study that suggests that chelation therapy *may be* helpful in *preventing* cancer. And finally, EDTA can be used to remove elevated levels of heavy metals from the body's tissues.

Severe liver and kidney disease may prevent one from receiving chelation. Severe heart failure may also prohibit its use. Pregnancy is also a condition in which chelation would probably not be used except in extreme cases.

EDTA chelation therapy has been scientifically proven to help. Despite a few studies that suggest otherwise, there is a significant amount of accumulated medical and scientific studies that support the effective-

323

ness of this treatment. One study of 19,000 patients with peripheral vascular disease (clogging of the arteries of the legs, arms, neck or head) who received chelation demonstrated that 80% received substantial improvement.

In 1989 the FDA began scientifically controlled trials of EDTA chelation therapy, and while the results have yet to be released, the FDA concluded that "safety was not an issue" with EDTA. Over the past thirty years, approximately 600,000 patients have had 12 million EDTA infusions in this country, and the FDA could find no evidence of any significant toxicity. In fact, no deaths from EDTA chelation have occurred when the treatment was properly administered and supervised.

The risks of serious side effects, when properly administered is less than 1 in 10,000 patients treated. By comparison, the overall death rate as a direct result of heart bypass surgery is approximately 3 out of every 100 patients undergoing surgery, varying with the hospital and operating team. The incidence of other serious complications following surgery is much higher, including heart attacks, strokes, blood clots, permanent brain damage with personality changes and prolonged pain. Chelation is more than 300 times safer than bypass surgery.

The biggest concern for chelation is on the kidneys. There are past reports that chelation may be toxic to the kidneys. However, this occurred with higher doses than are currently used today. Furthermore, kidney function is closely followed and the dose reduced on any one with kidney weakness or disease. A more recent study on 383 patients revealed that proper doses of chelation actually *improved* kidney function after chelation. Occasionally a patient may be unduly sensitive and thus kidney function is followed very closely.

Another potential side effect is thrombophlebitis, which is soreness and redness of the vein (inflammation of the vein in which chelation was given). Thrombophlebitis usually resolves with local heat treatment but may form a blood clot which potentially could break away and travel to the lungs. Thrombophlebitis occurs in less than 1 of 100 patients and blood clot formation in even rarer. Other side effects may include lower blood sugar, low blood pressure, nausea, diarrhea, numbness and cramps, headache, fever, and skin rashes. All of these can be avoided and easily treated with proper technique and following preventive instructions before chelation is given.

Specific testing is needed prior to starting chelation therapy. The first essential step is a complete and full history and physical examination by one of our staff physicians. Basic blood work includes a blood count, complete blood chemistry profile with special attention to the liver, kidneys and electrolytes, complete urinalysis, thyroid function tests. Hair test and blood test for minerals and heavy metals are also indicated. An EKG is also considered essential. Other tests that may be needed include an exercise (treadmill) test, vascular ultrasound, glucose tolerance test, heart echocardiogram, and other tests of the heart or vascular system.

EDTA chelation is very simple and easy to administer. Treatments are generally given every week to total 20 to 40 treatments. This schedule is of course dictated by the nature and severity of each person's condition. The principle medication, EDTA, is mixed in an intravenous bottle with additional vitamins and minerals. A very small needle is inserted into an arm vein and this mixture is slowly infused into the arm vein over 2 to 3 hours. During the treatment you are able to relax in a reclining chair, read, watch video tapes or talk to others. The atmosphere is pleasant and relaxing and few experience any further pain after the insertion of the needle. Our staff is highly trained and skilled in this specialty area to provide you with the best possible care. You are free to return home immediately after the treatment.

Special dietary and supplementation guidelines are extremely important to follow in order to prevent any mineral losses from chelation and to best treat the underlying medical condition.

These recommendations and supplement guidelines will be individualized after the blood and other testing is completed and tailored as needed.

Mercury Toxicity and DMPS Chelation

While EDTA is used for heart, vascular problems and to remove heavy metals such as lead, cadmium, aluminum and iron, DMPS is specific for removal of mercury and arsenic overload conditions. Mercury is one of the most poisonous elements known to man. The total amount of mercury from all chemical species has grown in our world environment to the point that chronic mercury toxicity is now an endemic disease. The sources of mercury and the amount absorbed into our systems is noted as follows by the World Health Organization (1991):

Exposure Source Micrograms of mercury absorbed per day

Dental Amalgam Fillings 3.0-17.0
Fish or Seafood 2.34
Other Food 0.25
Water 0.0035
Air 0.001

It is readily apparent that metal dental fillings, most of which are 50% mercury mixed with silver, nickel and other metals, are the chief source of mercury exposure today. In addition, mercury is still used in many medicines as a preservative. The highest mercury levels in seafood are found in fish caught from the Everglades, Great Lakes and Lake Washington. The types of fish that contain the highest amounts of mercury are blue marlin, bluefish, swordfish and fresh water fish. Tuna, shark, red snapper and grouper have intermediate amounts of mercury.

Mercury accumulation in the body has been recognized to contribute to a wide variety of symptoms. The American Dental Association admits to the following symptoms resulting from mercury accumulation:

> "Tremor, depression, fatigue, irritability, moodiness, inability to concentrate, memory loss, insomnia, nausea, diarrhea, loss of appetite, birth defects in offspring, nephritis, pneumonitis, swollen glands and tongue, ulcerations of oral mucosa, and dark pigmentation of the gums and loosening of the teeth."

Furthermore, mercury has been shown to be more toxic to the nervous system and brain than lead, cadmium or even arsenic. It also prevents hormones from working properly. For example, when mercury is present it prevents progesterone from binding to the cells and it also interacts with adrenal and other fat soluble hormones including thyroid hormones.

Mercury is one of the most toxic elements present in our modern world and mercury dental fillings and other exposures may cause ill effects in those people who are not necessarily toxic but are merely sensitive. However, not everyone with mercury exposure will have symptoms or become ill. The degree of mercury's toxic effects not only depends on the dose and duration of the exposure, but also on the genetic, environmental and nutritional factors that regulate our internal self detoxification systems.[1]

DMPS, Sodium 2,3 Dimeraptopropane-1-sulfonate is the chelating agent used to remove mercury from the body. DMPS is manufactured by Hyle in Germany and is imported to the United States to compounding pharmacists. It is a different medicine than EDTA and is much more effective for mercury and cadmium. DMPS is obtained through proper and legal channels. It does not have a drug patent in this country and does not have full FDA approval. DMPS can be prescribed by a Medical Doctor or Doctor of Osteopathy for the use of mercury removal under the Medical Practice Act of the State of Pennsylvania. At

---

[1] Refer to the Appendix A for further information on this subject.

this time DMPS is being investigated as an agent to remove mercury from the body's tissues.

DMPS has been researched for over 40 years in Japan, Germany and the former Soviet Union and has been used for treatment in these same countries for over 25 years. Safety research has shown it to be very safe and without side effects at the doses of 3.0 milligrams per kilogram of body weight. According to the manufacturer, DMPS has been shown to be safe when used according to instructions and given by the intravenous, intramuscular and oral routes. It's side effects may include, but may not be limited to, pancreatitis, nausea, headache, muscle pain or weakness, gastrointestinal symptoms, rashes, sensomotor neuropathy, decreased urination, cardiac arrhythmias and allergic reactions. According to the manufacturer, these symptoms are rare and are believed to be caused by the actual detoxification process. However, if you experience any of these symptoms please inform us immediately. We are unaware of any deaths or permanent injury from the use of DMPS. The effects of DMPS use during pregnancy is not fully known, but there are no known birth defects from its use. Lastly, DMPS will remove good minerals from the body along with the toxic heavy metals. For this reason, careful nutritional status analysis and supplementation is critical to ensuring the safety of this form of therapy.

DMPS is given as a "push" through the vein over 10-30 minutes. After DMPS is given, large amounts of mercury and other heavy metals are dumped out through the kidneys over the next 24 hours. These intravenous injections are given every 3 to 6 weeks until the mercury analyzed in the urine drops to zero. The series of intravenous injections must be given after all of the mercury fillings have been first removed. However, DMPS can also be given as a "shot" into the muscle during removal of dental fillings to help the body's detoxification.

The Woodlands Medical Center is currently actively involved in a FDA approved clinical trial involving DMPS sponsored by the Great Lakes Association of Clinical Medicine. This protocol was devised to maximize the effect of DMPS on mercury and heavy metal detoxification while ensuring full safety. The program is detailed and involved, but we feel is worth the effort, especially in chronic, progressive conditions unresponsive to all other known forms of therapy.

Initial Phase

You must first meet with one of our staff physicians to determine whether you are a candidate for this treatment and to assess any other medical problems you may have. This appointment will include a full environmentally oriented history and detailed physical exam. Alternatives to DMPS treatment will also be given. If you wish to proceed with DMPS, a consent form will be given for you to review and sign.

A detailed laboratory profile will be obtained including but not limited to a hair analysis for heavy metals and minerals, blood work for chemistry profile, blood count, magnesium, iron, thyroid function tests and thyroid antibody tests, red blood cell mineral analysis, and two separate 24 hour urine collection for kidney function and urine heavy metals and elements. Additional testing may include adrenal analysis, liver detoxification profile, sex hormone analysis and immune system studies. In addition, skin testing will be performed to rule out allergy to DMPS and lidocaine or procaine. If sensitivity to DMPS is discovered, a neutralization program can be given.

A supplementation program is outlined to ensure adequate mineral replacement and to promote the body's detoxification process and immune system function. This will include but may not be limited to a multiple high potency vitamin and mineral supplement, Vitamin C, Antioxidant formula, Chlorella or Blue Green Algae and Garlic. Individual supplementation with zinc, magnesium, copper, manganese or iron may be needed if testing reveals deficiencies in any of these areas.

After all testing is completed and the results obtained, a DMPS "challenge" will be given and a repeat 24 hour urine collection to immediately follow. This will analyze how much mercury is "lodged" in the body's tissues and subsequently pulled out by the DMPS chelation. If NO mercury is found in the urine after a DMPS challenge, you need to go no further with this treatment (mercury toxicity or sensitivity is probably not a problem for you). This "challenge" test can be given before or after all of the mercury fillings have been removed. Each DMPS treatment must be followed by an intravenous mineral mix within 24 to 72 hours. A pregnancy test will be given to all premenopausal women prior to the DMPS injection.

Dental Phase

A dental examination[2] is then performed to determine the number of mercury fillings, replacement filling options that best meet your individual needs, a treatment plan and cost estimates. During the day of, but before the actual removal of any mercury filling, you will receive a "shot" of DMPS in the muscle. This will help "bind" any mercury released from the dental extraction process.

---

[2] We will recommend one of several dentists that work in close cooperation with the Woodlands Medical Center and are knowledgeable in this area of biological dentistry, amalgam removal and composite replacements.

As soon as possible after the filling extraction (that same day or the next) you will return to our office for a mineral and vitamin IV and a series of anesthetic injections called "neural therapy". Neural therapy helps open the lymphatic drainage for the brain and leads to a fast detoxification of the brain. These "trigger point" injections involve areas of the scalp, sinuses, and tonsils. The procedures of a DMPS shot, neural therapy and mineral IV will continue until all of the mercury containing fillings are removed. This process may take one visit or many depending on the number and location of your fillings.

Those people who have already had their mercury fillings removed prior to seeing us will not benefit from this treatment phase and will proceed directly to the detoxification phase.

Detoxification Phase

This will include a series of one or more intravenous "pushes" with DMPS, immediately followed by a 24 hour urine collection for mercury and minerals. A mineral IV will be given 24-72 hours after the DMPS push. This DMPS-urine collection-mineral IV series will be continued every 3 to 6 weeks until the urine mercury reads *zero*.

Follow Up Phase

A complete examination, and a repeat of the same initial lab tests will be completed 6, 12, 18 and 24 months after the initial exam and testing was performed. This phase is needed to ensure safety and effectiveness of the therapy. If other heavy metals are found that are not well chelated by DMPS, EDTA chelation may be required.

As is evident, DMPS therapy for mercury detoxification can be quite an involved process. It is, however, the best known therapy for directly removing mercury from our tissues. The natural healing arts do offer other ways to help the body detoxify heavy metals, including mercury. This process can be slower, but less taxing on the body's vital force. If mercury or other heavy metal accumulation, toxicity or sensitivity may be a problem for you, our centers can develop a program that is individualized for you, whether it be EDTA, DMPS or other natural detoxifying programs.

Sources of Heavy Metals

Heavy metals are being implicated more and more, especially in today's environment, as possible contributors to various diseases and medical conditions. These metals are usually unseen and with continued low level exposure, slowly accumulate in the body's tissues. Most heavy metals will become lodged in the glands and soft tissues of the body.

329

Some, like lead, are also stored in the bones of both adults and children. Lead has been implicated in learning disabilities in children. Mercury is known to be stored in the endocrine glands, brain, liver and kidney. Aluminum is known to be stored in the brain and nervous system.

There are many ways for heavy metals to infiltrate our environment, food and water supply. Most are unsuspected by us. Once these heavy metals accumulate in the body, they act as poisons to our enzymes and biochemical systems which can lead to a wide variety of symptoms and problems. Consequently, it is important to be aware of the sources of potential heavy metal exposure and take avoidance measures when possible.

Aluminum (Al)

Sources:
American cheese
Antacids
Antiperspirants
Baking powder
Beer
Beer, soda and food receptacles and containers
Buffered aspirins
Commercially prepared vaginal douches
Cooking pots and pans
Foil
Food additives and colors
Margarine and hydrogenated fats/oils
Municipal drinking water
Pickles (alum)
Salt (anti-caking agent)
Spirulina
Tobacco smoke
Toothpastes with fluoride and flurositan
Water: some soft waters
Vitamins/minerals with fluoride

Occupations Exposures:
Aluminum mining, bar mills, and grinding mills

Arsenic (As)

Sources:
Beer
Colored chalk
Defoliants
Drinking water
Food supplements: bone meal, dolomite, kelp
Laundry and cleaning aides
Paints: decorative and gold leaf
Pesticides
Salt
Seafood
Seaweed: agar agar
Tobacco smoke

Occupational Exposure:
Cosmetic industry workers
Insecticide manufacturers

Cadmium (Cd)

Sources:
Carbonated cola drinks
Cigarette smoke
Contaminated drinking water
Dust and pollution
Fungicides and pesticides
Galvanized pipes
Instant tea and coffee
Plastic food containers
Plastic water pipes
Plastic wrap
Refined and processed foods
Shellfish
Silver polish for cutlery
Soft drinks
Superphosphate fertilizers
Tin or metal containers for food

Occupational Exposure:
Battery manufacturers

Industrial smoke, exhaust and wastes
Oxide dusts or fumes
Paint manufacturers
Welding

Copper (Cu)

Sources:
Beer
Copper cookware and utensils
Copper intrauterine devices (IUD)
Copper tubing and plumbing
Excess copper in vitamin/mineral supplements
Insecticides
Pasteurized milk
Oral contraceptives (Birth Control Pills)
Self tanning lotions and creams
Water: municipal or well

Occupational Exposures:
Copper mining/smelting
Electric wire manufacturers

Fluoride (Fl)

Sources:
Fluoridated water
Fluoridated toothpaste
Fluoridated mouthwash
Foods and beverages made with fluoridated water

Iron (Fe)

Sources:
Baby formula
Black olives
Commercially baked goods
(enrichment of white flour products)
Iron enriched foods
Iron pots and pans
Powdered milks (some)
Vitamin and mineral pills
White flour and its products

Various types of iron:
Ferric Ammonium Citrate
Ferrous Ascorbate
Ferrous citrate
Ferrous lactate
Ferrous sulfate
Ferric Oxide
Iron Peptonate
Sodium Ferric Pyrophosphate

Sources of Assimilable iron:
Blackstrap molasses
Black beans
Leafy greens and leafy green vegetables
Organically grown animal liver
Organically grown eggs
Prunes and prune juices
Raisins

Lead (Pb)

Sources:
Automobile exhaust
Bone meal supplements
Canned baby formula can seams
Canned fruits and fruit juice can seams
Canned food cans seams
Dolomite supplements
Eating snow
Fertilizers
Hair dyes for both men and women
Insecticides
Lead-glazed pottery
Liver
Mascara
Old water pipes/plumbing
Paint- older houses with lead paint
Pewter tableware
Plastic food containers with PCV
Tobacco leaves (lead arsenate used as an insecticide)
Toothpaste tubes

Vegetables grown near a road
Water
Wine

Occupational Exposures:
Hot lead typesetters
Lead miners and smelters
Photography developers
Toll collectors for bridges and highways
Traffic directing officers

Manganese (Mn)

Sources:
Vitamin/mineral supplements in excess
Air pollution from mining, mills and factories
Industrial exposure
Manganese mining

Mercury (Hg)

Sources:
Calomel-containing body powders & talc
Chlorine bleaches
Cosmetics
Dental amalgam fillings
Diuretic injections
Fabric softeners
Fish- blue marlin, bluefish, swordfish, fresh water fish,
tuna, shark, red snapper, grouper
Fungicides
Grains and seeds containing fungicides
Mercurochrome & Merthiolate
Organomercurial pesticides
Oral thermometers (if broken)
Paints, some water based
Plastics
Printer's ink
Sewage sludge fertilizers
Shellfish
Skin lightening cream

Tattooing
Thimerosal (used in soft contact lens saline solutions)

Occupational Exposures:
Agricultural nurseries using mercury-containing sprays
Dentists and dental workers
Electrical Equipment testing
Felt hat manufacturer
Fluorescent light tube manufacturer
Manufacturers of organic mercury compounds

Nickel (Ni)

Sources:
Cigarette smoke
Dental metal fillings
Hydrogenated fats and oils
Refined and processed foods
Stainless steel cookware (especially with acid foods)
Superphosphate fertilizers used in growing foods
Skin allergies caused by clothing zippers and closures; coins, detergents; jewelry; utensils and tools

Occupational Exposures:
Casting manufacturer
Chemical industry
Duplicating machine employees
Dyes: manufacturing and applying
Electronic & computers
Ink making
Jewelers
Nickel mining and smelting
Rubber workers

Selenium (Se)

Sources:
Mineral supplements in excess

Occupational Exposure:
Electronic equipment (some)

Photocopy machines using xerographic method
Photoelectric equipment
Word processor machines

Zinc (Zn)

Sources:
Mineral supplementation in excess

Occupational Exposure:
Zinc mining/smelting/plating
Galvanizing

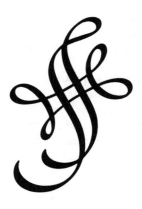

Chapter XXIII
Allergies and Environmental Illness

Just about everybody knows someone who suffers from allergies. It is estimated that 33% or more of the American population have allergies of some kind. And yet these figures do not even include food allergy and chemical sensitivity. Asthma in children has increased over 200% in the past twenty years. We believe this increase in allergy seen today is the result of the assault on our immune systems from today's chemically laden environment. We feel that the refining of foods, the use of food additives, the use of infant formula, the widespread use of and contamination of our food and water with pesticides and insecticides, heavy metal accumulation in our body's tissues, the constant and daily exposure to volatile organic solvent type chemicals in our homes, schools and offices, and societal stress all play a role in the development of allergy and environmental sensitivity. Our modern "21st Century" environment essentially bathes us in a sea of chemicals and the resultant effect is environmental illness.

There is also a genetic component to developing allergies. It appears that those with the hereditary pre-disposition to develop allergy will manifest symptoms to the degree of environmental insult they happen to incur. For instance, someone born with a mild predisposition to develop allergy will need a higher dose of environmental triggers than one who is born with a large predisposition to develop allergy. It is important to understand this concept so you can best modify your environment to meet your own unique genetic influences. We are all dealt a personal genetic "deck of cards" to be used our entire life. Although we cannot obtain a different deck, we can alter our lifestyle and behavior, thus shuffling our deck to find the best possible hand it allows; the better our hand, the better our health. Our Centers specialize in finding ways to shuffle your deck and modify your environment and health behaviors to maximize your personal strengths and minimize your hereditary weakness. This approach best describes Environmental Medicine.

Environmental medicine is the practice of directly correcting or improving environmentally triggered problems with the minimal use of drugs and toxic therapies. Environmental medicine takes a two pronged approach: find and then reduce your particular harmful environmental exposures while at the same time building up your body's natural ability to deal with these exposures. This is best understood as the total load concept. Our immune and detoxification systems can be compared to a

337

barrel. The larger our barrel, the more environmental insults it can hold and the less symptoms and reactions we incur. However, once our individual threshold is reached, our barrel then overflows and we manifest symptoms. The smaller our barrel, the quicker it can overflow when environmental triggers (exposures) are poured into it and the sooner we develop symptoms. We thus see the importance of reducing our exposures and environmental triggers (keeping our barrel as empty as possible) while at the same time trying to support and strengthen our immune and detoxification systems (increase the size of our barrel).

As we review the types of allergy and sensitivity, the many different testing methods and treatment modalities, keep in mind this barrel and total load concept to best understand the concept of environmental illness. There are only 500 physicians currently trained in Environmental Medicine at the time of this book's publication. In the Commonwealth of Pennsylvania there are only 14 environmentally trained physicians, only two are family physicians and the Woodlands Medical Center is the only fully integrated multi disciplinary family medical center offering this approach to health care.

Much confusion and misunderstanding centers around the word "allergy." The word allergy is derived from two Greek words meaning "altered reaction." The substance which provokes a reaction in an individual is called an "allergen" or "antigen." This can be dust, mold, pollen, food or other substances.

When medicine began to scientifically understand allergy in the 1930's, they discovered a biochemical pathway in the body that caused the typical Hayfever symptoms we all know so well. This involved an immune compound in our blood and tissues called Ig E and was responsible for an immediate allergy reaction: exposure to animal dander caused sneezing, itching and watery nose. It is this definition of allergy that became accepted by the medical community. As time and medicine progressed, it was discovered that other pathways in the body also lead to specific symptoms and could produce delayed reactions. Whereas immediate reactions occur within minutes to several hours after exposure to an allergen, delayed reactions can occur anywhere from 12 to 72 hours after exposure to an allergenic substance. These delayed pathways are still not well understood and are probably the mechanism by which chemicals and other substances produce physical symptoms. Unfortunately, this does not fit into the classic example of "immediate type Ig E allergy" and thus the concept of chemical allergy has been very difficult for the medical community to accept. Consequently, we prefer the word "sensitivity" to describe any reaction to a chemical, food or other sub-

338

stance that does not fit the classic "immediate type Ig E allergy" mechanism.

There are many clinical pictures of the person with allergy and sensitivity. We can, however, list five basic categories:

•**Inhalant Allergy:** those that have essentially nose and respiratory allergy symptoms to common airborne substances such as dust, mold, pollen, grass, trees, and animal dander. The symptoms may be all year long or just at certain seasons (ie., spring and fall). Hayfever is an allergy to ragweed and is the classic example of an Ig E inhalant allergy.

•**Food Allergy:** those that have predominately food allergy. They usually do not have seasonal variations in their symptoms but the symptoms vary depending upon their exposure to the foods that cause reactions. The reactions and symptoms may be immediately apparent or be delayed for up to 3-4 days after eating the particular offending food.

•**Chemical Sensitivities:** those who have a variety of both physical and mental symptoms upon exposure to chemicals such as perfume, gasoline, tobacco smoke, cleaning products, pesticides, detergents and many other chemical compounds. They may not have inhalant or food allergy. Some of these patients may even be sensitive to electromagnetic fields. It is important to understand that chemicals can cause both injury and toxic reactions and at the same time cause sensitivity reactions in our bodies. Most chemically sensitive individuals also have some degree of chemical injury. This may have occurred from a single large exposure or from a long term low level exposure to one or many chemicals. Chemicals that have such disrupting effects on the body's hormones and metabolism are called "xenobiotics;" "xeno" meaning chemical and "biotic" meaning biological action. In our extensive experience in this field, we have found that nearly all individuals with significant chemical sensitivity have other concomitant allergies, weak digestive function and hormonal imbalances, especially the adrenal. This leads us to the next category.

•**Multiple Allergy and Sensitivity:** those who have a combination of inhalant, food and chemical sensitivities. There are an infinite number of these combinations, varying in degree and severity, and largely dependent on the genetic makeup of the individual (size of their barrel) and the amount of exposures they have incurred. The majority of those with environmental illness fall into this category of multiple allergies and sensitivities.

•**Universal Reactor:** those with such severe allergies and environmental sensitivities that they seem to react to "everything." This condition is the deterioration of the above person who has multiple allergies and sensitivities. They usually have many health problems and are often labeled as "crazy" or "depressed" by their doctors and peers. They often need to take extreme avoidance measures to stay well and require the best the environmental medicine can offer them.

We can now see that environmental illness is the result of adverse reactions to substances in the air we breathe, the food we eat, the water we drink, the medications we take and to substances found in our everyday home and office. These reactions can be mild, moderate, or severe, and can involve just about any organ or system in the body. This includes the nervous system and brain, immune system, endocrine (hormonal) system, reproductive system, urinary system, gastrointestinal system, respiratory system and musculoskeletal system. Those organs that show symptoms upon allergen or chemical exposure are known as your "target organs." Your target organs may stay the same over time or change as your condition changes. Environmental illness can also be the underlying factor in many diseases and medical syndromes seen today such as depression, anxiety, high blood pressure, diabetes, auto-immune disorders like rheumatoid arthritis, lupus, asthma, bronchitis, frequent ear infections and sinus infections, attention deficit, hyperactivity and learning problems in children, colitis, irritable bowel syndrome and many other conditions. Because environmental illness often masquerades as other types of diseases it is often undiagnosed or misdiagnosed. Herein lies the critical need for an environmentally trained practitioner.

Testing

Testing for allergy and environmental illness may be quite simple or involve many innovative laboratory and radiographic testing. Unfortunately, there is of yet no one test that can diagnose environmental illness or chemical sensitivity. The following is a partial list of possible testing techniques that can help one suffering from allergies or environmental illness.

•**Environmentally Oriented Interview:** The first and foremost essential in diagnosing environmental illness is the environmental oriented history and physical examination. This is much more detailed than the typical medical interview that is directed to a person's current problem. A detailed search is made for the environmental triggers to the person's illness; questioning often starts with the individual's pre-birth history and then methodically reviews the entire past medical history looking for possible exposure events in that person's lifetime. The types of environmental exposures and stressors include exposure to pesticides, heavy metals, mercury (silver) fillings, volatile organic solvent type chemicals such as paints, petroleum products, natural gas, formaldehyde, phenols, and chemicals found in carpets and building materials. In addition, all aspects of the individual's health is evaluated in an attempt to find all of the factors contributing to his or her total load. This includes searching for physical stressors such as infection (viral, bacterial, parasitic, and fungal), poor nutrition, food and chemical reactions, allergies to inhalants, inadequate or too much exercise, hormonal imbalances, digestive disturbances, insufficient rest and sleep. Emotional stressors that contribute to the total load include: job stress and frustration, marital difficulties, divorce, financial difficulties and past or present abuse to include physical, emotional, verbal or sexual abuse. This is a time consuming process but well worth the effort once certain triggering events are discovered. Such information allows for more specific testing and treatment modalities that would best help the individual. To aid this process, we utilize a detailed medical history form that is required to be completed prior to the first interview.

•**Elimination/Challenge Diet:** This is a simple and no cost way to help uncover food allergies. We recommend all allergy and environmental patients undergo this 3 week home test no matter what other testing is performed. Instructions are given to eliminate the most common foods allergies for one week and then to add them back one item at a time. During this process, close observation is made by the patient looking for any symptoms or change in their condition. If there is a question of a food reaction, the item can be retested to see if a repeat reaction occurs. This elimination/challenge diet is recommended ONLY for unknown food allergies. Do not use this challenge test for known food allergies, especially those that are known to provoke serious symptoms. Refer to Appendix D for detailed instructions on this elimination/challenge diet.

•**Pulse testing:** An increase of the resting pulse after exposure to an allergen can be a simple and easy way to determine your individual sensitivities. It involves taking a resting pulse measurement (usually

341

somewhere between 60 and 90), eating a food or being exposed to a chemical or a certain room and then rechecking the pulse 15-30 minutes after the exposure. A rise of 20 points in the pulse rate may be an indication of a sensitivity to that exposure. Start by sitting quietly for 10 minutes and then take a resting pulse. Then eat one suspected food, expose yourself to a suspecting chemical or room in your office or house. Continue to rest and recheck the pulse 15 to 30 minutes later. Smoking, eating, chewing gum, emotional excitement and physical exertion must be avoided during the test. This test is simple, easy to do and has no cost. It can be done virtually anywhere and allows for testing of a wide range of substances and places. However, some people are not "pulse changers" and will not have an increase in their pulse despite being sensitive to the exposed substance. These people will not benefit from the pulse test.

•**Skin testing:** At the Woodlands Medical Center, we use two very specific types of allergy testing called serial endpoint titration (SET) and provocation/neutralization (P/N). These allergy testing procedures differ from standard allergy testing which places a panel of allergens on the skin and reads if there is a positive or negative reaction. It tests immediate Ig E reactions only. If positive, you are then placed on a standard allergy extract that is slowly made more concentrated over time. Everybody that reacts to a certain allergen is placed on the same program at the same starting dose. With SET or P/N you are not only tested to see if you are allergic to a substance, but also are tested to find the best starting dose for you as an individual. We are thus able to provide allergy therapy that harmonizes with your particular immune system and with less chance of a reaction. SET appears best suited to testing inhalants and the P/N technique is best suited for testing foods, however, we can use P/N testing for inhalants if needed. Chemicals can also be tested by the P/N method. The advantage of SET and P/N testing over standard allergy skin testing is that a treatment vial can be made specifically suited to the patient's testing results and immediately started. Furthermore, SET and P/N can assess some of those difficult to uncover delayed reactions.

•**Serum (blood) testing.** There are a number of laboratories that offer blood testing for foods and other substances. They can measure either immediate or delayed type reactions. The advantage to these tests is that they can evaluate up to several hundred items at one time. The disadvantage is their high cost and the only treatment one can offer from the results is avoidance of the food or substance provoking a positive reaction. This is not a problem if only a few items are found positive, but can become quite daunting if many foods and substances are found to be positive. Furthermore, we are unable to make any vaccine or immunotherapy from the results of the blood tests.

•**Chemical Assays:** Chemical assays of blood and tissue can be performed at special labs trained and certified to perform these delicate tests. Chemicals are usually found in the blood shortly after an exposure event. These chemicals are rather quickly stored in the body's tissues and are then difficult to uncover by blood testing. Sometimes tissue testing may be of help but this requires surgical removal of the body's tissue. If we are able to see the patient shortly after their chemical exposure we can utilize the blood assays; however, we frequently see the patient long after the exposure has occurred. In such cases the blood testing for chemicals would not likely yield much useful information.

•**Chemical Antibody Assays:** In addition to measuring the direct blood level of a chemical, we can also test for blood antibodies to chemicals. This test is better suited to those that are seen by our Centers long after their exposure. Investigations have shown that people exposed to environments containing out-gassed chemicals may produce antibodies to the chemical or to closely related chemicals. These antibodies can be detected using an ELISA technique. Furthermore, antibodies that are formed to attack a person's own tissues can be tested. This is called autoimmune disease and can be seen in the environmentally ill patient. Auto-antibodies to thyroid tissue, nerve cell tissue, muscles and connective tissue can all be measured.

•**Porphyrin Metabolic Testing:** A number of chemically sensitive people will have abnormal liver and bone marrow production of heme which is the primary component of hemoglobin in the red blood cell. Their lab tests can reveal abnormal activity in one or more of the eight enzymes involved in heme production. Chemically sensitive patients can have intermittent or constant disruption in these enzyme steps. The testing is very extensive and involves blood, urine and stool measurements for porphyrins. The timing of testing is crucial because it may be abnormal only during a chemical exposure and then return to normal once the exposure has cleared. Those most likely to benefit from this testing are chemically injured/sensitive patients with nervous system, psychological and/or skin symptoms that are triggered by chemical exposure and have at least one of the following: symptoms worse by sunlight exposure, symptoms worse by fasting, dieting or skipping meals, or the symptom of occasional red or dark brown colored urine that is not due to blood.

•**Triple Headed SPECT Scan:** This is a new brain imaging technique that measures the uptake of labeled glucose in the brain. Recent investigations have shown abnormal glucose uptake in various areas of the brain in people with chemical injury/sensitivity and chronic fatigue patients. There are only a few university centers that have a triple headed SPECT scan. This test may be helpful for those with nervous system, mental or emotional symptoms as part of their environmental illness. This test does not offer any treatment but may help establish a cause, especially if done before and after a chemical exposure.

•**Testing for Compounding Factors:** This includes testing for heavy metal overload, immune system assays, hormonal evaluation of the thyroid, adrenal, estrogen, progesterone and testosterone, Candida immune complex and antibodies in the blood; stool analysis for digestive function, bacteria, yeast or parasites; permeability testing for a "leaky intestine;" liver detoxification assessment; and vitamin, mineral and amino acid analyses. Any or all of these may be needed to take the necessary steps to decrease the total load and increase the size of the patient's "barrel."

To summarize, testing for allergy and environmental illness must be individualized to each person's unique problems. At our Centers, we make every attempt to choose those tests which will not only help diagnose the problem but then also offer specific treatment. Much of the tests just discussed are very expensive and do not offer any specific treatment. They are, however, helpful in proving environmental illness to employers, insurance companies, disability agencies and other legal agencies.

Treatment

The key to understanding the most effective treatment for allergy and environmental illness is to take as many measures as possible to reduce your total load and increase the size of your "barrel." The less frequently it overflows, the less symptoms occur and the more functional you can become. Anything and everything you can do to reduce your total load contributes positively to your health.

Avoidance: of offending allergens and reactive substances is the first and foremost treatment modality. It should always remain at the top of the list of all treatment measures. Avoidance therapy cannot be over-emphasized and recovery from allergy and chemical injury (toxicity) or sensitivity mandates avoidance measures to be taken to the best of one's ability. Those with inhalant allergy must take measures to avoid their particular offending allergens, be they dust, mold, pollens, grasses, trees or dander. Molds are frequently a problem in environmental illness and along with dusts will give symptoms all year long. Trees, grasses, pollens and weeds give seasonal symptoms only.

In some cases an allergy mask is required when inhalant avoidance is impossible. Those with known or suspected food allergies found by the elimination/challenge diet, blood or skin testing should completely avoid the offending foods for three to six months and at the same time rotate their safe foods on an every three or four day basis. Food allergy avoidance and rotation can be one of the most difficult parts of allergy treatment and it is for this reason we offer all of our expertise and support to our patients requiring this demanding but rewarding treatment. Our centers can help you find an allergy diet that is safe, enjoyable and nutritious while at the same time avoiding those foods that are making you sick. Refer to Appendix B for an example of a rotation diet. Avoidance of pollutants in air, food and water is key to decreasing unwanted chemicals from poisoning the body's biochemical pathways. Air and water filtration is frequently needed. HEPA air filters are recommended for pollens, dust and molds, while carbon block filters are recommended for chemicals and other substances. Ozone generators are also available to bind air borne allergens and chemicals in the environment so they can no longer provoke a reaction. There are many air and water filtration products on the market today and our centers can guide you in finding the best products to fit your individual needs.

Avoidance measures to chemicals also include substituting less toxic home cleaning supplies, art and craft supplies and home finishing materials for the usual toxic items. Natural methods of pest and fungus control are to be used instead of the very toxic home and lawn pesticides and fungicides frequently used today. In some cases toxic carpets and gas heaters and stoves may need to be replaced.

Pure drinking water is equally important. According to the National Resource Defense Council, July 1994, 50 million people are drinking tap water that is contaminated with heavy metals, pesticide residue or harmful bacteria. Of them, one million people have suffered some form of health consequence and 900 have died. The best source of pure water at this time is natural spring water found in glass bottles that has been tested for purity. Such water is very difficult to find today but is not impossible. The next best would include charcoal filtered tap water, and lastly, spring or distilled water found in plastic bottles.

Although avoidance measures may initially appear daunting and overwhelming, a combination of a commitment to wellness on your part, patience, and the careful guiding hand of our Centers can transform your present environmentally sick home, school and office to an oasis of health and healing. Refer to the end of this chapter for more help on taking avoidance measures and other resources to aid this worthwhile endeavor.

Immunotherapy: The Woodlands Medical Center offers immunotherapy for inhalant, food and chemical sensitivities. These desensitizing extracts can help control reactions to your particular offending substances by modulating your immune system to be less reactive to them. We have obtained the best results using injection therapy for inhalants and sublingual (drops under the tongue) for foods and chemicals. We can, however, use sublingual drops for inhalants, especially for children. Allergy shots are usually given weekly while drops are routinely administered three times a day under the tongue. Immunotherapy is usually continued for one to three years but some may obtain full benefit with less or more time required. When using immunotherapy for chemicals, it must be understood that we are treating only the "allergic" aspect of chemical exposure, not the toxic aspect of the chemical exposure.

We are anxiously awaiting the results of a new and exciting form of immunotherapy called Enzyme Potentiated Desensitization (EPD). This form of allergy treatment uses the aid of enzymes in the extract and only requires one shot every two months. If the final studies are as promising as the initial investigations, we will surely offer this "new and improved" immunotherapy technique to all those that may benefit.

Nutritional Therapy: Most individuals with environmental illness have nutritional imbalances, that if not corrected, significantly limit the potential for improvement. Proper nutrition is vital for your body's detoxification and biochemical pathways to function at their prime. Nutritional assessment and treatment must be individually based as each of us is genetically different from another. Truly, in terms of nutritional therapy, one man's meat is another's poison. The environmentally ill patient must obtain nutritional supplements that are of the purest quality, easily absorbed into the system, while at the same time not provoking a sensitivity reaction. At times, intravenous vitamins, minerals and amino acids may be needed to overcome severe deficiencies and intestinal malabsorption problems that are not responsive to oral supplementation alone.

Detoxification: Environmental patients universally have weak detoxification processes as the result of genetic influences or from chemical injury to these biochemical pathways. We feel that supporting the body's ability to detoxify from environmental insults is a prerequisite for successful treatment of this condition. Although nutritional therapy is a cornerstone to supporting and strengthening our detoxification mechanisms, additional measures are taken to fully accomplish this goal. For example, EDTA or DMPS chelation may be needed for heavy metal removal from the body's tissues. Refer to the Appendix A for a detailed explanation of our detoxification program.

Acid-Alkaline Balance: The majority of environmentally injured people are too acidic resulting from their overworked detoxification processes. All of our detoxification pathways run better in a slightly alkaline environment. The best way to achieve an alkaline body and blood pH is to consume adequate amount of vegetables to balance the acid forming proteins and carbohydrates. Consuming "green" drinks and supplements like barley green, blue green algae and sun Chlorella can also shift the balance to a more alkaline environment in a gentle and natural manner. Some environmental patients find acute relief from sensitivity and exposure reactions with the administration of alkaline salts. This can simply be accomplished by added ¼ teaspoon of baking soda to a glass of water and drinking several times until the reaction has subsided. One may also use standard formulas such as "Bi-carb Formula" by Vital Life or other tri-salt formulas. Bi-carb formula contains a balanced mixture of sodium bicarbonate and potassium bicarbonate. Calcium carbonate can also be used as a third type of alkalinizing salt.

Hormonal Therapy: We frequently see hormonal imbalances and glandular weaknesses in the environmentally injured and sensitive patient. It appears that chemicals in our environment have the ability to mimic some of our own hormones, especially estrogen, leading to a relative estrogen excess and progesterone deficiency in our bodies. Furthermore, these chemicals can also weaken and disrupt other hormonal functions such as thyroid, thymus and adrenal. This is so common that we universally consider the adrenal patient as described in chapter II and the environmentally ill patient "sister diseases" and treatment for one is treatment for the other. A careful review of chapter II will benefit all environmentally ill people. A careful hormonal and glandular evaluation is crucial to recovery of the environmentally ill patient.

Treatment of Infection: Allergies and sensitivities can develop after an infection and hidden, smoldering infections can intensify sensitivity symptoms. Any viral, bacterial, parasitic or other type of infection should be treated at the same time attention is given to strengthening the immune system. Intestinal infections with bacteria, parasites and yeast are perhaps the number one microbial burden to the immune system and must be eliminated for full recovery. The well popularized yeast syndrome is but one example of these intestinal invaders that can play havoc with the immune and detoxification systems.

Treatment of Digestive Dysfunction: A poor, weak digestive system seems to accompany nearly all of our environmentally ill patients. It appears that a downhill spiral occurs as environmental insults weaken the digestive function, so then a dysfunctional digestive system can intensify allergic and sensitivity reactions, namely to foods. As an example, food allergies can create inflammatory reactions in the intestinal lining that results in malabsorption and the "leaky gut" (see Appendix C) while at the same time the weakened intestinal absorption allows for the development of more food allergies. Treatment efforts are directed towards avoidance of offending food and chemical allergens while supporting the digestive functions with well tolerated, nontoxic digestive supplements.

Treatment of Dental Toxic Burdens: As discussed in chapter 22, metal dental fillings that contain mercury can lead to health problems and may be another load to the immune and detoxification systems. Trace amounts of infection hiding in old root canals can also be a hidden source of infection. We work in close association with several biologic dentists that are not only aware of these hidden problems, but can offer you the best dental care in treating them. If mercury toxicity is determined to be a problem, then a specific detoxification program can be administered after removal of these noxious fillings.

Osteopathic or Chiropractic Manipulation Therapy: As discussed in a previous chapter, musculoskeletal conditions and malalignments may be part of the environmental patient's total load. By evaluating and treating such problems, the total load is reduced and one step closer to recovery is taken.

Homeopathy: Constitutional and acute homeopathic treatment can be a boon to the environmentally ill patient who frequently cannot tolerate medications and often supplements. Because this therapy offers only help without side effects or creating other total load burdens, we encourage all environmental and allergy patients to consider homeopathic therapy. Refer to chapter 15 for a more complete description of homeopathic medicine.

Rest and Exercise: A careful balance must be achieved between the needed rest for recovery of the adrenal glands, immune and detoxification systems with the benefits of a slow, gradual, graded exercise program that can be an essential part of the environmentally ill patient's treatment. This balance must be carefully obtained through the guiding hand of your Center physician.

Mental, Emotional and Spiritual Treatment: As stated in chapter II, stress, regardless of its origin, adversely affects the adrenal endocrine system, immune system and just about all other functions in the body. Autogenic training, deep breathing techniques, visual imagery, humor, laughter, and developing and nurturing a positive, productive attitude all aid in stress management and improve health. Because most medical providers are not familiar with environmental illness and its effects on the nervous and emotional systems, many individuals are inappropriately labeled with a mental health disorder by their orthodox physician and prescribed some sort of psychiatric drug in a futile attempt to mask symptoms. On the other hand, some environmentally ill patients also report past or present mental, emotional or spiritual traumas, that if unresolved, may be a part of their total load and interfere with recovery. Our Center practitioners are uniquely qualified to help you with these issues and are trained to be most discreet in such matters. The road to recovery from environmental illness is truly one that travels via the path of the spirit.

The success of your treatment and the length of your recovery is extremely variable and dependent on many factors. Namely, the number of allergies and sensitivities you have; your unique inheritance factors; the length of time you have been ill; your nutritional state; other diseases present and the degree of chemical injury received. It is for this reason we must take an individual treatment approach to accomplish the detective work needed to reduce the total trigger load and increase the size of your "barrel." We cannot accomplish this without addressing the individual as a complete whole: body, mind and soul. This way of healing is a rebalancing process which often takes time. This time of healing, however, should not be looked upon with impatient resentment, but embraced as the necessary means by which you may learn, grow and develop in every aspect of your being. Dr. Marshall Mandell has said that in order to treat our ills, we "look for magic, but must in the long run settle for hard work." We are ever willing to be a guiding force in your effort to recover from allergy and environmental illness.

Chemical (Xenobiotic) Avoidance Measures

We don't have all of the answers on where environmental xenobiotics are found and how they are absorbed into our systems. However, the following are some recommendations on what you can try to do to lower your exposure.

Source of Chemicals and Action to be Taken With Food

The key for safer food is reducing the number of chemicals that could contaminate it. Whenever possible, as budget and availability allow, buy organically grown, unsprayed, fresh, whole food. Some farmer's cooperatives and supermarket chains are using private companies to test their produce for pesticide residues. Look for certification.

Thoroughly wash fruits and vegetables in a mild soapy solution (bit of ivory soap in a pint of water) or use a commercial fruit and vegetable wash designed to remove pesticide residue. Then wash off the washing solution. Discard outer leaves of lettuce and other leafy greens.

Buy locally produced foods and avoid foods grown in other countries they may be imported with possible pesticide contaminants that are banned for U.S. use. Out-of-season fruit is usually imported and is twice as likely to be contaminated as domestic fruit.

Eat fewer and smaller portions of fatty foods, including animal products as many of the xenobiotic chemicals are stored in fats. Trim off fatty portions of meat as much as possible.

Choose minimally processed and packaged foods. Peel waxed produce. Wax is often mixed with fungicides and cannot be washed off.

Preventing Plastic Chemicals From Migrating into Food and Water

Chemicals in plastic tend to migrate into fatty foods, especially hot fatty foods Plastic wrap should never come into direct contact with fatty food in the microwave. Do not use left-over margarine or yogurt tubs in the microwave. Use ceramic or glass cookware instead.

350

When possible, replace plastic cups, Styrofoam cups and other eating utensils that come into contact with hot fatty foods with glass or metal. For example, instead of buying a plastic thermos, consider a metal one.

As much as possible, avoid food, water and other beverages sold in cans, plastic containers and plastic bottles. For example, try to buy water from distributors who can deliver large glass jugs in convenient dispensers.

Reducing Inhalation of Chemicals

The newer the plastic or synthetic product, the more it will release or "out gas" chemicals.

You can speed up the out gassing process of some products, such as a new shower curtain, for example, by baking them out in the sun for a few days. It may help to wash new plastic, such as children's toys, with washing soda.

Consider buying used products, such as a used car, instead of a new one. Avoid heating plastic, unless you are purposely "baking it out." For example, ensure that electrical cords aren't resting on top of heating elements, and if you live in the country don't burn trash at all (and ask your neighbor to stop, too). Use as much ventilation as possible when new appliances such as computers and hair dryers are switched "on." Choose untreated natural building and home furnishing supplies.

Pesticide Control

Reduce your exposures to pesticides. Don't use them yourself at home or in the garden, and pay attention to where you or your family might be exposed to them—on the golf course, in the office, or from neighbors.

There are good alternatives to pesticides for pest control. Integrated Pest Management (IPM) is a pesticide control system which minimized pesticide use and was established by the US Dept of Agriculture under President Carter (see B.I.R.C. below). Check your supermarket for IPM grown produce when you cannot obtain organic food.

351

Resources

Mother's and Others for a Livable Planet, Inc. 40 West 20 St., NY NY 1oo11. A nonprofit organization dedicated to translating environmental concerns to everyday life through information and education.

The Bio-Integral Resource Center (B.I.R.C.), PO Box 7414 Berkeley, CA 94707 Publication and service nonprofit organization for least toxic pest management (IPM)

Americans for Safe Food, Center for Science in the Public Interest, 1501 W 16TH ST, NW, Washington, DC 20036-1499. Can provide a list of mail order suppliers of organic food.

Less Toxic Living, 5th edition. Carolyn Gorman. Environmental Health Center, Dallas, TX. 1993. (215-236-1890). Excellent paperback book listing of safer home and office products and where to obtain them.

Nontoxic, Natural and Earthwise, Debra Lynn Dadd. Jeremy Tarcher, Inc. 1990. List over 400 inexpensive do-it-yourself formulas to protect yourself and your family from harmful products. It also lists over 600 mail order sources of less toxic products for the home and office.

The Whole Way to Allergy Relief and Prevention, Jacqueline Krohn, M.D. Hartley & Marks Pub., 1991. This book is a must for all environmentally ill individuals. It is a practical encyclopedia and a complete guide to treatment and self care of environmental illness.

Success in the Clean Bedroom, A Path to Optimal Health, Natalie Golos and William Rea, M.D. Pinnacle Publishers, 1992. A step by step approach from your bedroom to your kitchen helping you create a nontoxic home and office. Excellent information and practical pointers.

Staying Well in a Toxic World, Understanding Environmental Illness, Multiple Chemical Sensitivities, Chemical Injury and Sick Building Syndrome. Lynn Lawson. The Noble Press, 1993. The best book on describing and understanding environmental illness and chemical injury.

US Consumer Product Safety Commission's hotline: 800-638-2772

Chapter XXIV
Miscellaneous Diseases and Treatments

To keep this book a respectable length, we are grouping together in this chapter a variety of methods that aren't necessarily related but that have all proven useful in "healing the sick." I realize it is impossible to describe in one book all the techniques we use, but those discussed are typical of the work we do. If you have a problem not mentioned in this book, feel free to write or call us on our toll free line and we will reply promptly to let you know if there is a natural method of overcoming your difficulty.

Leg Ulcers and Unna's Boot

A type of therapeutic aid known as Unna's Boot is without a doubt the most useful aid I've seen for helping to heal leg ulcers and other conditions of the legs caused by interference with the return of blood *from* the legs to the heart. If the circulatory problem in the legs is due to poor blood flow *to* the legs, usually the chelation method (see Chapter **) is the preferable therapy, but if the problem is centered on an inadequate return flow to the heart because of varicosities or other inabilities of the veins to properly convey the blood, Unna's Boot therapy has proved invaluable.

The easiest way for the physician to use this device is by the use of a special gelatin-coated bandage, which can be ordered from most medical supply houses. Three or four-inch widths are used, depending on the size of the legs. The affected leg is wrapped from toe to knee very carefully and evenly with the gelatin bandage. When the gelatin bandage dries, it produces a moist non-rigid but inelastic leg cast, which helps support the collapsed veins in a way that support hose and even heavy elastic stockings can not. As the patient walks, the massage action between this bandage and the veins greatly increases the venous blood flow. The increased blood flow enables the body healing mechanism to function more normally and most leg ulcers heal within a relatively short time once the Unna's Boot treatment is initiated.

It may be possible at first to leave the bandage on only a day or two if the leg is very sensitive and in some extreme cases we have had to replace the bandage daily until the circulation improved and pain diminished. Once the sensitivity is reduced, however, the bandage may be left on for a week or two between replacements, although for best healing

I prefer not to leave it on longer than one week because after this time it dries out too much to provide its most beneficial therapeutic effect.

A patient with the Unna's Boot should always be encouraged to walk while the bandage is in place. The milking of the veins that occurs during rhythmic walking effects the healing, rather than the bandage itself.

This method is not unique with our Centers, or even to our profession. It was developed by a medical physician and is available to all general practitioners. However, in our forty years of practice we have found very few physicians who use or who are even familiar with this therapy. Perhaps, because it is messy and somewhat tedious to put on, many physicians eschew it for antibiotics and various salves and ointments. The prescribing of these, rather than applying the Unna's Boot certainly does save time for the physician, but in our experience doesn't always benefit the patient.

If you have leg ulcers or similar inflammatory states due to varicose veins or other vascular difficulties, I suggest you look into the Unna's Boot. It is entirely natural, harmless, inexpensive and extremely effective in almost all instances.

Recently, we have added the **MicroLight 830 LLLT** therapy to that with the Unna's Boot. By treating the leg ulcer just prior to the putting on the Boot, we have been able to hasten healing.

The Jobst Machine

While on the subject of leg difficulties, I want to mention the Jobst Company of Toledo, Ohio, which devoted almost its entire efforts to appliances that aid the circulation and overcome swelling of the legs and feet. Although this company makes a variety of excellent elastic stockings and related products, it is their reciprocal pneumatic machine for reducing leg edema that we want to describe.

The Jobst machine, which is designed to help drain the various forms of water or edema from the legs and arms of patients so afflicted, consists of an automatically controlled air compressor unit and a rubber and cloth boot that goes over the affected extremity. The boot is built like a balloon, and a small tube from it fits onto the compressor. The compressor inflates the boot so that it applies pressure evenly on all parts of the treated limb. After a short preselected time, the pressure is released and the boot collapses for a specific interval. This alternating cycle is repeated as long as is desired, usually fifteen to twenty minutes per part.

By this intermittent compression and decompression, the blood and lymph are greatly aided in their passage from the affected limb. If these treatments are properly given, combined with other efforts to remove the cause of the vascular congestion and edema, the patient will receive great help in overcoming the edema.

The Jobst machine can't cure because it doesn't remove the cause of the condition. However, when the congestion is overcome, the cause can often be more readily attacked by our other natural methods.

The Webber Technique

In my work, I come into contact with many fascinating people; high on this list was H. C. Webber. A chemical engineer by profession and an organic gardener by desire and avocation. Webber has one of the most astute medical investigative minds that I have ever encountered. In his formative years he examined the whole procedure of the chiropractic and osteopathic adjustment. At that time he formulated certain personal conclusions that were contrary to those generally held by other investigators in this field, but that he believed to be valid. In order to implement his discoveries, he helped to develop a specific type of adjusting table that he thought more physiologically designed than any he had seen previously. With this table, he produced a variety of manipulations that were different from any then or now in vogue.

Unfortunately, Webber had no degree in medicine, so when he attempted to use this therapy to help the sick, there was a complaint, an investigation and finally an injunction preventing him from continuing his clinical research. There was no restraint, however, preventing him from teaching this method of therapy to licensed practitioners and he graciously and patiently trained me in his method manipulation.

The basic Webber technique consists of a specific gentle adjustment to open the various articular surfaces of the body vertebrae. Most chiropractic and osteopathic treatments are designed to replace malpositioned vertebrae. This method attempts to free the nerve, blood and lymph supply by freeing jammed or fixed vertebrae not necessarily out of alignment. Webber contended that his method has the effect of balancing and normalizing many of the endocrine glands, particularly the pituitary glands.

The treatment takes only a minute or two and is never harmful, so we use it routinely in many cases and most patients feel that it plays an important part in their recovery.

The specific table used in administering this therapy is designed to counteract the various adverse effects of gravity on the segments of the spine and their attendant nerves. It is rare and we are fortunate to have one of the few remaining tables approved of by Mr. Webber for his unique therapy.

Two conditions have been especially helped by this therapy: Intractable headaches of cervical (neck) origin and lumbar disc compressions. The latter cases sometimes obtain almost miraculous relief by this therapy.

Urinary Problems and Natural Treatment

Orthodox treatment for kidney problems, other than infections, has always been less than satisfactory. Because the kidneys act as filters for many of the toxic end products of drug therapy, if they become diseased, chemical medication may easily aggravate kidney disorders. Medical treatment for severe kidney diseases therefore usually consists of transplantation or kidney dialysis, in which a machine takes the place of the kidney. Very little has been done medically to help regenerate or rebuild the kidney.

Chronic kidney disorders in the earlier stages can be helped greatly by natural therapy. We don't limit ourselves to any single specific method. Because this is such a vital organ complex, we use everything at our disposal to encourage the vital force to heal the diseased kidney. If the condition has not already progressed too far, our success is usually most gratifying. Even in severe disorders, natural methods offer help; although a *complete* cure isn't to be anticipated, it isn't beyond the realm of possibility.

Alkaline Urine

One of the more common urinary problems starts as a simple burning and irritation during urination and can develop into the various forms of cystitis. This condition is generally more common in women and in, our experience, stems more often from urinary alkalosis than from any other cause. As long as the urine is slightly acid (pH 6 or less), most bacteria can't proliferate, because the acid medium isn't conducive to such growth. On the other hand, if the urine exhibits a pH above 6 (pH of 7, 8, and even 9 are possible), it then provides an acceptable medium for bacterial growth. A strongly alkaline urine can by itself, even in the absence of infection, create sufficient irritation of the urinary tissues to cause a frequent desire to void small amounts of urine.

Because urinary alkalosis is so common, we make it a policy in our Centers to check the pH of the urine in every patient complaining of frequency or burning of urination, bedwetting in children or any form of urinary disease in which there is a semblance of difficulty that might be related to the urine itself.

On the market there are several pH testing papers for selftesting. You should be able to find such papers at almost any drugstore and for those plagued by urinary difficulties such pH examination may well provide a clue to an irritating problem. Be certain that you obtain pH papers that are designed for urinary testing. You want a rather narrow range of pH (From 5.0 to 8.0 or 9.0). Wide range papers are not accurate enough to show the subtle changes in pH needed by most of our patients. We always carry the proper pH papers in stock, so if in doubt ask for them at our one of our Centers.

The treatment of urinary alkalinity is usually very simple. Dr. D. C. Jarvis recommended apple-cider vinegar and honey for the correction of urinary alkalosis. However, I don't think that acetic acid is a good compound to use in the body; in our own work, we recommend not vinegar, but cranberry juice, unsweetened or sweetened only with honey, to change urinary alkalosis in patients. Cranberry juice has proven so successful that more and more urologists are recommending it, this being one instance in which a natural product has proven more effective and successful than any of the drugs available.

Mild and infrequent cases of urinary alkalosis can be treated at home by the use of this method. We usually recommend a pint to a quart of cranberry juice a day and abstinence from milk and citrus fruits during the treatment, because both milk and citrus fruits tend to increase the alkalinity of urine.

Urinary irritation, if caused by alkalosis, should leave shortly after treatment is begun. If the irritation persists, if it occurs more than once or twice a year, or if it is improved while taking the cranberry juice only to return when the cranberry juice is discontinued, home treatment is not adequate, and you should call our Center promptly.

Digestive Disorders

At one time, it was necessary for man, like the other animals, to search long and hard for his food. Usually he was pleased to obtain sufficient food to assure basic sustenance. At that time, man, as most wild animals now, probably had few digestive disturbances. For many centuries, however, man has been so resourceful in providing for himself that food for most is readily obtainable, not only in amount but also in such variety that it boggles the imagination. While the imagination may be boggled, the digestive apparatus is disturbed. In general, today, we tend to eat too much of too many things from too many areas, too often and under the wrong circumstances.

One has only to watch TV commercials to discover what ails us. Commercials for Alka-Seltzer, Bromo-Seltzer, Tums, RollAids, Maalox and a variety of other substances to help us when we eat "not wisely but too well" fill the screen. Recently, even these have not seemed adequate to quell the complaining digestive system and so the FDA has seen fit to allow the over the counter use of the much stronger anti acid drugs like Tagamet. While this move is a bonanza for the Drug Cartels we cannot help but be concerned just what it will do, long term, to the digestive systems of Americans. Commercials for these products alternate with those trying to sell us something for our headaches, which, too, are often caused by improper diet, or something for constipation which is almost always caused by bad diet. A good two-thirds of the drug commercials on TV are for products that are directly or indirectly connected with our digestion.

At our Healing Research Centers, we treat a great many digestive disorders. The first fundamental of all such treatment is to correct the patient's food intake. Most patients can be greatly helped by simply placing them on our Basic Maintenance Diet, a diet designed and balanced to help the digestive system correctly handle the food that enters it. In many specific disorders however, such as gastritis, peptic ulcers and colitis, specific diets must be given at least until the basic pathologic disorder is overcome. Along with these diets, nutritional remedies are prescribed that aid in healing the patient's disorder.

Many herbal and homeopathic remedies are designed for overcoming digestive disturbances. These disorders, which are so rife in humanity, often respond poorly to orthodox drug therapy because the drugs, since they are not basically natural to the body environment, often aggravate the condition when used over a long time. The natural nutritional remedies and herbs are readily accepted by the system, as one might welcome an old friend returned from a long journey.

Many digestive disturbances are basically of nervous origin rather than due to specific organic causes. There is a large nerve center behind the stomach called the celiac, or solar plexus. If this nerve center becomes disturbed, which can easily happen if the emotions are upset, the whole mechanism of digestion can readily become disoriented. I find that, when this has occurred gentle fingertip manipulation of the nerve reflexes on the abdomen and over the solar plexus does much to relieve this nervous disorder. In fact, this is the only therapy that some patients receive at our Center and it has been known to completely cure many nervous digestive disorders. In addition to the manual manipulation of the Solar Plexus, we are now beginning to use the LLLT on this are with good results.

In severe digestive disorders, we aren't afraid to use our whole armamentarium of natural methods. The herbal colon therapy, diathermy, sine wave, Magnatherm, manipulation, spinal therapy, LLLT and the

Webber treatment all have their place in certain problems. Most digestive disorders are caused, however, by improper diet and emotional irritability. Whenever we find these problems in our patients, we attempt to correct them before serious pathologic disorder results. In doing this, we can make the Beverly Hall Corporation Healing Research Center live up to its name.

Hemorrhoids (Piles)

Some disorders, like the fruit "prunes," bring a smile to our lips whenever they are mentioned. This is true unless you happen to be a grower of prunes or are afflicted with the mentioned disorder. Hemorrhoids obviously fall into this last category. You will never see a TV doctor treat hemorrhoids; they don't make for great drama, but more pain and discomfort can stem from this disorder than from a great many of the more "respectable" diseases.

Most cases of hemorrhoids are caused by congestion of the hemorrhoidal veins, which may result from several circumstances: (1) hereditary weakness of the venous tissues; (2) constipation, which puts pressure on the hemorrhoidal veins, interfering with the proper drainage; (3) any form of liver congestion, because the hemorrhoidal veins drain into the portal circulation, which passes through the liver before reaching the heart; and (4) various forms of colon and rectal disease, which may cause irritation and weakness of the tissues in this area.

The usual medical treatment for hemorrhoids is surgical removal. Some years ago injection treatments and negative galvanism were popular, though at present most of these non-surgical methods have lost favor and most physicians simply recommend the knife. What most physicians don't tell their patients is that the recovery period from this operation can be very painful because the rectal area has many sensitive nerve endings. It is also a rare physician who tells his patients that unless his habits are changed the hemorrhoids very likely will return necessitating another operation.

There are some patients in whom an operation is probably the therapy of choice; however, many cases of hemorrhoids respond very well to natural methods. In all cases, it should be the naturalist's duty to remove the cause of the disorder.

Constipation should be investigated; the general diet should be arranged to remove as much stress as possible from the liver; the patient should be warned about the use of highly spiced foods; alcoholic beverages should not be used, particularly wines and cordials; and sugar should be restricted to healthful limits. More fresh fruits and vegetables should be eaten and any local disorders of the rectum or associated areas that can be treated without surgery should be corrected. If the foregoing regimen is carried out in conjunction with herbal and specific nutritional supplement support, surgery can be circumvented in many instances. Where an operation must be performed, such a regimen at least should prevent the recurrence of hemorrhoids after the surgery.

For mild disorders, I can recommend a home treatment that has truly proven useful and sometimes almost miraculous in its curative capabilities. This is what I call my garlic and honey method.

The patient is asked to obtain some untreated and unpasteurized honey and several bulbs of garlic. Each night before he goes to bed, he is to remove one clove from the garlic bulb, strip off its papery outer covering and make a few small scratches in it with a paring knife. This clove of garlic is then dipped in the honey and inserted into the rectum as high as the index finger can push. The clove is left in place and will be voided with the next bowel movement, usually the next morning. Garlic oil is one of the most powerful healing agents known for rectal and hem orrhoidal irritation.

The garlic should be used for four nights in succession; then on the fifth night the raw honey should be warmed until it just loses its viscosity and runs freely. This honey is then drawn up into an ear syringe and injected into the rectum. The following night the garlic is again used and thereafter the honey and the garlic are alternated each night until a complete cure has taken place. Such a cure may take anywhere from one week to a month, depending on the severity of the inflammation.

It is important for the patient using this method to watch his diet and also to follow the general recommendations made for all hemorrhoid patients.

Here too, of late, we have been adding the LLLT with very good and sometimes near miraculous results.

The Marvelous Red Beet

The method I am about to describe is one I knew nothing about when I began to write this book. It all came about in this fashion: A short time ago I treated a woman for an abscess of the breast. Although our treatment was helpful, the disorder kept recurring, and even my most valued natural methods didn't seem capable of stemming its course. Out of desperation, the patient took antibiotics. Although this controlled the immediate reaction, it didn't prevent a recurrence. During the last exacerbation, the patient was visiting an old physician friend of hers in California who suggested that she try slicing a red beet and putting the raw slices over the abscessed breast. He told her that it was a method he himself had just learned recently and so far he found it very successful for such disorders. She tried it, and within a few days the abscess was cured and hasn't returned since.

After returning to Pennsylvania, the patient told me of her experience and suggested I try this method. Because I am always eager to test new natural methods no matter from what source, I told her I'd try it at the first opportunity. A week or so later, a patient of another physician showed up on a day when he was off. Upon examining her, I found a large boil on her left thigh that hadn't come to a head but was large and very painful. I suggested that she put the raw sliced beet on the boil just as my patient had described to me. I told her to get in touch with me within a day or two for the boil should then be ready for lancing.

I didn't hear from the patient for about a week and then one day she dropped by. I asked her if she wanted me to lance her boil. She just said, "What boil?" I said, "The boil you have on your thigh." She said, "Do you want to see?" In an examination room she showed me the spot where the boil had been. The skin was absolutely normal. I could see no sign that a boil had ever been there. I was happily surprised and asked her to tell me exactly what happened.

She said, "I went home that night and I told my mother just what you said, and I never saw a woman laugh so much in all my life. She said, 'My God, what kind of an insane doctor are you going to? Tomorrow I'm going to take you to my doctor and we're going to have that boil taken care of and you're not going to any of these quack doctors again.' Then I asked her, 'Can I put on the beet tonight?' and mother answered, 'I guess it's nothing that's going to hurt. But tomorrow we get that boil taken care of!'

" So that night I put the beet on just as you told me and went to bed. When I arose in the morning, I took a look at my leg and called my mother. I showed her my leg. When the beet was removed, the boil had completely vanished. There was only a small red mark remaining. Both mother and I were amazed. Within a couple of days even the red mark had vanished and now there isn't a sign of the boil." I then asked the patient, "What did your mother do?" She said, "What do you think? She called up all her girl friends and told them about it."

The results with boils and abscesses were so dramatic that I started using the beet slices for other staph infections. One of the most common forms encountered in daily practice in that of severe acne, and I suggested the beets for several of our worst cases. In almost all instances, the most severe lesions disappeared overnight. One patient told me that within two hours after putting on the beet, the pustule had vanished.

Although "beet therapy" isn't a cure-all for acne, since it works only on the surface lesion, it is a great help and certainly far more natural and physiologic than the various suppressive creams, antibiotics and other more or less toxic substances usually used for this purpose.

What is it in the red beet that performs this miraculous function? I don't know. I only know that it works with amazing consistency and regularity. We are now in the process of testing the raw beet and the raw beet juice in a variety of other conditions and as this investigation proceeds, we shall report on more on this in future publications of our Healing Research Centers.

I wish to diverge from my subject for a moment to comment on the use of natural agents. Boils and red beets have been with mankind for many centuries and yet only now we are using the one to cure the other. With such a common condition, miraculously aided by such a common vegetable, being undiscovered by mankind for these many centuries, one must wonder how many other serious diseases could be helped by simple natural methods if only the time and energy were taken to investigate them. Our government spends millions of dollars annually to investigate disease and yet, until just recently, not one penny of this was spent studying natural methods. All this money goes into the continued research of orthodox medicine's destructive methods. If only a small portion of these funds was advanced to study natural methods, who can say how many beet-and-boil relationships we might find?

Hyfercation

This method, like the Unna Boot, is not unique to our Healing Centers. It is a basic medical treatment, but it isn't well known to most patients.

Hyfercation is a method by which small skin growths such as warts, moles and papillomas can be removed by the application of a high-frequency electrical current. In common parlance, the skin defect is "burnt off." Such a method was quite popular at one time, though in recent years it seems to have lost much of its popularity; most physicians use either surgery or other methods such as freezing for removing these small skin growths.

In each instance—hyfercation, surgery, or freezing—one is destroying the tissues. Because the destruction is approximately the same with each method, theoretically there is little reason to prefer one over the other. In practice, however, they differ. There are several reasons why we prefer the electrical method in our Healing Centers.

It is simple and speedy. A small mole or wart can be removed in just a few seconds. While for most small growths, we don't find anesthesia necessary, a topical (local) anesthetic can be used. Usually we merely place a small ice bag on the site to be hyfercated for a minute or two before treatment and this numbs the area sufficiently for all except the most complicated cases. Rarely is the pain encountered during hyfercation objectionable to the average patient, and it disappears almost immediately after the treatment. In my experience, both freezing and surgery are less painful at the time but more painful later. The hyfercated area needs little after-attention and most patients rapidly forget that the treatment has even been given.

Hyfercation, by the nature of its heat and desiccation, tends to kill any malignant cells as it removes the offending part, whereas the scalpel may cause such cells to pass into the bloodstream, even though a large section of the offending object is removed. There have been no incidents known to us of malignant material being spread by hyfercation.

The use of this method is, of course, a matter of opinion. We at the Healing Research Center use it almost exclusively for removing small skin encumbrances, and we have never yet had a dissatisfied patient.

Skin Diseases

Practically all skin diseases respond very well to natural therapy. In fact one of the first great natural physicians, Father Sebastian Kneipp, considered the skin to be the major organ of disease elimination and he did much of his work to treat this portion of the anatomy.

In natural healing, we look upon skin conditions in a different light than do our medical contemporaries. We believe that most so called skin diseases are merely the body's attempt to eliminate a disease toxicity through this organ with the largest area in the body. Therefore we generally treat this condition from the inside out—that is, we work to overcome the internal disease process so that the skin elimination will no longer be necessary and the skin can then clear and become supple and smooth once again.

The medical treatment of skin conditions is usually by what we call the suppressive route, in which various substances are used to suppress or drive the skin eruption into the body. This action, according to naturopathic and homeopathic theory clears the skin but forces these toxic substances back into the body fluids, where they can do great harm that only becomes apparent later.

The natural healer will treat the skin as well, but it is always with a form of treatment that hastens the removal of toxic products and never leads to their suppression.

The LLLT has proven to be of surprising value in skin conditions. It seems to aid the body in its eliminative efforts and in this way is in full harmony with natural therapeutic law. Several miraculous cures have been affected by its use in recent months.

"Poison"

We work and live in Pennsylvania Dutch country and one of the most common skin disorders here is what the local folk call "poison." This is usually an attack of contact dermatitis from poison ivy, oak or sumac. We use various homeopathic and specific natural remedies with great success in the treatment of this very aggravating condition, but a therapy I nearly always recommend is very simple and can be used by anyone anywhere. This is the parsley tea treatment.

To prepare this properly, 2 quarts of water are brought to a boil and then removed from the heat. Fresh cut parsley is spread liberally on top of the water, a lid placed over all, and the potion allowed to steep for half an hour. The liquid is then poured off and refrigerated. Two tablespoonsful of the tea is taken each hour until the condition is healed. Even the most severe cases of "poison" can be helped with this therapy, although for the best results you should consult a Center physician for the proper nutritional and homeopathic remedies to accompany the parsley treatment. .

Few conditions are so exasperating to most physicians as those of the skin. We in the health field believe this to be true because physicians usually attempt to treat them in direct opposition to Nature's efforts. In our work we trust Nature and try to aid her in her efforts. We are almost always well rewarded by her and by our grateful patients' thanks.

Foot Problems

The big problems with foot conditions is that it is difficult to rest the affected part and still carry on any kind of a normal life. Very facetiously I tell patients who want to know how to relieve the pressure on their feet to, "Learn to walk on their hands."

In all seriousness however, there are few things more distressful than painful feet. Many of these problems can be avoided if the proper measures are taken early on in life.

Excepting congenital deformities, most of our are born with good feet. It is what we do to them as we grow and mature that causes us most of our later problems. The villain, assuming there is a villain, is not our unnatural appetite, our indolence or even the Medical Profession (how rare) but Dame Fashion. The natural foot is narrowest at the heel and from there widens until it is at its widest at the toes. Fashion, for centuries, has declared that this is not attractive; or worse yet, not sensual. Dame Fashion tells us that our footware needs to come to some form of a point in the area of the toes. Thus dictating a footware form that is in direct opposition to that of nature.

When fashion is observed, the foot suffers first and then, as the various forms of foot conditions develop from the long term unnatural pressures placed on the foot, the fashionable wearer suffers for the rest of his (or her) life. Thus, the vast majority of foot deformities that occur in our mature citizens can be laid at the feet (with her bunions, hammer toes and the like) of Dame Fashion.

What to do about it. The various foot problems can be helped by natural means. The new LLLT is helping many of these sufferers, but in truth the main reason for this section is to make a plea to mothers and fathers to see that their children are not forced to suffer as so many of us have. Look at your children's feet and insist that they are fitted with shoes that match the anatomy of the foot. Let's not feed any more foot victims to Dame Fashion. We were able to put the deforming corsets of the last century behind us; why not the deforming shoes of this century?

Interestingly, there are shoes that are made in the form of the foot. They are made by special firms who cater only to those individuals with severe foot conditions. If these shoes are a part of the cure for such people, are they not the prevention of foot deformities also?

One last comment before we leave this subject. Even though you may have good shoes with a wide space for the toes to work, you can undo some of the benefit of them by the improper use of stockings. After you pull on your stockings, grab a hold of the toe of the stocking and pull it away from the foot. This is to give the toes some room in the stocking. It seems a simple thing but it can make the difference between deformed toes and good toes.

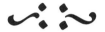

Chapter XXV
A Few Gracious Comments
On Some Old Friends

We are all too often drawn to that which is new, different, or unique and tend to ignore that which is common, old and familiar, even though these old friends may have served us well, without flinching, for many years. In this chapter, I want to say a few kind words about some old methods of therapy that have served us well over the years, but with which most patients may be unfamiliar.

Short-Wave Diathermy

To the patient, the short-wave diathermy is a "heat machine." The diathermy however, is not a heating pad. The heating pad heats because of a heat-producing coil within its inner substance. As the electricity passes through this coil, heat is produced by friction of the electrons and the pad itself becomes hot. This heat is then transferred to the patient's skin by conduction. The blood vessels under this heating pad dilate, bringing more blood to the area to carry the heat to other parts of the body so that the affected area doesn't become overheated. The heat from a heating pad rarely penetrates more than a few millimeters because the circulation rapidly carries it off. Because this surface heat stimulates certain reflexes, it is useful in many instances.

The diathermy functions on the principle of electromagnetic wave energy and, in essence, it is a small radio transmitter that produces heat by passing radio waves through various tissues of the body. As the wave passes through the body structures, heat is generated deep within the muscles and bone; if sufficient radio energy is given, temperatures up to 107° F may be produced for a few minutes in these parts.

It is thus possible to produce a selected area of fever in the body to treat certain diseases by a method similar to that which the body itself uses when it produces a temperature to overcome infective disorders.

In our Centers, the diathermy is used most commonly for relaxing the muscles of the back and other areas that may be tense. Diathermy is an excellent preliminary therapy for most of our manipulative work. Also, we find that ultrasound and other specific therapies are more effective if diathermy is used first to increase the circulation and tissue activity in the treated area.

In many muscular conditions, diathermy alone is an adequate treatment; and in these cases, diathermy produces a quicker and more satisfactory cure than the newer, more expensive modalities.

Diathermy may also be used for a variety of chronic and acute infections. One must be careful, however, not to use diathermy when the body is making a completely adequate inflammatory response on its own. Used in this instance, diathermy may interfere with the body's attempts at overcoming disorders by causing an over dilation of the involved vessels, causing stagnation instead of the desired increased circulation.

Chest congestions due to colds and flu, bronchitis and the many disorders in which mucous builds up in the bronchial tubes respond well to short-wave diathermy treatments. In fact, diathermy is almost specific for these conditions and good results are usually to be expected. The patients are usually all too eager to tell you how much better they feel after the first diathermy treatment.

Many low-grade chronic infections can also be helped by using short-wave diathermy. Discretion must be used in these cases, however, for the objective is to use just enough heat to stimulate the circulation of the organ involved. If one overstimulates, one may aggravate the disorder, though this should never occur in competent hands because it takes a considerable degree of over treatment to cause trouble.

Sine Wave Therapy

Sine wave has been used therapeutically even longer than diathermy. While simple in make-up and low in cost, it is nevertheless invaluable in natural healing.

Sine wave is an alternating electrical current used to produce muscle contractions. The current that comes from your house receptacle is a 60-cycle sine wave and although it is too low in frequency and too great in amplitude to be useful medically, it also acts as a muscle stimulant. Anyone who has ever gotten a good jolt from a house outlet won't forget the way the muscles contracted.

This muscle stimulation is the only known effect of most sine wave machines on the body. Therefore in order to make sine wave therapeutically useful, it is necessary to vary the character of this contractibility so that this energy can be used for a variety of physical therapeutic purposes.

If we turn the sine wave current on and off, we produce surging sine, the muscle will contract, then relax, contract, relax, and so on. A muscle treated in this fashion will strengthen and grow in physical size. Such therapy can prove useful in rehabilitating victims of polio, stroke and diseases in which muscle atrophy plays a part. In pulsed sine wave, the alternating off and on periods are very rapid (three to four a second), acting less to strengthen the muscle than to eliminate toxic substances from the muscle and allied tissues by the constant milking effect produced by the pulsing wave.

The steady or unaltered sine wave is called a tetanizing current; it is used to reduce pain and to detect hidden inflammatory areas in certain circumstances. These three forms of sine wave enable one to produce a variety of effects in the tissues for therapeutic purposes. For instance, the tetanizing sine wave tends to reduce pain in the area because of its nature to overstimulate, thereby exhausting the pain producing components, causing them to relax and rest. In this way a particularly painful spastic muscular problem can be reduced almost instantly.

For conditions of muscular weakness, common in many low back problems and in some upper-back difficulties, we usually use surging sine wave. This strengthens the muscle and ligamentous structures in the treated area better than exercise, because a specific area can be treated so that no adverse strain is placed on the patient. Often patients with low-back problems also have other disorders that might be endangered by exercise. Here surging sine wave treatments are of great help.

Pulsed sine wave is most useful when there is a congested area we want to de-stagnate so that the blood and lymphatic fluids once again may flow freely.

In many patients, the three aforementioned conditions can occur simultaneously—that is, a muscle spasm with pain and tissue fluid stagnation. In these chronic problems, all three forms of current— tetanizing, surging and pulse—may be useful at various periods in the treatment. One of the manufacturers of sine wave equipment has produced what they call an automatic model, which alternates at minute intervals between these three forms of therapy. We use this sine wave machine exclusively at our Healing Research Center, and though the machine is expensive, we find that nothing else can take its place, and the therapy is frequently requested.

The Myoflex

The Myoflex is a form of sine wave but differs from most in that it is designed to produce an electrical wave that is supposed to be similar if not identical to that produced by the human nerve itself. In this way it is able (so says its inventor) to send constructive nerve impulses to affected body parts to aid in their healing or regeneration. Does it work? Thousands of our patients declare it does. Who am I to tell them no?

Galvanic Current

With the exception of static electricity, galvanic current (direct current) is the most ancient of all electrical forms of therapy. This current is the same type produced by a flashlight or an auto battery. It differs from sine wave in that it has polarity—one pad is positive and the other pad is negative. Because of the polarity, galvanic current has a chemical effect on the body rather than a muscle-stimulating quality.

Galvanic current produces a variety of chemical effects at its poles, which are distinctly opposite one from the other. For instance, one pole releases oxygen; the other releases hydrogen. One pole tends to soften tissue, the other tends to harden tissue. One subdues pain; the other stimulates. In general, the positive pole is used more for acute conditions, and the negative for chronic problems. For the acute state, the positive pole tends to subdue pain, reduce congestion, and stimulate the resolution of inflammatory reactions. On the other hand, the negative pole tends to soften tissue, stimulate inflammatory reactions, and dissolve calcium deposits.

You may ask why would we ever want to increase inflammation or cause inflammation? In chronic joint ailments, such as an arthritic knee or calcified shoulder bursa, we have what is known as a "cold" condition. There is little inflammation left in the area, the tissues have been inundated with calcium and the joint is stiff but not overly painful unless we try to move it beyond what the mineral deposits will allow. To heal this area, we must first dissolve the calcium, and then stimulate an inflammatory state so that the dissolved calcium will be removed and the tissues enabled to return to as normal a condition as possible. Remember it is by the process of inflammation that the body heals itself. No inflammation, no healing.

While positive galvanism is very useful in acute conditions, the negative form of galvanism can do some things that no other known form of therapy can do as well. In many chronic calcium disorders, it is a sovereign remedy in the true sense of the word, which is unfortunately little used today and almost completely ignored by orthodox medical practitioners.

Ionophoresis

Owing to the polarity of the galvanic current, it can also be used to "drive" various forms of medicinal substances into the tissues under treatment. This therapy—ionophoresis—is always used in conjunction with the basic positive or negative effects of the current.

It isn't practical here to mention the various substances that can be used with galvanic current in ionophoresis. The selection must be left up to each natural healer. I do hope, however, by this discussion of galvanism to reawaken an interest in this great remedy, which is not only effective and harmless, but is also inexpensive. This combination is very rare in medical equipment today and has never been common at any time in medical history.

Ultra Violet Therapy

Another form of therapy once very popular and now seldom used even by natural practitioners is ultraviolet light. It has suffered somewhat the same fate as galvanic therapy and, like it, should be rediscovered.

Ultraviolet light is similar to sunlight but only in a narrow band of light energy. The ultraviolet rays are tanning rays and they also are strongly bactericidal—they kill bacteria. They also cause vitamin D to develop in the skin. When there is no sunlight, as during winter, rickets can be prevented in children with ultraviolet therapy. Nowadays, of course, we use a vitamin D tablet and the same results are accomplished with less effort. I believe, however, that there are beneficial effects on young children from ultraviolet light, in addition to its ability to produce vitamin D. As the years pass, I use whole-body ultraviolet radiation more and more on my young patients who exhibit low resistance during the winter months, and I find most of them benefit greatly.

Besides the general body regenerative effects of ultraviolet radiation, it is a specific for several skin disorders—so much so that it rapidly cures many disorders that resist the best efforts of some dermatologists. In days past most dermatologists used variations of ultraviolet therapy in their practices, but it seems the siren call of the drug houses has reduced this use by the younger practitioner.

Full body irradiation is done with the hot quartz UV lamp but a cold quartz UV lamp can also be used for certain other conditions. Skin conditions frequently respond better to the cold quartz. We also use in our Centers a small cold quartz applicator that can treat many areas of the body, with these healing rays of the sun, where otherwise the sun doesn't shine.

Sunlight, even in this artificial form, apparently is a tremendous healing agent and although anything can be overdone, surely ultraviolet therapy, carefully and properly administered, deserves a place high on our list of timehonored natural methods.

Infrared Radiation

Infrared radiation probably has less effect on the physiology than any of the methods we have heretofore described. Basically, infrared radiation is produced by a long-wave heating unit. There are no chemical or electromagnetic effects known from its energy. The unit should be considered mainly as a heat lamp. As such, it serves its purpose day in, day out, relaxing patients, soothing their bodies, and preparing them for more specific therapies. It is like a servant who has only a relatively small task to perform but who performs it with skill, dedication and never failing allegiance. What more can be asked of any servant or therapy?

Interestingly, the light energy given off by that new wonder, the Low Level Laser, is in the infra red spectrum. Maybe this faithful servant had a few tricks up his sleeve that we did not know about.

Joint Manipulation

Various forms of manipulation of the bony frame have been used since earliest times. At various periods in history, man has systematized such manipulations and given the procedures titles and names. At present in this country, the most familiar methods are called osteopathy and chiropractic.

For many years after the inception of these two therapies, their practice was belittled by the more orthodox physicians. In recent years, however, the effectiveness of manipulation has so proven itself that the tone of the medical world has changed and today these therapies are gaining more and more adherents.

In our Clinic, we find that most patients have some form of mechanical bony malalignment in conjunction with whatever other condition may exist. If this mechanical condition isn't corrected, their cure is always prolonged and may be incomplete. This structural component is usually corrected by manipulation in the early stages of treatment. In this way all our other forms of therapy function better than if such corrections weren't made.

Manipulation is such an integral part of patient treatment at our Centers that we almost take it for granted. Yet, in patient after patient referred to us by other physicians we find that a cure is often obtained by using his treatment, but with manipulative therapy added. In other words, we often find that manipulation is the catalyst that enables our other therapeutic methods to function to their best advantage.

A Few Parting Words

In this chapter you have met some of our old friends. When patients come to our Centers, and see the vast array of equipment at our disposal, they often stand in awe, and perhaps sometimes wonder if all this is really necessary to get people well. The answer surprisingly is "no." All you really need to get people well is a knowledgeable physician with the skill and desire to heal. All the equipment and devices are simply aids and tools that enable us to work more speedily and efficiently. This isn't to disparage any of our instruments; they serve a purpose. A good carpenter tries to have the best tools, but he could still build a house with poor tools. It would take him longer, and the results might not be quite as good, but it could be done.

Healing comes from within. All our instruments are simply extensions of our hands and eyes to speed the curing procedure. Although we have great admiration and faith in all our new fascinating instruments, the old tools still fit well in the hand and rarely, if ever, fail us.

Patients also ask us, "Don't the new drugs make all these things obsolete?" My answer is this: Man has built a chemical house of cards for himself and his progeny. These chemical compounds, not occurring in nature, will eventually cause the body to so rebel that they will have to be abandoned. At that time the world will be very thankful for these and other natural forms of healing to help relieve them of their suffering.

Chapter XXVI
A New Look At Marital Problems

(Thirty years ago, I began work on a text entitled *One Flesh*. In this work I developed a new and somewhat unique manner of examining the sexually differentiated emotional responses of men and women. The ideas presented in this book form the basis of much of the marriage counseling that is done at our Healing Centers. The book, *One Flesh*, was never published because other work took priority, but its philosophy was preserved in this chapter of *It's Only Natural* in 1975 and again in 1986 in a work entitled *A Guide for the New Renaissance*. This present chapter will draw from both of these previous efforts in order to give you the best possible view of this effort to help both men and women to understand each other better.)

After years of counseling those with marital problems, it became apparent that there were severe discrepancies in the complaints voiced by the individual parties. The problems that upset a wife were hardly ever noticed by her husband and vice versa. At times it was difficult to realize they were both discussing the same marriage. The events in the marriage were recognized by each, but their personal evaluation was radically different.

Gradually I began to detect a pattern of predictable responses from the wife, and later a similar set from the husband. As a result of these observations, an investigation was begun into the emotional responses that could be distinctly linked to the gender of the individual. The medical literature on this subject was negligible. Many vague allusions and comments were made on the theme but no systematic dissertations were available. Most modern authors seemed to be of the opinion that there were no real differences between the male and female emotional responses. My own observations, however, wouldn't allow me to accept this conclusion, so I continued my search into philosophical and literary works. Here my efforts were better rewarded. It soon seemed obvious that the artist was more observant of his fellow man than the scientist. Although I still found no book expressly on the desired matter, the analytic minds of the great writers provided much help in formulating the theories and practices presented here.

From this extensive investigation and personal observation, I concluded that not only are there common individual gender-oriented emotional responses, but also that the causes of these can be found and categorized. This work has also shown me that an understanding of these causes can greatly help the individual to understand himself (herself) and his (her) marital partner.

The purpose of this work is therefore twofold. First, to describe in detail the causes, character and functioning of these sex-oriented incentives and, second, to show how a knowledge of these incentives can help in individual and marital contentment. I realize this is a demanding objective. If the reader won't allow his preconceptions to interfere with his search for truth, I believe he will find my enthusiasm not altogether unwarranted.

In researching my subject, I have always tried to keep the law of cause and effect uppermost in my mind. Because I believe this to be an orderly not a chaotic universe, I have always sought a practical reason behind any theoretic emotional incentive I might postulate. It was therefore necessary in beginning this study to investigate the basic differences between male and female and particularly their distinctive purposes in Nature's plan.

For Creation to continue and prosper some form of gender is necessary so that the various species may be perpetuated. At times, as in the case of some trees, the entire process is encompassed in one unit. In most animal forms of life, the reproductive functions have been separated and the male and female forms evolved.

In the instance of complete sexual units one can say that each is like the other, as the function of a tree is like other unisexual trees. Once the individual parts of reproduction are separated, however, this similarity no longer exists. Because the purpose and nature of the male unit of reproduction is different from that of the female (and vise versa), a different set of rules and incentives was necessary to regulate each. I feel that these incentives were logically devised to help ensure the continuance of each individual life form. Therefore, by examining the incentives that would, in the case of each gender, best fulfill this demand for procreation, we may begin to discover the individual inborn incentives present in the male and female.

These incentives—inborn intuitive natures—aren't directly related to the mental or moral fiber of the individual. They are simply drives placed within his or her being to carry out the design and demands of Nature. Because the natural needs and demands for the male and female are different, it only makes biologic sense that the emotional nature of the male and female must vary to meet these distinctive demands.

The most important natural laws at this level of existence are those for the conception, growth and final maturation of the young animals. Because of certain physical laws that must be considered. in the fulfillment of these objectives, Nature has established certain patterns in the animal kingdom that, although altered in certain species, are sufficiently stable to enable us to make some general conclusions.

In most forms of higher female life, the egg (ovum) necessary for fertilization is discharged at only a few specific periods during her sexual maturity. In the human, this is usually about once a month, while in some animals it occurs only two or three times a year. We therefore have a variable fertilization factor in one of our sexual partners.

If the male had a similar cycle—if his sperm was only present at a certain time during the month, or year—much difficulty might ensue, attempting to make these two times coincide. Therefore to ensure fecundation, and the perpetuation of the species, it was necessary for the male to have a constant supply of sperm so that fertilization might be possible whenever an ovum was ready. It was also necessary that the male should have a readily-awakened desire for this cohabitation, because when the female's time arrives, no matter how short it may be, there should be a male available to use her fertile period advantageously. The only practical way that this could be accomplished would be to have the male (more or less) ready at all times.

Because it is only necessary—or practical from Nature's point of view—for the female animal to allow coitus at the time of her ovulation, Nature gave her desire and acquiescence only at this time. The male, on the other hand, in order to fulfill his biologic purpose, must be capable of desire at any time. These dictates of Nature for the animal world, to a large extent, are carried over to the human world. Although we, as the superior species of the earth, don't particularly like comparison with the lower animals, it is nevertheless true that the same need for the perpetuation of the species that Nature demands of them is also demanded of us. It is therefore only practical to expect conservative Nature to put the same or similar incentives in us as well as them.

From this discussion, we may surmise that the first sexually differentiated incentive is that given to the male animal, which creates in him, in his youth at least, a constant or nearly constant desire to cohabit with the female of his species, thus helping to perpetuate his own kind. In most animals, when he has performed this duty, the need for his services is over and he can go his way. The biologic demands on the female, however, are now just beginning, for it is she who must bear the consequences of impregnation through the long months of intrauterine maturation of the offspring. She must pass also through the trials of birth and aftercare until the progeny is mature enough to be on its own. The intuitive drives necessary to see that this program of Nature is carried out in the best interests of the species are obviously quite different than those previously ascribed to the male.

377

In the average female of the upper animal species, an actual biologic desire for sexual relations isn't necessary. Acquiescence alone is adequate. Pleasure isn't denied her, but it isn't essential for fertilization.

The main natural incentives that she must have are those producing love, affection and the desire to be a mother to her offspring. These must be so strong that she is willing to give her own life to protect the products of her womb. This must be carried forth by a drive within her that she follows intuitively, so that she may care properly for this infant until it is strong and intelligent enough to subsist without her.

Thus, in Nature, there is need for two entirely different and distinct biologic incentives. First, we must have on the part of the male a strong, unvarying and unswerving desire to cohabit with the female. This desire must be so compelling that whenever she is ready for cohabitation, he will not only be physically prepared, but also psychologically and emotionally eager to enter into such an act. She, on her part, need only have enough feeling and desire to acquiesce to this sexual invasion of her privacy. It isn't necessary that she enjoy such an embrace, although such isn't denied her. From this time on, however, assuming that fertilization has taken place, her own biologic incentives begin to take precedent. All her instincts directed toward the care and nurturing of the creature growing within her are brought to the fore. After the emergence of this small replica of her species, she is flooded with maternal impulses that don't abate until all progeny have left her protecting care. From Nature we are therefore provided with the basis of the first two sexually-oriented and differentiated instincts .

Primary Sexual Incentives

With this background, we can transfer these principles to humans. These basic incentives are present to a great degree in most of this planet's races, even though their forms may be greatly disguised by our civilized ways. The innate purpose of these incentives in the animal world is also a requirement in the human and so we shouldn't be surprised to find close similarities. The two incentives discussed above concern basic reproduction, birth and infant care. I have therefore labeled them Primary Sexual Incentives (PSI). The PSI in the human male is, as far as I have been able to ascertain, nearly identical to that of the lower animals—it is the crude biologic urge for sexual relations with a female of his species.

The Male PSI

The mechanism for this incentive is based on the very nature of his sexual structure. In the male, two glands—the testicles— begin producing spermatozoa at puberty. The sperm henceforth will be produced each day until senility overtakes him. Along with the sperm is produced a thin fluid carrier, which with the various lubricating fluids from the prostate, Cowper's glands and other glands along the urogenital tract complete the male sexual secretion. When the secretion accumulates to a certain extent, there is a desire for release. Whether the simple pressure of the secretions brings about this desire or whether there are still more complicated unknown reasons is not a point to be discussed here. That it does occur, however, and that it is a physical and biologic fact can't be denied. This call for release has little to do with morality, goodness or anything of an intellectual nature. It is designed to fulfill a natural demand. If, after a time, it isn't released or utilized in some manner, Nature will release it as a nocturnal emission. This intrinsic production of pressure helps to establish the biologic base of the male PSI.

Nature builds the mechanism and gives man the necessary desires. What man does with it is up to him. Nature is not moral. She merely wants a continuation of the species. It is up to man to say how, when and under what circumstances this perpetuation can or should take place.

I don't want to intimate that the desire for copulation in the male is based strictly on the physiologic pressure of his sexual fluids, although this is certainly an important component of his libido. The way in which the forces producing the male PSI operate are quite complicated and can be greatly modified by certain mental and moral concepts he may have developed during his life. Yet there seems little doubt in the minds of most physicians and scientists that the continual production of sperm and seminal fluids by the various male glands (along with male hormone production of course) certainly does participate in producing the male sexual appetite.

Even though love is an attribute respected by all, it isn't necessary for the continuance of the physical forms of the race. Although a strong libido is essential in man, love is not, and it is therefore not a part of the male PSI. There are few moral or ethical restrictions placed on the male PSI by Nature; man must provide these himself.

The Female PSI—Love and Affection

The female PSI is much more complicated than that of the male. From our foregoing studies, this should be rather obvious.

To say that a woman doesn't exist who inherited desires similar to those of a man would be making a very broad statement. Undoubtedly, such women do exist, but in a true form, I have found them to be very rare. In my experience, most women who act in this manner are simply making a deluded attempt to appear appealing to male escorts because they think he may find such actions intriguing and interesting. They usually successfully achieve what they deserve.

In the normal woman, a different incentive occurs. After rather extensive research, I believe that at about the same time the biologic urge is developing in a boy, an urge of an entirely different form is incubating in the young adolescent girl. It is a rather strange feeling that is far more difficult to discern than that of the boy's simple sexual drive. Young girls become possessed with a need for affection and a desire to give affection that is different from anything they have heretofore understood as a child. It manifests itself in many ways—affection for teachers and older people that they may like, the desire to cuddle stuffed animals and the love of pets. This is, it seems, actually a forerunner of the mother love that is to come. It is, of course, related to the same love of progeny and desire to care for them that seems to manifest in all of the higher forms of female animal life. Like it or not, the innate demands on a woman are almost identical with those of her lower female counterparts.

There is no need for the woman to have any pre-coital desire for sexual intercourse per se. There is no biologic reason for her to enjoy this act. All that is needed is for her to allow the union to take place. However, once copulation has occurred and impregnation is accomplished, there is a need for very complicated emotional and instinctive incentives. She now must have the emotional stability and desire to carry the result of copulation to its fulfillment and then to love and care for the resultant child until it is mature enough to care for itself.

I realize that this view seems as if I am dehumanizing womanhood. Nothing could be further from the truth. I am simply categorizing certain drives and emotions that all women manifest. This is not the complete woman. This is only a small cog in her makeup, but it is a very necessary and important cog that will remain with her throughout her whole mature life.

To many, it may not seem necessary for nature to place within the breast of a woman this strong desire to care for and rear children. It is true that civilized humans should realize the necessity to perpetuate the species, but do they? During the long history of mankind, there have been many great and famous men of varied professions who have disputed this obvious duty; and had some of their ideas prevailed, it is possible that the human race would be extinct today.

The mind can rationalize almost any type of activity, no matter how heinous or contrary to the better instincts of mankind, if it believes it is of benefit to the self in one way or another. Actually, even often worse than the selfish despot is the misguided "do-gooder" who fervently believes that it is his "duty" to force men to live according to his rules.

One has only to look at the various forms of torture and inquisitions down through the ages to see what man is capable of doing in the name of expediency. I believe that Nature fully realizes what would happen if the perpetuation of the species were left to human integrity. Nature takes no such chances. She believes in force and so placed this strong direct incentive for the perpetuation, nurture, and love of the species within the breast of every normal woman.

The female primary sexual incentive, therefore, instead of being a desire for copulation as it is in the man, is a desire for love and affection—both to give and to receive. This desire is at first more or less unobjectified—that is, she loves everything. She has affection for everything and for nothing. It is simply a vague feeling that blooms within her at puberty. As time goes on, it becomes more and more centered on the male sex and, we hope, finally in one man. First, a friend, then a lover, next a husband, and finally the father of her children.

The female PSI is much less understood than the male PSI, not only by men—who not possessing it can't possibly understand it—but also by women, because of their lack of knowledge. While the male PSI is advertised all over the whole world— because it is a commercially saleable commodity known as sex—this female drive for love and affection isn't as exploitable and therefore is generally ignored.

How many men complain of their inability to understand women? When this happens, nine times out of ten, the woman is responding to her PSI and because a man doesn't have this characteristic in his PSI or any real desire to understand hers, he is completely mystified by her actions. Here we have the seed of a great many difficulties in marriage (If not the majority). If men could only learn to understand the nature of the female PSI, learn to live with it, accept it and utilize it to the fullest extent of their ability, marriages would become increasingly more joyful, divorce rates would drop and it would be possible to create a true heaven on earth in place of the chaos that now all too often prevails.

The PSI—both male and female—is basic to our existence. Without them neither you nor I would be here. Let us thank Nature for her thoughtfulness but also pray that each sex, in time, is able to gain a better understanding of the other's primary incentive.

MCD, A New Incentive

Man, so the Bible says, does not live by bread alone; it also seems to be true that man does not live by PSI alone. There is a strong biologic force in PSI and it will drive him to various activities throughout his life. However, except in perverted and abnormal men, it isn't the prime compelling instinct of his existence. There is another almost as strong. This second male force is perhaps the most fascinating of all discoveries I have made in my research.

I call this second male incentive Masculine Creative Desire (MCD). To understand it fully, let us review a moment. The feminine PSI is a rather broad and inclusive component of her life. It begins in her early love and affectional nature, becomes creative with the bearing of children, continues with the rearing of her family and ceases its expansion only in death. Her PSI is not only sexual; it is also creative. Although the creative nature of many women can be satisfied with the birth and care of their family (Although more and more women want more than this.) as a natural fulfillment of their love and affectional incentives, this is certainly not true of the average man. I have yet to find a man who felt that he had fulfilled his creative reason for existence by the propagation of children alone. Man does has a creative sphere, but it lies elsewhere.

It's a Man's World

It has been said of the woman that her natural creative sphere exists in the womb and because this can never be true of man, it could follow that his creative world is everything else outside the womb. God and Nature, in the just proportioning of the work of the world, have given woman the right to produce the greatest and most sublime creation possible—a human being in the likeness of God. To man, in compensation, has been deeded the right and ability to create in every other sphere of activity. We often hear, "It's a man's world." Outside the womb this is true, for man has been given the rest of the world as his creative playground and is provided by nature with a distinct masculine incentive toward this end—the MCD.

This MCD seems to be within all men, in differing degrees. It is the desire that pushes them ahead to create all the sublime and inane things produced in our world. It propels the scientist who will spend his whole life investigating and cogitating on the habits of the common flea. (No woman in her right mind would ever do such a thing; women are far too rational and practical.) It also has created for us music and art whose sublimity is almost beyond contemplation. This male MCD has produced almost every good man-made thing about us and every despicable man-made creation as well. Like most forces given to man, the MCD is not good or bad; it simply exists. It is up to man to properly direct it.

MCD is completely and entirely separate from PSI. The average man lives two lives. He lives the life of his MCD—his work or creative sphere. He also lives the life of his PSI—his home, family and sexual existence. These two can be entirely separate. They may work together, but by nature they are not joined. They almost never blend. This is some-

382

thing most women find difficult to understand. Her PSI and creative nature issue from the same source, his from separate sources.

Nature of MCD

When I first undertook this research project, I felt that MCD was centered in a man's job or work—that is, whatever he did to make a living was the exercise of his MCD. I soon realized that while this may be true in many instances—if his work is creative and fulfilling—many men don't find a creative outlet in their employment. The MCD is therefore not so much what a man does as it is a driving force within him to create, or to produce something that was not on earth before him. Unfortunately, many of the things a man must or can do for a living aren't motivated by MCD. Thus, he may find his work dull and uninteresting. He is then working only to make a living at a job that doesn't necessarily stimulate his creative desire. This is an unhappy man. If he would only listen to the promptings of his MCD and follow where this strange piper leads, he would be more contented and the world would be much more satisfying to him and with him.

MCD also creates in a man certain unique faculties. One is the ability of concentrating his attention, sometimes his whole attention, on a subject that has very little short-range practical value to himself or to humanity. He will do this simply because there is a drive within him forcing him to create something original in this field. You may have heard of various artists, writers or painters who have spent their lives in poverty rather than produce works the public wanted, but which they felt no desire to create. If they had changed only a little and given way to the fashion of the world, they might have become rich and famous. This they couldn't do, for something within them forced them to produce that which they must. Most such idealism is MCD based. Perhaps this is what the Bible means when it speaks of the talents within each man. I am not a Bible student, but as a scientist, I do know that there exists in man this strong compelling force I call MCD.

It can be so strong that at times it will overcome his PSI, as all too many wives and sweethearts realize. Often women want to talk of love when their men want to talk of baseball, hunting, cars or anything else that at present is stimulating their MCD.

MCD has many avenues of manifestation. It is usually not directed along just one line; in fact, it can be directed along several lines at the same time. A man can have MCD about hobbies, sports, world affairs and of course about his regular work all at one and the same time. There are many manifestations of the MCD, yet there is one fundamental activating force behind all MCD—the creation of something new or the improvement of a condition. Fixing a leaky faucet and writing a symphony can both be MCD-oriented though few women could ever understand the connection.

One interesting and exasperating characteristic of MCD is that it isn't necessarily practical. Women also create—oh yes, many women love to create—but almost always they have a rational reason for doing so. Women also work, but again for a reason. They usually work to advance themselves or their family. They work for things that they want or so that they will be appreciated. There are many reasons why women work and create, but almost all of them are well founded and eminently practical. Women are too pragmatic for MCD. It is almost unheard of for a normal woman to do anything without a practical purpose behind it. Women are basically rational and practical. Men are dreamers and idealistic, despite reputations to the contrary.

Most men will understand what I mean by the impractical nature of MCD. It is this incentive that makes men climb mountains simply because they are there. It is incentive that forces men to want to create music that may never be played in their lifetime. MCD forces men to create, not for accolades or monetary remunerations, but simply for the pure love of the creation itself. When man has created his entity, he is satisfied (for the moment). If others appreciate his work, this is all well and good, but at times this can detract from the creation. The true creator can't stop for appreciation; he must go on to further efforts because he is only happy when creating.

In trying to explain MCD to women, I have encountered great difficulties. It's like trying to explain the female PSI to a man. The only analogy I have been able to give a woman is that it is similar to her desire for a child. There may be no practical reason; she simply wants to be a mother and I think most women who have been mothers understand this sensation. Somewhere down within her, she wants to be a mother and feel a child within her. Man's MCD is similar. Many women don't feel complete until they have borne a child. Many a man can't feel complete until he has followed his MCD and is successful in his own creative world. Many stories in history and literature are based on this fact. Many great authors have described the nature of this drive although they never gave it a name.

Is There an FCD?

But what about the woman? Does she have anything similar to MCD? Yes, in a way. At first, her PSI is only for love and affection, but as her life involves a lover, husband and then children, her PSI expands.

This love and affection metamorphoses in the creative instincts necessary for the bearing and nurturing of a family. The growth of this incentive knows no end because it is based in the manifestations of creative love that is unfettered and untrammeled.

For the unmarried woman, a sublimation must take place; her PSI must be directed at some worthy but asexual objective. Even here, however, her creative sphere and her PSI are simply an expansion of one another.

It has been said by a man far wiser than myself, "Love to a woman is her whole being; to man, a thing apart." Love, as such, is an outgrowth of a woman's PSI. The greatest part of her entire world is bound up in it. Her whole life becomes an expansion of this simple primary PSI. It expands and grows, but it doesn't change. It simply encompasses more and more. She has one real life and that is a life of love in all its many manifestations. It matters little whether this is in the business world or in the home; unless her life is based on love, it is wasted and sad. This is not true of her husband. He has two lives. He has his PSI (his family), and he has his MCD. The two are separate and distinct. Actually, this separation of his MCD from his family and PSI is quite necessary because only in this way can the work of the world be done. Much of business has to be done coldly and calculatingly. It has to be done without emotional instability and it therefore shouldn't have within it the elements of sentimentality that go along with love and affection that are so common to the feminine nature.

The SSIs—the Equalizers

The various incentives I have just described are important (if not vital) to the perpetuation of the human race and to its constant efforts to make this earth a heaven (or hell) for all its inhabitants. We find in all men two unique incentives—first the Primary Sexual Incentive (PSI), which is a strong biologic urge for mating; and second, an innate drive that I call Masculine Creative Desire (MCD). This latter forces him forth into all avenues of activity that can come to his mind and heart.

The woman has also a PSI, which is not a biologic urge for sexual expression but rather a desire for love and affection. Each of these attributes is necessary for the perpetuation of the species. The male PSI is necessary to induce him to fertilize the female. The male MCD is necessary to give him the incentive to be the provider and the protector of the family that will result as a consequence of this fertilization. The female PSI, expanding into mother love and even beyond, is necessary for the creating, nurturing and the maturation of the family.

Nature has chosen her incentives well. She leaves nothing to chance or the good intentions of her beings, for she knows all too well that they are never to be trusted in important matters. She believes in strong incentives that all but force humans to follow a certain course to produce the ends she deems essential.

Do these same incentives also satisfy the physical and emotional needs of men and women? If we examine these incentives carefully, we find that Nature has left some very serious gaps that humans must fill through various means if they desire to live happy and fulfilling lives.

Perhaps the first and most obvious gap is the absence of an incentive that is common to both men and women. Because of this lack, it is easy to explain why each sex finds it difficult to understand the other. How can a woman understand the desperation and potential for evil that may be contained in the male PSI when she has no comparable feelings? How can a man understand her need for love and affection, her desire for tenderness and gentleness when he has no feminine PSI to aid his judgment? How can any man understand her feelings about children or married life, when his own natural incentives are so different?

On the other hand, how can any woman fully appreciate the demands of the masculine MCD? Isn't it difficult for her to understand why he spends his time trying to create something, working on it perhaps night and day, even though it may bring to her or to their family no money or practical usefulness? What good does it do him to tell her of his internal drives when she can't understand this inherent demand on his nature?

In the normal man/woman relationship we have the strange paradox of two people who need each other very much and yet who, by nature, understand each other so little.

For the proper exercise of his PSI, man needs a woman. For the complete fulfillment of her PSI, woman certainly must have a man. The man, of course, can fulfill his MCD without a woman and yet any victory achieved through his MCD is often hollow without someone to share it with. Though they have a strong need for each other, there is still little direct understanding between most couples.

Because of these incentives, people come together and marry. Later because of them, they may separate and divorce. (Up to fifty percent in some of our states.) They can't live without each other and they can't live with each other. When I arrived at this point in my research, I began to look for other incentives that could bridge this gap. They weren't readily forthcoming but, in time, two new—though somewhat vague— incentives were discovered.

These incentives apparently weren't developed by Nature because some people have them in abundance, some only meagerly and others seemingly not at all. Still, in these new and elusive incentives, I hoped to find an answer to marital happiness—a bridge of understanding between man and woman.

I like to call these factors the humanizing incentives, for as far as I have been able to ascertain, they are present only in the human or at least are only capable of being developed to any degree in normal men and women.

These drives differ from the primary set in that they aren't automatically developed by Nature, nor are they necessary for her design of species perpetuation. They are, we might say, a gift to mankind. They are latent or potential incentives that men and women may develop if they so desire.

Nature may not need these incentives, but man needs them desperately because they make of him a true human being instead of just another animal of the field. Because of their nature, I have called these latent drives Secondary Sexual Incentives (SSI). That of the woman is more easily developed, although it is poorly understood and only rarely brought to its highest potentiality. That of the male is more difficult to develop and is therefore more highly prized. These incentives are secondary to their primary counterparts, the PSIs. Man's SSI seems to be directly related to his PSI, as is the woman's. Even after the secondary incentive is developed, it is apparently necessary to have the primary incentive still in full force for the secondary to operate at fullest efficiency. If it comes to a showdown between the secondary and the primary sexual incentive, all too often the primary incentive seems to dominate unless a great deal of effort is exerted by the individual to prevent this reversion.

Character of SSI

After lengthy study and research, it seems that these latent factors (SSIs), are, in each case, basically the same as the primary factors of the opposite sex. That is, the secondary sexual incentive in woman is a desire for sexual congress, per se—a biologic urge for a sexual release within her. The SSI of the man is the growth of a love and affectional nature. It is a feeling of love, similar to that of a woman; it is not lustful or selfish but a true humanizing component that can be developed by all men. It is that, nearly alone, that can make of man more than an intelligent brute.

Female SSI

The female SSI, as stated, is a direct analog of the male PSI. In the average woman, the desire for sexual release, per se, is a latent or developable incentive. The reason this desire is held in abeyance in the young girl is not hard to ascertain if we understand Nature's needs. It isn't necessary for a woman to desire sexual congress to participate in cohabitation. It is only necessary for her to have a feeling of love and affection toward the man she marries and who completes sexual congress with her. Actually, it would undoubtedly be very detrimental to Nature's needs if women did have a male-type PSI before marriage. For remember, man's PSI is needfully so strong and potent at times that he will risk life and limb to accomplish its directives.

One can readily imagine what might happen in the world if both men and women were imbued with this same constant sexual drive. It is doubtful that many children would see the light of day, for the demand wouldn't be for progeny but only for pleasure. Thus, the human race would soon die out in one monumental orgy.

(Since this was written some twenty years ago there has been a change in the life of many young women. Since it has proved "commercial" for the media to foster the concept of what we can only call "female lust" as a normal component of womanhood, many young girls today feel that they must develop their SSI long before its natural time. This is one of the major reasons for the chaotic and lewd sexual situation in America today as well as one of the main reasons for the many new sexual diseases now afflicting so many of our teenagers.)

Once a woman has married, however, and come under the protection of her husband, such a sexual urge could be allowed if properly controlled and subordinated to her PSI. When she has, through her love and affectional nature, virtually laid down her life for the man she loves by exposing herself to the dangers of childbirth, it seems only fair that she now have the right to pleasure and satisfaction from sexual intercourse. Woman, it seems, is so physiologically constituted that although Nature doesn't develop within her a desire for sexual relations, per se, this feeling can be awakened by the stimulation of her love centers by her husband. This awakening is the prelude to a continuing growth of physical and psychologic sexual maturity, if she hasn't been preconditioned (by family, custom or church) to reject such development.

I certainly feel that developing her SSI is of great importance to any woman's marital happiness. If it does evolve, there can emerge a deep bond between the couple; if it does not, as unfortunately is too often the case, then the marriage can never be anything but a mockery and must eventually come to a sad end—either by divorce or, worse, by a continued growing disgust that erodes all love in the partnership.

The fact that the female SSI does exist and is not as easily developed as one might believe, offers an explanation for much of the statistical frigidity of the American female— estimated to be fifty to eighty per cent, depending on the definition of frigidity. I think that most of these women are not inherently frigid but that they just have not been able to develop an adequate SSI.

While the SSI usually develops owing to the stimulation of sexual intercourse, it is not automatically so accomplished. If a woman has had certain inhibitory training in her life, such as an overprotective mother who has produced a deep fear of sexual intercourse, or if she has perhaps been tangled in the Freudian web of clitoral and vaginal orgasms, or involved in religious sophistries about intercourse, it is very possible that she may be retarded in developing her SSI. If it has not bloomed within a certain period, she may believe she is frigid and as a defense mechanism may psychologically stop within herself any further attempts toward development. To keep from being frustrated further, she may divorce herself from any expected pleasure or desire during intercourse or attempt to sublimate it into many secondary forms. ("All I ever think about is my garden.")

There are times when the female SSI is very slow to develop but is not fully inhibited and does emerge late in life. All physicians have female patients in their late 40's and even 50's who are just beginning to feel the sexual sensations they should have experienced shortly after marriage. Unfortunately, just as they start to feel a desire for sexual activity, they find the sexual capabilities of their husbands start to decrease. This problem of male sexual weakness with age can be helped by your Center physician. You have only to ask.

The Male SSI

Of all the incentives herein described, the male SSI will probably be the most disputed. By its very character, it is the most vague, abstract and difficult to develop or even understand. In many ways, it is a luxury rather than a necessity in comparison to the other incentives. A woman can live in peace with a man who has no SSI if she knows no better, but after exposure to this enigmatic incentive, it is doubtful that she would ever again be willing to tolerate its absence.

The male SSI is the most civilizing of all these drives. A man having a strong SSI is incapable of the heinous acts so frequently representative of his sex. Through it alone can emerge the true "One Flesh" marriage. Only by its force can a world ever be free and safe for all life. Through the union of love, called marriage, men and women are given the opportunity to complete their natural being,—she, by the osmotic assimilation of masculine positive and sensual characteristics and, he, by the gradual

389

and usually unconscious growth in him of the love and compassion that is such a natural part of her being. As with all such things, the bad are not made good by wedlock, nor the stupid, bright. However, the chances for each person to better his own qualities are usually increased by marriage. Nature and the Almighty have conspired to produce a situation in which their human offspring could prosper and evolve; if such does not happen, it is not necessarily the instigators who are to blame.

To understand the male SSI, it is essential to comprehend man without it. Man, by nature, is full of positiveness, strength and agressivness (The result of his hormones if nothing else). These are his masculine characteristics. The more of these he has, the more he manifests manhood. It's a great and wonderful thing to stand on your own two feet and to be a man; yet there is something still greater and that is the possibility of becoming an advanced human—a near-God, if you will. To accomplish this goal, a man must not only be full of strength and positiveness and possess a strong creative ability, but he must also possess gentleness, understanding, forgiveness, compassion and true non-individualized love. A man who is merely a mind or virile sex force is rarely loved or revered by his contemporaries. A man, to gain the approbation of all about him now and in the future, needs to be much more. The men we eternally admire usually have a strong love and affectional nature along with their other masculine characteristics. This love nature is a female characteristic, I must admit, but it isn't a characteristic that feminizes a man. Rather, it produces in a strong man greater strength and force—that which no weak man can develop.

The male SSI is secondary to his other incentives. A man does not and should not lose his primary incentives by developing his SSI. This is why he doesn't take on more negative feminine traits. A woman's love and affectional nature can lead her astray through over sentimentality, whereas a man's MCD should prevent such a consequence on his part. The male SSI rounds the rough corners of his PSI and MCD. It should not be allowed to alter their positive and useful functioning.

The greatest example of male SSI we have in Christendom is that of Jesus. In other religions we have Buddha, Moses, Mohammed and the various other messiahs who have come to earth in love and self-denial to help mankind.

More recent examples would be men like Abraham Lincoln, a man certainly not effeminate and yet one renowned for the strength of his love and of his great compassion. We may honor an Einstein and we may even revere a Steinmetz or an Edison, but we love a Lincoln and adore a Christ. Few of us will have the opportunity to serve our fellow man as these, yet the force of our own example should not be belittled.

How does man obtain these attributes? How does he develop this loving nature? Admittedly, there are other ways besides the method I shall mention, but this one seems the most common and perhaps the most natural.

It is possible for us to develop traits that we don't already possess by first observing these in others and then trying to develop the same actions and movements within our being. Because women are the embodiment of love and affection, man usually develops his SSI through contact with women. By their constant example, women help men to unfold their budding love and affectional nature. But far more than mere example is present in the one-flesh marriage. Here the whole structure of the union, including the physical sexual exchange, aids in this worthy objective.

Think back to your own experience. How many times have you known a bachelor who changed for the better (in your opinion of course) after marriage? If he was an old carousing buddy, you may have not cared for the change, but the world appreciates it because he is undoubtedly now a much finer and more refined person. Not all men are equally affected, of course. But he is a brute indeed who is left untouched by a good woman's tender graces.

While almost all men are unknowingly civilized to a degree through marriage, it is far better if they can do so consciously. The rational husband will realize that these attributes of love and affection that are so much a part of his wife can become a useful force in his own life. These attributes will detract nothing from his strength of character and positiveness as a man, but they can greatly modify his more brutish tendencies. Therefore, he loses nothing of value and gains much in graciousness and effectiveness as a man by fostering this development.

The Danger in the SSIs

In developing an SSI (male or female), one must allow it to flourish without destroying the primary incentives. If a woman allows the SSI to predominate, to cause her mind to become dirty and lustful like that of some men, then it destroys all the finer parts of her own character and individuality and it would be better if she had never developed it at all. This is also true of a man who allows married life to make of him a wishy-washy, hen pecked, sentimental fool lacking all positiveness and strength of character. Every new attribute brings with it corresponding responsibility and this certainly applies to the characteristics of the SSI in both male and female.

391

The PSI comes on us whether we like it or not. The MCD is thrust upon all men to some degree. They are not good or bad; they simply exist and become a part of his nature. On the other hand, the SSIs must be developed and as far as I can ascertain, there is no limit to their development.

A woman's SSI is unlimited because it isn't based on physiologic factors, as is its counterpart—the man's PSI. The female SSI can grow throughout life and become stronger and of a more satisfying nature as a woman grows older if it is properly nurtured. This is also true of the man's SSI. His developable love and affectional nature knows no bounds. It can extend from an almost invisible amount to that which brings the adoration of the whole world for centuries to come. As far as I can determine, nature limits neither of the SSIs.

Those of us who have worked with SSIs are greatly enamored of them because we realize this kinetic force can help form the happiest of marriages, the most satisfying of relationships, and the most powerful family units. Almost everything that has to do with love, sexuality, marriage, and family can be strengthened and brought to complete fruition through proper use of SSIs.

Ingeniology

In this chapter I have presented what I have discovered of the emotional differences between man and woman. I call this effort "Ingeniology"—the science of instincts or incentives.

If you can understand the differences between men and women, you can understand the basis of attraction and repulsion. Life in our world is the art of understanding and functioning with others. The Buddhists say: "To know all, is to forgive all." If you can understand what is behind people's actions, then not only is it possible to forgive them, it is possible to love and help them. Once you can do this, you have expelled hate from your own nature and have started on the road to becoming "perfect as your Father in Heaven is perfect". When you can do this, you have started living the life of the "One-Flesh" concept, not only with your mate, but with all humanity.

If you can understand these incentives, you will know much about every human. The one-flesh concept is based on the natural laws of man and not on a psychoanalytical sophistry that is constantly changing. It is a teaching that eliminates guilt and future recriminations by preventing the acts that cause such feelings and not by some posthumous psychologic mumbo jumbo.

Marriage, as we know it, has often failed—not because the state is wrong, but because it hasn't been properly understood or utilized. Those who, because of the apparent failure of marriage have advocated a looser structure of relationships, have not shown their practices to be advantageous. The one-flesh concept shows us the error of the latter and the perfecting of the former. Marriage, properly and fully expressed, is man's most advanced state. With this work I hope to offer a beginning guide toward this desirable objective.

Postscript: The following is taken from a book I wrote some ten years after the above chapter was originally penned. It offers some specific suggestions for the One Flesh marriage that we all thought could be helpful to our married patients (or those who would like to marry). I trust you will find the information of value.

In the book *A Guide for the New Renaissance* form which this selection is taken, the healing and regenerative nature inherent in the sexual fluids exchanged during non-obstructive coitus is discussed at some length and so this is taken as an important fact in the following narrative.

The Nature of the Marriage

Once a worthy marriage is achieved, the couple can turn their attention to the nature of the One Flesh sexual union itself. The first consideration here is that the marital act is performed in such a way that full benefit of the magnetic fluid and emotional exchange is achieved. If this does not occur, most of the benefits of the One Flesh marriage will remain illusive and the couple may well spend their days in discouragement and disenchantment.

The basic law of the One Flesh sexual union is that: *Nothing must prevent the normal exchange that takes place in the vagina between the seminal fluid of the man and the vaginal secretions of the woman.* This even excludes various chemical substances used as spermicides. Although they may not prevent the admixture of the fluids as some forms of contraception do, they will have an injurious effect on the constituents of the normal fluids and tend to neutralize the desired benefits of the exchange.

There are two corollaries to this basic law that are vital to the perfect union. The first is: *There must be love in the hearts of each partner for one another or the fluids exchanged will react adversely and tend to destroy both the husband and the wife instead of building as they should.* For this reason, loveless marriages can become destructive to both parties and the sexual relationship tends to become more and more infrequent in such a union. Abstinence becomes a form of ego self-preservation for each.

The second corollary is: *If the couple is to be able to make full benefit of the one flesh potential, the exchange of sexual fluids is necessary on a regular basis*. In general, this should be at least once or twice a week. In the young and vigorous it may be more frequent, but it usually takes two to three days for the husband to build up a full supply of the various components of the seminal fluid.

In older couples this seminal fluid build up may take even longer but if a good natural diet and proper health habits are followed the One Flesh union can be continued far into ole age.

Selecting a Contraceptive Method

When all these factors are considered, some surprising conclusions may be drawn. Many of the common methods of contraception do not allow for the proper One Flesh sexual exchange and, therefore, are to be avoided. The condom, oral ejaculation, anal sex, withdrawal and any other form of sex that does not allow the semen to be deposited in the vagina is destructive to both body and Soul. Various forms of chemical agents such as foams, jellies, creams or sponges are not acceptable because they adversely alter the fluids necessary for the proper functioning of the One Flesh union. Although the intrauterine device and the "pill" do not have the detrimental effects described above, they are such hazards to health that they can be recommended only under very special circumstances. Rhythm and other time-of-month methods certainly fit the criteria for the proper vaginal exchange, but often do not fit well within the needs for regular sexual union.

For most couples the best compromise, when contraception is required, is the use of the latex diaphragm with a non spermicidal surgical jelly instead of the usual toxic spermicide used on the rim of the diaphragm (spermicide may be used on the portion of the diaphragm that is against the cervix since this will not interfere with the exchange and absorption of sexual fluids. A cleansing douche should be used after the removal of the diaphragm, however, to remove all traces of the spermicide from the vagina since some of these can be irritating.) If the diaphragm is properly fitted, there should be no effectiveness problem when used in this manner. For those who like the sex act without encumbrances the diaphragm can be used only during the unsafe times of the month and the rest of the time they can go a la natural.

In my many years of medical practice I have seen several couples who for various reasons could not effectively use the diaphragm method. For these, some other variation was devised. However, these are always chosen to fit into the basic tenets of the One Flesh marriage. If this is a problem that you have feel free to discuss this with your Center physician.

394

Some Important Last Words About the One Flesh Incentives

When the One Flesh concept was first made known over thirty-five years ago, it was opposed by many women's groups as being sexist, because they felt it was an attempt to degrade woman's place in the world at large. Nothing could be further from the truth. The problem was that these groups tended to misunderstand the differences between intelligence, talent, human creativity, and these incentives, particularly MCD.

The male creative incentive does not necessarily give men any particular intelligence, wisdom, talent or creativity that is in anyway superior to that of women. It does tend to direct qualities men possess into certain areas that Nature finds useful for women's purposes. It is entirely possible for a woman, by her desire and will, to enter these same fields and to succeed where many men have failed.

Many men have a strong MCD but not the intelligence, talent, or desire to do anything productive with it. These are some of the world's most miserable beings. It is a misery no woman can truly understand any more than a man can comprehend the urge within a real woman to have a child.

Perhaps this difference would be better understood if we were to compare the incentives of birds to that of a human aviator. Each year the birds take off at a certain time to make a long flight to a specific spot in a southern clime. This is done year after year without fail or deviation. It is regulated by the incentives placed by God (Nature, if you will) in these beasts at their conception. These incentives were placed there for one reason: To assure the preservation and evolution of the species. This it has done and will continue to do unless man interferes.

For many centuries man envied the birds' ability, but now by the power of his talent and creativity he has the wherewithal to emulate the flight of creatures. But he has one great advantage: He can now fly where and when he wishes, because he is not governed by the limited incentives of the birds.

So it is with human creativity. There is in both men and women an inborn incentive to create. The objectives of this creativity are distinct with each sex and are given by Nature in an effort to perpetuate and idealize humankind. However, both men and women, since they were given by their Creator the two great boons of intelligent thought and free will to execute the desires of that thought, have the ability either to harmonize themselves with these incentives or to change them to whatever purpose they desire. We see this throughout our world today.

Women decide that they do not want to be mothers but would rather enter the world of men and beat them at their own game. Men are willing to stay home and take care of the house because they really enjoy it. It is a common trait of human nature to think that the grass is greener on the other side of the fence. We have been given this right by God to come to a fuller understanding of the correctness of His original incentives by the suffering and sorrow we create through our deviations. In essence, we all are prodigal sons and daughters of our Heavenly Father and must some day return to Him, realizing that His ways are best, after all. But, like our biblical counterpart, we will first squander nearly all our sacred inheritance in riotous living.

There are, of course, many legitimate reasons for the repression or sublimation of these incentives, but even this is not to be accomplished without a certain amount of effort and loss. In some religions, the officials, both men and women, are expected to subjugate their sexual desires and expression. Unfortunately, no one told Nature about this and she keeps placing the same old incentives into the bodies of these individuals. This fight between man's conception of Spirituality and Nature's truth has been going on for many centuries and as yet neither side is showing any signs of giving in. In such a fight it is well to put the money on the side of Nature, for she has always, in the past, proven her superiority in such matters. Some day we believe that men and women of wisdom and perception will realize that a religion that prevents their best men and women from procreating is doomed to retrogression and ultimate extinction if such a practice is allowed to persist.

Before we leave these incentives, one point must be made as plain as possible: These are incentives. They are not commands. If you don t like them, you have the right to attempt to ignore or sublimate them. On the other hand, it has been my experience that to ignore or deny their existence is to possibly court problems in life. We have come to Earth to learn and to experience and to do this we must be willing to examine all the possible influences in our lives. Certainly these incentives are one of these influences.

The variations of human activities in relation to One Flesh incentives is truly endless. It has not been possible to delve beyond even the surface of this subject here, but enough has been given for the ardent student of human nature to have a field day watching the actions of his fellow earthlings as they go about their lives being directed by these incentives, but ever eager to deny such external influences.

Chapter XXVII
Whole Being Regeneration Service

Most individuals go to see a physician because they have some sort of symptom that bothers them. They want the physician to correct the problem so they can get back to living their life as before. This approach is certainly understandable and is that carried out with most of our own patients as well.

However, in the early days of the original Clymer Health Clinic we realized that this was not enough for many patients. They wanted more. They wanted us to help them to optimum health, not just the absence of disease symptoms. Also, as we began to handle more and more patients who came to us as a last resort, we found that these patients could not be helped without a near complete realigning of their health habits and thinking.

In order to serve both these needs we instituted the *Whole Being Regeneration Service*. In this endeavor, every facet of the patient's life is taken into consideration, so that needed corrections can be recommended if required.

This service is divided into two distinct parts: investigational and therapeutic. The purpose of this service is to help all who participate therein to achieve the best state of health possible.

The Investigation

The investigational stage is designed to ascertain the complete mechanical, chemical, electrical and emotional balances of the body to the extent that our present technology allows.

Some of these methods are discussed in Chapter II. However, in these individuals, because of the very selective care given, it is possible to use diagnostic measures that are in the extreme forefront of medical technology. Since these are always being newly developed, they cannot be described here.

The Treatment and Regeneration

The therapeutic phase, of course depends on what is found in the investigational phase. Very specific dietary instructions are given these patients according to the findings. The nutritional supplementation is also individually arranged by the patient's physician in accordance with the findings of the investigational stage.

Each patient will have several lengthy interviews with his Center physician in which his personal needs on all levels will be carefully discussed. In this way, the Whole Being Regeneration Service is as close to having one's personal physician as is possible to establish in the present medical milieu.

Not only is the physical body given the most careful scrutiny and indicated therapies, but also the whole emotional and spiritual nature of the patient is surveyed and specific advanced therapeutic methods are available if the patient needs or desires them.

A Dream Come True

Almost since the beginning of the Clymer Health Clinic some twenty seven years ago, one of the few honest complaints has been the patient who says, "I wish I had more time to talk to you, doctor." In order to run a clinic economically and still not charge high office fees, it is necessary for the physicians in a large clinic such as ours to see many patients every day. With proper regulation and the understanding of his patients, the physician can still provide completely adequate care for these patients. However, some desire more than adequate care. They want the finest and most extensive care possible. It is for this rather select group that we have established the Whole Being Regeneration Service.

Such a plan, we admit, cannot be inexpensive. However, our Centers are founded on humanitarian principles, and all the professional men connected with the Clinic have come here because they want to devote their lives to helping their fellow men. Personal aggrandizement is not a consideration with our staff, so although the price of this plan must be sufficient to pay for tests, remedies and a reasonable fee for the attending physician, it is not exorbitant and definitely within the financial ability of the average middle class family.

Because only a few patients can be handled at any one time with this service, it is necessary for all those interested in the Whole Body Regeneration Service to contact us several weeks in advance to obtain a reservation for a specific physician. If one's time is more flexible, it's often possible to obtain a reservation much earlier, but we can't guarantee this.

Chapter XXVIII
The Final Healing Ingredient

One day, many years ago when I was practicing in Seattle, Washington, a patient of mine brought her sister from New Jersey to my clinic. After the Easterner had dressed, she came out into the clinic hall and encountered the usual procession of happy chatting women, laughing youngsters and smiling nurses and said, "This isn't a doctor's office; it's a three-ring circus." Our office was apparently so different from the usual staid professional atmosphere she was accustomed to that she was rather flustered at first and didn't know quite how to take us.

Within a few minutes, however, she was running up and down the halls like everybody else, laughing her head off and having a great time. When she left, she said to me, "I haven't had so much fun in a doctor's office in all my life. The only problem is, I really don't know how I'll ever go back to Jersey and face those other doctors again. I'm afraid you've spoiled me for life." That was the last I saw of her, but when I left Seattle in 1969 to take over the directorship of the Clymer Health Clinic, I tried to bring this atmosphere with me. I believe I have succeeded. In fact, if anything, it has become more pronounced here than it was out West. In our Beverly Hall Corporation Healing Research Center we believe that we have taken this ambiance to a new plateau.

I like to think of this pleasant atmosphere as the final elusive ingredient in our cures. It is nothing more nor less than a happy optimistic outlook about the whole spectrum of life and health. It isn't an outlook we describe to the patients, nor is it something we suggest to them. It is a way of thought and life that permeates every person connected with our Healing Centers. We attempt to create, in the atmosphere around and about our Centers, vibrations of love so strong that they would melt the heart of a Scrooge.

We attempt to instill in our patients a true sense of love and realization that we humans weren't put on this planet to suffer, but rather that we are here to be healthy and useful. True, at times suffering may be our lot, but this suffering is only for the purpose of guiding us toward the proper road so we may learn to live within the laws of God and Nature.

People get well at our Healing Centers because we won't let them do otherwise. It takes a very determined person not to improve under our care. We exude such strong, healthy, happy vibrations that our patients are lifted right out of their doldrums and improve in spite of themselves.

Nothing about this final ingredient is new and all rational physicians agree that a constructive, optimistic outlook benefits the patient, yet how much is done in most medical establishments to produce such an outlook?

The reason we perpetuate such an atmosphere is that everyone connected with our Centers deeply believes in what we are doing. We all know that our methods are good. We all know that, given an opportunity, we can help almost any patient who crosses our doorstep. With this thought, it is easy for us to be happy and positive. It is easy for us to be optimistic because this optimism is based on the results of our past efforts.

At our Healing Research Centers, we sincerely and truly love each and every one of our patients. Each patient is to us a rare and individual jewel. Some are highly polished, some are a little more rough, but all have the potential of being of inestimable value. This love is the capstone of the final ingredient. Happiness, joy and the vibrations created by these emotions can give the patient a feeling of belonging and can give him a sense of assurance that he is going to get well. But love, true love, for these children of God, alone can carry the cure to its final completion. So in the last analysis, we find that this great secret of our Centers is simply to follow the admonition that Jesus gave his disciples when he last departed from them: "Love ye one another."

Appendix A

The following three monographs have recently been made available to the patients of our Healing Centers. Since they offer up-to-date information about subjects discussed in the body of this book, we felt it was important to include them.

Will Detoxification Help Me?

Introduction

Many people are burdened with so many symptoms that it is difficult to separate them from each other, let alone trace each one to a single cause.

Attempting to treat each symptom with a different drug or even a different natural supplement often can lead to a further burden on the body's already overloaded defense and detoxification systems. One of the most insidious causes of symptoms is an overload of toxins, chemicals and biochemical debris that our bodies are unable to discharge. This cumulative toxicity is a direct result of our modern "20th century" diet and "better living through chemistry."

Our detoxification system can be related to a sanitation or janitorial service. The "sanitation engineers" (intestines, blood and lymph) collect our trash and take it the main plant (liver) where it is either burned or compacted and then sent off for disposal (kidneys, lungs and skin). If there is too much trash (external and internal toxins) or if there is a breakdown in the system, we see a build up of internal debris causing intoxication and a disruption of the body's normal functioning.

Although our ability to adapt and survive is amazing, it is becoming increasingly apparent that our detoxification ability has its limits. When these pathways are too heavily burdened, they are unable to complete their "clean up" tasks and the overflowing chemical and toxic load then damages the normal functions of our cells leading first to warning symptoms and then, eventually, to organ damage (disease).

Two scenarios are often the result. The first occurs when the detoxification abilities of our body become overwhelmed and we subsequently become more and more sensitive to ever smaller amounts of environmental toxins, foods and inhalants. This invariably leads to what is termed "environmental illness" or "chemical sensitivity." The longer this process continues the more symptoms that develop. The second (and more insidious) scenario is that which produces a chronic low level but long term overload of our detoxification systems.

This assault may eventually lead to cancer, heart disease or many of the other degenerative diseases seen today. Genetics and other circumstances often dictate which path a person travels on this dangerous toxic freeway.

Recent research has shown a tremendous variation from person to person in our ability to detoxify. On one hand, we find those with a "bull-moose" constitution who can detoxify up to 60 times better than those who inherited a "canary" like constitution. Those in this latter category have detoxification systems that are easily overwhelmed. The reason for this discrepancy appears to be genetic differences in the liver's ability to perform its detoxification work. Thus we see that as a consequence of genetic uniqueness, some people may be much more susceptible to external or internal toxins than others.

Nature Cure to the Rescue

There is, however, hope for those with a stressed detoxification system and its resulting problems. An old but recently "rediscovered" method is now available to address these seemingly difficult and impossible to treat problems. This detoxification program is based on the principles established by early Nature Cure practitioners over a century ago. The human body, however, is the same now as it was then and these well established methods are just as effective today as when they were used by the legendary Father Kneipp and Henry Lindlahr.

We, at the Beverly Hall Corporation Healing Research Center, have thoroughly investigated both the classical and more recent detoxification programs and have drawn upon the best and most successful to create and implement a program we feel is second to none.

What are the Sources of Toxins?

Xenobiotics—Xenobiotics is the name given to describe foreign chemicals in the body. These chemicals are found in the air we breathe, our food, our water and are present in our home and work place. They include organic solvents (formaldehyde, phenols, plastics, air fresheners, cleaning agents), pesticides, insecticides, heavy metals (such as metal dental fillings) and even over-the-counter and prescription medications. A subset of these "xeno-biotics" can even mimic hormone functions in the body (especially estrogen) and are thus called "xeno-estrogens." These chemicals are easily absorbed through our lungs, skin and digestive tract and are stored in our fat and brain/nerve cells. Once stored they become hard to dislodge. However, they are released under certain conditions and, once released, unless they are properly and promptly excreted they circulate in the system to again cause symptoms.

Food Allergies and Injurious Habits—Substances such as alcohol, caffeine, tobacco and other "recreational drugs" readily contribute to the toxin overload.

Chronic Bacterial and/or Viral Infections—the body's attempt to fight them off produce toxic by-products along with the toxins produced by the germs.

Intestinal Bacteria, Yeast and/or Parasites—are a major load of toxins that are released and after being absorbed are sent directly to the liver. They can reside in our intestinal reservoir for quite some time and literally "have a party." This is a major source of hidden toxic load in many people today. The well popularized "Yeast" or "Candida Syndrome" is only one of these intestinal invaders that can cause problems with your detoxification system. The current term to describe the imbalance or overgrowth of such intestinal interlopers is Intestinal Dysbiosis. The toxins that are released from them are called endotoxins. Even treating and killing these microbes may create a toxic condition termed "die off."

As we have described, there are many factors, both inside our bodies and in our external environment, that, added together, may contribute to our toxic load. If our bodies detoxification abilities match or exceed our load, we experience few if any symptoms. If our detoxification system becomes overloaded by the accumulated toxins, symptoms and disease result.

How do Our Bodies Detoxify?

Intestinal Tract—This is the first and critical stage of detoxification and one of the major areas of elimination in the body. The intestinal lining surface is actually as large as that of a tennis court (if stretched out). Its job is to not only digest and absorb your food and nutrients but also to keep harmful substances and toxins from reaching the blood stream. The lining of our intestines are covered with immune type cells that are ready to ward off germs and other harmful substances. If this protective intestinal barrier breaks down from infection, toxins or other causes, the resultant condition is termed Leaky Gut Syndrome. This "leaky gut" now allows a multitude of toxins through the barrier which head straight for the liver. (See Appendix C)

Liver—The liver is akin to the trash processing plant described in our earlier example. The liver has three main functions (according to present knowledge). (1) Filtration of the blood of toxins and packaging them for excretion. (2) The formation of bile that is then stored in the gall bladder. (3) The metabolism of protein, carbohydrates and fats along with storage of vitamins and minerals. As can be seen, the liver is an intricate, complex and remarkable organ.

It appears that the liver has two stages or phases of detoxifying, termed Phase I and Phase II. Both are important since they each perform distinct essential functions. Phase I is called the P450 system and the enzymes produced in this Phase are the first to break down and transform harmful toxins derived from the blood and intestines. After this initial processing the toxin is sent to the next station or Phase II. In transition between Phase I and Phase II the toxin is called a "toxic metabolite" or "free radical" and in some cases is a more powerful toxin than before it went through Phase I. In Phase II, this toxic metabolite is neutralized by being "bound-up" and "packaged" ready to be delivered to the excretory systems. Finally it is either excreted through the bile to be deposited in the intestines for elimination or sent through the blood to be excreted through the kidneys (urination), skin (sweating) or lungs.

We can immediately see several scenarios that might cause dysfunctional liver detoxification. Phase I can be weak, Phase II can be weak or both can be weak. Both can be functioning well but have to deal with just too many toxins. One scenario, however, can be particularly troubling. This occurs when Phase I is "hyperactive" and is dumping its toxic metabolites to a weak Phase II. This activity generates "super toxins" and can lead to many of the problems seen in our patients today. This person has been termed the "Pathological detoxifier."

Substances which "hype-up" Phase I and thus lead to the buildup of toxic metabolites include alcohol, barbiturates, pesticides, exhaust fumes, high protein diets, paint fumes, sassafras, saturated fats, steroid hormones, certain medications like sulfa, antibiotics and antidepressants (Prozac, etc.) and charcoal broiled meats.

In individuals with a leaky gut and/or dysfunctional livers, toxic wastes accumulate in adipose (fatty) body tissue, including the brain and central nervous system. Stored toxins also can recirculate in the blood and may contribute to long-term health problems. This includes damage to the immune, endocrine and nervous systems. Conditions that have been related to impaired liver detoxification include Arteriosclerosis (clogging of the arteries), allergies, Arthritis, neurological diseases, Fibromyalgia, environmental sensitivities and Chronic Fatigue Syndrome (Adrenal Syndrome.)

Excretory organs—The excretory organs include the intestines, kidneys, skin, lymph system and lungs. These organs have the responsibility to remove or discharge all the toxins that the liver and other body cells package up for disposal. The importance of regular bowel habits (thus preventing constipation), good water intake to promote kidney flow, proper bathing,* exercise and deep breathing are all apparent once detoxification is understood.

How Do You Test for Detoxification Problems?

Comprehensive Digestive Stool Analysis—Anywhere from one to three stool samples are taken and sent to a laboratory for a detailed analysis and examination. Not only is the digestive function determined but a thorough search is conducted to find any abnormal intestinal bacteria and/or parasites or any imbalance of those normally found. If pathological invaders are found, they are tested to see which remedies will provide the best treatment for that particular type of germ. Such an analysis is critical to taking the guess work out of clearing Intestinal Dysbiosis. This test is crucial in assessing your "internal toxins."

Intestinal Permeability Test—A simple test where the patient ingests a mixture of two sugars (lactulose and mannitol) that are not normally absorbed by the intestines. Afterwards a urine sample is taken. If either of the two sugars are found in the urine we have evidence of a "leaky gut," the severity of which depends on the amount found. The leaky gut can be a major source of toxin overload to the liver in addition to playing a major role in food allergies and many inflammatory diseases.

Liver Detoxification Profile—This is a simple harmless non-invasive test in which a weak solution of caffeine and benzoate is taken and both urine and saliva are collected to be analyzed to determine how well Phase I and Phase II liver detoxification enzyme pathways are functioning. This test can help determine if you are one of the "pathological detoxifiers."

Urine Organic Acid Analysis—Urine is collected for 24 hours and analyzed for certain type of metabolic compounds called organic acids. This test is an adjunctive indirect test to determine the liver's detoxification ability and the toxin load it is attempting to process.

Other Tests—Hair Analysis and specific blood and urine tests may be indicated in certain individual circumstances to assess the level of external toxins that may be overloading the detoxification pathways. Some of these toxins include heavy metals, pesticides, organic solvents, formaldehyde, phenols, etc. Food allergy testing may also be needed. This can best be accomplished by the Elimination/Challenge Diet, skin or blood testing or a combination of these.

Diet and Nutrients Helpful in Supporting Detoxification

Diet—We stress a low allergic diet that emphasizes sufficient protein for cellular repair, proper food combining for the least digestive strain and naturally grown un-sprayed and unprocessed foods as much as possible. Sulphur containing compounds found in cruciferous vegetables (broccoli, brussels sprouts, and cabbage) have been found to support both Phase I and Phase II of liver detoxification. Beans, split peas, lentils, garlic and onion also perform this same function. Beets have had a long recognized value in supporting liver function. No specific diet is useful for all patients, however, since so many food sensitivities may manifest in patients in need of Detoxification. Your Healer here at the Healing Research Center will carefully go over your diet with you and help you to ascertain just what is best for you.

Intestinal Cleansers—Bentonite clay acts as an adsorber of toxins and harmful intestinal by-products. It works best when combined with pysllium fiber, which acts like a gentle scrub brush to help clean and detoxify the intestine. Specific natural "antibiotic" like substances to kill harmful invaders include liquid Caprylic Acid for yeast, Citrus Seed Extract for yeast and bacteria, Gentian Extract for yeast and bacterial, Garlic–Pro for yeast and bacteria, Tricycline for parasites, Colloidal Silver for infections and other products that are less stressing on the body than prescription medication.

Phase I Liver Nutrients—Iron (if deficient only), molybdenum, riboflavin, niacin, magnesium, vitamins A, C, E, carotenoids, selenium, and flavonoids.

Phase II Liver Nutrients—Glutathione, L-cysteine, N-Acetyl cysteine, zinc, copper, manganese, thiamine, taurine, glycine and methionine.

Flax Seed Oil or Fish Oils—These also support liver detoxification, immune function and decrease inflammation.

Phosphatidyl Choline—This compound has also has been shown to prevent liver damage from free radical toxins.

Liver Healing Herbs—Milk Thistle (Silymarin), Dandelion (Taraxacum), Artichoke (Cynara) and Tumeric (Curcuma) are also very potent liver protectors and stimulators of bile production and flow in the "sluggish" liver.

Blue Green Algae, Chlorella and Barley Greens—These and other "green" foods have established a track record for being helpful agents in a detoxification program. They are very dense in vitamins, nutrients and other cofactors as well as being powerful antioxidants and probably perform other functions we have not yet discovered. They can be an important part of any detoxification program, no matter what toxin involved.

Our Healing Research Centers Detoxification Program

This is a general guideline only and is meant only to serve as a starting point. Each individual has a unique genetic background and is exposed to different environment and social conditions that prevent forming "one program for all." The key is determining the individual uniqueness of each person and then designing a program that best fits that patient's condition. We have spent the last forty years bringing this need into realization.

1. Testing—Each situation will be analyzed and testing as described above will be individually determined. Some people may need very little testing, others may need an extensive evaluation.

2. Diet—Diet is crucial for many reasons. Unbalanced diets frequently promote the growth of intestinal germs (Dysbiosis), which leads to the development of internal toxins. Food allergies must be controlled by the best means possible. This usually means some form of Elimination and/or Rotation Diet. The digestive function should be relieved of any heavy burden and following guidelines on food combinations is very helpful in this area. Naturally grown foods should be consumed as much as possible to minimize the amount of pesticides ingested. The majority of our good "fresh" fruits and vegetables today contain disturbing amounts of pesticides and other external toxins. Your Healer here at the Healing Research Center will help you select the diet that is best for your specific present needs.

3. Water—Your drinking water should be as pure as possible. The best would be certified and tested spring water in glass bottles, certified and tested well water or good filtered water. During detoxification, it is imperative to consume 8-10 full glasses per day of the best quality water that can be obtained. This will flush dislodged toxins ready for excretion through the kidney and urinary system.

4. Xenobiotic Avoidance—To the best of one's ability, it is wise to avoid common volatile organic solvents and other xenobiotics in the environment. This action is critical for those with environmental illness and chemical sensitivity and is best accomplished by "cleaning up" your home and work. There are several books we recommend to help assist and guide you in such an endeavor:

Less-Toxic Living, by Carolyn Gorman
The Whole Way to Allergy Relief and Prevention, by J. Krohn, M.D., pages 156-161
Clean and Green, Annie Berthold-Bond
Nontoxic, Natural and Earthwise, by Debra Lynn Dadd
Success in the Clean Bedroom, by W. Rea M.D. and Natalie Golos.

407

Volatile Organic Compounds are solvent-type commercial chemicals that are highly prevalent today and react as extremely dangerous xenobiotics. Exposures come from occupational use of these chemicals, breathing contaminated air inside buildings and some instances direct absorption through the skin. All such solvent-type chemicals are fat or lipid soluble and therefore have an affinity for the brain and nervous system (because of their high content of lipid/fat compounds). In addition, they are absorbed by our cell membranes and fat tissues. They tend to remain in these areas of the body for long periods of time.

5. **Exercise**—This is important to stimulate blood flow and promote excretion of toxins through the skin. The exercise prescription will be given as determined by individual conditions and circumstances. As a general rule you should attempt to walk 20-40 minutes per day, three to five days per week so that body processes can function normally. Those with adrenal syndrome or heart conditions must always consult their Center Healer before exercising.

6. **Stress Management–Autogenic Training**—Balancing the nervous/emotional centers in the body is very important to promote the detoxification process. The autonomic nervous system controls the blood flow to the entire body. If an imbalance in this system is present (as it is in most of those today), then blood flow is interrupted to all the vital organs, including those of detoxification.

Over the years we have found that helping our patients to transmute (change) "emotional toxins" like worry, anxiety, anger and resentment into love, compassion and understanding can lead the way for the body's chemical detoxification. We have long realized that when people are "tied up" emotionally, they don't release body toxins but instead these remain in the body and can act as the nidus of a serious disease process.

Your Healer here at the Center is ever ready to help you with these problems. Feel free to discuss such matters with him. He is especially trained to not only be helpful but most discreet in all such consultations.

7. **Intestinal Cleansing**—For this purpose we use Bentonite Clay, Psyllium Fiber and other agents specific for any microbe that may need to be treated. In some patients the "Internal Bath" may be an essential part of the Detoxification. Only your Healer is to make this determination. If he decides that such a treatment is in order he will personally give you all the details. Do not attempt such a treatment on your own during Detoxification.

8. **Liver Support**—Anti-Oxidant Formula: 1 tablet 3 times per day to support Phase I and II of liver detoxification. Liv-Rinse: 3 a day to give added support and to stimulate bile flow (methionine, dandelion,

beet root, black radish, golden seal, choline, inositol and milk thistle) S.A.T.: (Milk Thistle, Artichoke, Tumeric), 1-2 per day. And (if needed) Amino Acids of Glycine, Taurine, Glutamine, Ornithine, Serine and Histidine. Where these remedies are too overwhelming for the over-worked liver we often begin Detoxification with Homeopathic Natrum Sulph and then gradually add Betafood or A,F & Betafood as the patient is able to tolerate these compounds. As these nutrients become well tolerated we will administer C-C-H, an herbal extract made to the Center's own formula.

9. **Kidney Support**—Drink 8-10 glasses of water per day as described above. 1-2 cups of kidney tea may count toward this total. Healing Research Center Kidney Tea: 1-2 cups each morning. Arbu Tone: 1-2 caps, three times per day (if required)

10. **Skin/Lymph Support**—Lymph/Skin Rub: Use a bristly shower brush, loofah or skin brush and rub the two following areas of your skin for several minutes while showering or bathing: Outsides of both thighs (stimulates lymph flow from large intestine). Chest area (stimulates lymph flow from kidneys, liver, pancreas, stomach and gallbladder).

Massage, Chiropractic or Osteopathic Manipulation Therapy: To work out "tissue sludge" and promote toxin removal from the muscles and soft tissue. To be done weekly if possible.

Detoxifying Soak Baths: The methods outlined here have been shown by researchers to be helpful in persons made ill by toxin exposures. Since treatment should always be individualized, your Center Healer will tell you which of these measures is best for you. Soak baths have the advantage of being convenient since they can be performed in your home at little cost compared to sauna treatments. On average, they should be performed 2 to 3 times per week but this will vary according to the patient and conditions, therefore, always follow the instructions given you by your Center Healer. Any given bath should be terminated at the first sign of dizziness or weakness and your Center Healer notified before subsequent baths are attempted. Begin with 10-15 minutes and work up to one-half hour if well tolerated. Water temperature should be comfortably warm. Hot water can be added to the bath water from time to time to maintain a relatively constant temperature.

The following is the general order of these baths. If there is any deviation from this procedure you will be so directed by your personal Center Healer:

1. **First:** 8 baths: 2 pounds of baking soda added to the bath water.
2. **Second:** 8 baths: 2 pounds of Epsom salts* per tub of bath water.
3. **Third:** 8 baths: use 2 pounds baking soda and 2 of Epsom salts.

4. All subsequent baths: use two to four pounds of Epsom salts.*

Use the loofah sponge or rough cloth during the bath. Drink an eight ounce glass of water during the bath. Follow each bath with a shower of lukewarm or cool water as tolerated to stop the sweating and scrub the skin thoroughly to remove any accumulated toxin debris deposited on your skin during the bath.

Since electrolytes and minerals may be lost during these baths, it is best to replace them with the following formula:

    1. ½ teaspoon of sea salt added to the food during the day

    2. Take a dose (500-1000 mg.) of Vitamin C before and after bath. You may also take one Antioxidant tablet before the bath.

    3. Approximately ½ cup of Natural Toxoid Formula to be taken following the bath. This is to replace zinc, potassium and other minerals.

    4. Tracelyte, 1 teaspoon three times a day or other equivalent trace mineral formula that your Center Healer may determine is best for your needs.

    5. At least 8 glasses of water should be drunk during the day. Good filtered or tested bottled water is preferable.

11. Other Supplements: These are to be used only on the recommendation of your Healer.

A: Oral Vitamin C—It is encouraged to take oral vitamin C, either as ascorbic acid or buffered vitamin C, starting with doses of 3 grams per day (3,000 mg.) and slowly increasing up to 6 or 10 grams per day if tolerated. If you develop abdominal cramps or diarrhea, dosages should be decreased until symptoms disappear. Doses should be divided into three or four separate doses throughout the day such as mid-morning, mid afternoon, and late evening. This, of course, is flexible and will be modified by your Center Healer as needed.

All symptoms must be discussed with him. If plain ascorbic acid (not buffered) is used, it should be taken in a capsule, as it tends to erode the teeth when there is direct exposure.

B: High Nutrition Vegetable Oils—We recommend 1 tablespoon of Flax Seed Oil and 1 tablespoon of cold pressed Virgin Olive Oil per day. These oils support the biochemical pathways in the body involved with detoxification and inflammation. They also slow down the assimilation of toxic chemicals from the intestinal tract.

C: Blue Green Algae, Green Vibrance or Barley Green— Experience has shown these to be of value in certain instances. Your Center

---

* One may wish to substitute in full or in part Dead Sea Salts for the Epsom salts. They are more expensive and can be obtained at most local health food store.

Healer will recommend one of them for you if he feels they are necessary for your recovery.

D: Multiple Vitamin and Mineral—Ultra-prevention III, Livec or another similar product as recomended by your Center Healer.

E: Niacin— This nutrient helps detoxification by increasing blood circulation in the lipid tissues. It is used by your Center Healer only as required. Under no circumstances are you to take Niacin without the specific approval and direction of your Center Healer.

12. Intravenous Vitamin C: Vitamin C is a powerful detoxifier and when given intravenously, it can add a great deal to the effectiveness of all our other measures. It is more effective if given slowly over a period of two to three hours. It is most effective if given following the Detoxifying Soak Baths. For the best results they should be administered three times per week. Other nutrients may be added to the drip to increase the effectiveness of vitamin C.

New Insights for Your Healing

Today in our nation, we are faced with one of the most insidious health hazards to ever plague mankind. The reason there is such danger and insidiousness is, since no one dies from the condition and the objective symptoms of the disease are few, most doctors and almost all Government health agencies completely ignore its existence.

I first encountered this condition nearly forty years ago and at that time, for want of the better term, I named it Adrenal Syndrome, since most factors pointed to a diminished functional ability of this gland in my patients. I first shared my experiences with this condition with the medical community in 1975 in my book *It's Only Natural*. This work was followed in 1983 with an entire work, *Adrenal Syndrome*, devoted to this enigmatic condition. The latest rewrite of this work was issued in 1994 and was retitled *Chronic Fatigue Unmasked*.

While this last printed effort to make this dehumanizing condition understood and appreciated for what it is, and for what it is not (that is not malingering), is very thorough, there are further new and vital insights that I would like to address here. The most important of these is a new look at the different types of reactions patients may have in the various stages of this condition and the use of Passive treatment in the care of patients in all stages of this disease.

The Resistance Phase

When I first began to treat Chronic Fatigue, the great majority of my patients were in the early or fatigue stage of the disease. Therefore, most of the treatment patterns described in my books on this condition deal with this stage. However, as the causes of this condition* continue to proliferate I find more and more of my patients in the later or resistance phase.

Surprisingly, we find that one of the reasons for this greater number of patients in the later stages of Chronic Fatigue is the fact that it is being treated by more and more physicians now that it has belatedly been accepted as a real condition. Prior to this new acceptance, patients with Chronic Fatigue would usually be told that there was nothing wrong with them, that their symptoms were all in their head and to go home and stop worrying. The patient had no other alternative (unless they came to us) but to just go home and rest since they had strength to do little else. This forced rest usually kept the patient in the earlier stages of

---

*The underlying cause of this condition is long term unremitting stress. Where such stress has reduced the vitality of the body it can often only take one more severe stress incident to throw the individual into the full blown Chronic Fatigue state. While this last stress is the one that usually gets blamed for the condition, it is only the "straw that broke the camel's back."
Each of us has our own breaking point dependent upon the vitality of our glands and immune system. Some individuals have inherited such a weak immune system that they will suffer from this condition no matter what measures they take to prevent it (Even these can be helped with passive treatment, however). On the other hand there are still a few left whose systems are so strong that they will never develop this condition no matter what may come along. The great majority of us lie somewhere between these two extremes.
In my opinion the reasons that this condition is now the fastest growing epidemic in our nation can be laid at the feet of the modern dictum, "Better Living through Chemistry." The traditional stresses of physical strain, emotional strife, bacterial and viral invaders, trauma, natural poisons, etc. have been with us since the earliest days of mankind and yet we have few verified cases of Chronic Fatigue during these years. What has changed in our lives today is the explosion of man made toxic chemical substances for which the body has had no time to create the needed internal antidotes. A list of these assaulting agents would have to include pesticides, water pollutants, air pollutants, almost all modern medical drugs, multiple vaccinations and food additives. As each new generation has its collective immune systems assaulted by an increasing number of these "unnatural" substances the children are born with ever weaker immune systems and so the predisposition to this condition grows exponentially with each new generation.

this condition since they were not able to force themselves to those activities that would move them into the later stages.

Once the medical profession accepted the condition, however, this scenario changed dramatically. Patients in the early exhaustive stage of the condition were recognized and treated symptomatically. That is, if they were exhausted (and consequently depressed) they were given medication to "perk them up." All too often this medication only acted as a whip to the weakened glandular system and so the patient did not rest as in the past but attempted to go back to their "normal life." The end result of this treatment seems to be a much greater number of patients in the later resistance phase of this disease.

On the last page of this brochure you will find a detailed chart by the legendary Dr. Hans Selye,* one of the real pioneers in this work. Here you can see the stages of this condition from normal to final collapse. Please note that in the reactive stage the patient may feel somewhat normal but is actually much closer to final collapse than in the early exhaustive stage. Our work is to bring the patient back to the normal stage and not leave them in the seductive but dangerous reactive stage as do so many physicians today.

Passive and Active Treatment

Most medical treatment and even the large majority of Alternate Treatment is of the Active type. By Active treatment I refer to that form of treatment that depends on some action of the body to react to the treatment to actually treat the disease. For instance, most drugs depend on the body to react to them in such a way to create the desired effect. The drug is a stimulus to create a body reaction. The same is true of many alternate therapies. Most certainly the Chiropractor depends on the patient's nervous system to react in a certain manner so that his adjustment is effective. We may even consider nutritional supplements as Active treatment in that they require the body to make special efforts to digest and metabolize them.

For most patients there is no reason not to suggest Active treatment. It is the bulwark of most healing therapy. Unfortunately, many Chronic Fatigue patients have such weakened systems by the time they come to us that their bodies are not able to react properly to many types of Active treatment. This includes even the most natural and gentle. This fact was first encountered by us many years ago and at that time we instituted the protocol of Passive treatment for these patients. In Passive

---

*Dr. Selye's chart is to be found in chapter two of this book.

treatment, the healing does not require the patient's body to react, only to graciously accept the energy and vitality given to it. Most of the various modalities ("machines") that we use are Passive treatments. In our experience, they are able to help even the most sensitive Chronic Fatigue patients, even those commonly known as "Universal Reactors."

In our usual course of treatment we begin with the Passive treatments and then as the patient grows ever stronger we gradually add the Active treatments. This procedure has proven effective for over thirty-five years and has allowed us to successfully treat a vast number of patients who had been rejected by other physicians as "hopeless."

Herbal Signatures

Many Phytotherapists (herbal physicians) who have an abiding faith in a Universal power greater than ourselves also believe in the existence of plant "Signatures." A plant Signature is a marking on the plant that gives the experienced investigator an idea as to how that plant can be used to relieve human suffering. This faith in "Signatures" is based on the belief that a loving God would not allow a disease to plague mankind without also making available a cure from His storehouse. It is merely up to the dedicated Phytotherapist to learn to read the language that God placed on His plants.

We are fortunate to have Phytotherapist George Benner on our staff. George has spent decades studying plant "Signatures" and brings this dedicated and spiritual insight to every herbal specific he creates. We have found that when even our most reactive patients cannot use the ordinary supplements or herbal remedies they can use these "Signature" based specifics.

Alterative Therapy
The Royal Road to Health

One of the most interesting, most misunderstood and most under used healing agents in all of medicine is what is known as an Alterative. In *Webster's New International Dictionary* an Alterative is defined as, "A medicine or treatment which gradually induces in the patient a change from a morbid or diseased state to one of health."

An Alterative is not a pain killer; it is not a tranquilizer; it is not an antibiotic; it is not a powerful "miracle" drug; it is rather a mild natural agent that helps to reverse the morbid disease process. An Alterative rarely works rapidly because the chronic disease processes it is designed to help are not capable of such sudden change. Note the use of the word "gradually" in Webster's definition. This word is used knowingly and specifically. A true Alterative works slowly because it works on the underlying disease processes and not simply on the surface manifestations, as do most of our modern "miracle" drugs.

Almost all of the remedies and treatments used at the **Beverly Hall Corporation Healing Research Center** are used in an Alterative Mode. This includes the various physical medical treatments with the **Magnatherm, Myoflex** and the other similar therapies. It also includes the carefully selected Nutritional Remedies we use to augment our hands-on therapies. Except in emergencies, we always attempt to use natural high biologically active supplements in low potency so as to better obtain their Alterative rather than drug-like effects.

Many of the most powerful Alteratives are to be found in the plant kingdom. These, in the form of Extracts or Homeopathic Medications, are used in the Alterative treatment of almost all of our patients. As mentioned in a earlier paper (New Insights for Your Healing), we search for certain plant "Signatures" to help us in choosing the proper herbal Alterative for our patient's needs. Frequently, we discover that several different Extracts are required to help the many conditions from which a patient may suffer.

However, from our long experience in this field, we have found that it is usually not wise to attempt to use Alterative Therapy to treat all these conditions at once. With such a plethora of Alteratives working, the body may not be able to respond as desired because of a lack of needed vitality to work with all these beneficial agents at the same time.

Therefore, it is usually more expedient for the Phytotherapist to select only one Alterative at a time for any particular stage in a patient's healing process. Once the therapist feels that this initial Alterative has fulfilled its objective, he will add other agents (in turn) for further healing. In this manner, each of the patient's conditions is addressed by the most effective Alterative without overstressing the body's healing forces. Even using only one herbal Alterative at a time, the dosage, in sensitive patients, must be carefully monitored so as to keep the healing process from being forced to move faster than the body can accept.

We use this same caution with all our other Active Alteratives such as the MC and the new **MicroLight 830** Low Level Laser. We find, from our research, that these units also act as powerful Alteratives and, as such, must be carefully configured to the specific needs of the individual patient. You can help your therapist to determine your ideal dosages by reporting any unusual effects or reactions you may experience following these treatments. For obvious reasons, such experiences must be reported to your therapist prior to your next treatment. Ideally, you should have little or no adverse symptoms if your treatment dosages are as desired. Healing of chronic conditions can not be hurried. As a wise old physician told me, "You cannot push a chronic patient to health, you must take them by the hand and gently lead them to health."

Your Partnership With Us

In working with Alteratives, it is absolutely essential that the patient establishes a working partnership with the therapist. It is mainly from the patient's feedback that the therapist is best able to determine the effectiveness of the various Alteratives used. This patient participation is particularly vital when it is time to make a change to a new or supplemental agent. It is also very important that the patient be as objective as possible in this partner relationship. As we frequently tell our patients, "Do not be nice to us." That is, do not tell us you are improving unless you really are. We must have your uncolored objective feelings and symptoms concerning your condition if we are to give you the best care of which we are capable.

As mentioned, an Alterative is something that gradually alters the course of a disease condition to a healthy state. As this alteration takes place, obviously the symptoms of the patient will change. These changes may occur for a variety of reasons and it is essential that your therapist be informed of all these changes so that he can decide just what they mean and whether or not he needs to change your treatment to better take advantage of the altered course of your condition. Sometimes the Alteratives may be acting too rapidly and need to be moderated but more likely you may be experiencing a "healing event" and slightly modified treatment may be required to take full advantage of this propitious situation.

It is well to always remember that therapy at our Healing Research Center is not something we do to you. It is something that we do together. It is the healing of the future in which the patient assumes his or her own responsibility for the cure along with the dedicated therapist. We are here to guide every step you make toward vibrant health but you must take the steps. No one else can walk the path to health for you.

A Carriage With Many Horses

The early Nature Cure exponent, Henry Lindahr, M.D., used to compare this method of healing to a horse-drawn carriage. He equated

Homeopathy, Osteopathy, Chiropratic and Allopathy (orthodox medicine) to a one-horse carriage since they depended on one basic philosophy to effect their cures. Nature Cure (Naturopathy), on the other hand, he stated, uses everything that is good in all these fields and therefore is like a carriage with a full compliment of horses pulling it. Such is the functioning of our Healing Research Center.

We are ever ready to use every known (and a few that are generally unknown) type of Alterative Treatment to help move our patients from a morbid diseased state to one of health. Our carriage has many horses to help each of you gain the healing and health you desire. In your healing, we will combine the best of the known Passive and Active healing procedures (see New Insights for Your Healing). With your constant feedback, we will use each of the many therapies at our disposal where it can best accomplish the desired result.

God and Nature Do the Curing

An old saying goes, "Nature and God cure the ailment but the doctor takes the fee." All the greatest of physicians can do is to give the body an opportunity to heal. That is exactly what Alterative therapy is all about. We do not cure you. Your own body must do that. But we are dedicated to applying the necessary Alterative Therapies to allow your healing to take place. In this process your body can be moved only as fast as its nature allows. If we attempt to move it faster than it can accept, a reaction may occur. If we move it too slowly, final healing may be delayed.

Your Beverly Hall Corporation Healing Research Center physician constantly works to achieve that happy medium by which your healing takes place as rapidly as your body can accept without undesired reactions. In this process, you are a vital link since you have important "inside information" to help him in his efforts. By keeping your Healer fully attuned to your body's signals, you can be an invaluable aid to your own healing.

Appendix B

Diets

The Basic Health Maintenance Diet

The Basic Health Maintenance Diet, if followed faithfully, aids in restoring health where lost and in continuing good health in those so blessed.

First thing upon arising, take a full glass of warm water with a pinch of sea salt added. Half a lemon may also be added if troubled with constipation. One half hour later breakfast is taken.

Breakfast #1

Only fruit is taken. One may use as much as desired. The following are particularly recommended: apples (juice, raw, baked, or as sauce), apricots, bananas (very ripe), berries of all kinds (best raw), canteloupes, cherries, grapefruit (Indian River brand best), grapes, lemons*, limes*, oranges*, papayas, peaches, pears, pineapples, coconut (fresh best, drink milk), plums, rhubarb*, tangerines*, and melons of all kinds.

Dates, prunes, figs and raisins may be used if they cause no trouble, but they are more sugar than fruit and should be restricted during colds, flu, and similar disorders.

All fruit should be washed well and rinsed, preferably in one of the products sold at healthfood stores, to remove chemical sprays. If at all possible, try to buy fruit from a private party or healthfood source so that it hasn't been sprayed. One of the following may be added to this breakfast, if desired or felt necessary: nuts, seeds, lean fish, or meat. These supply sustenance to the meal without disturbing the digestion.

Breakfast #2 (Nonfruit)

Although a fruit breakfast is recommended, some may find it insufficient at first, or they may want some diversification. The following may be used in this case.

Cereal. Any whole-grain product may be used. Wheatena, steel-cut oats, millet, mates, seven-grain cereal, and other such products.

Milk or Cream. Raw milk or cream is preferred. Some may be used on the cereal and the rest drunk. Cereal coffee or herb teas may also be used.

---

*These foods should not be used if you have arthritis, bursitis or related diseases.

Bread. Whole-wheat toast, whole-wheat or cornmeal (undegerminated) muffins, whole-wheat waffles, pancakes, or cornbread may be used.

Raw Vegetables. Raw vegetables should be taken with the above because these foods are all acid-forming and raw vegetables are needed to control this condition. Raw celery or carrots are sufficient.

Dinner and Supper

Dinner and supper have similar construction. One meal (either dinner or supper) will be smaller than the other, but the type of foods used is not altered, only the amounts.

Protein

Provide only one protein at each meal (small portions of two proteins from the same group may be used). Proper proteins may be chosen from the following:

Group I Dairy Products: Milk (raw), buttermilk, home-made ice cream, cottage and natural cheese (no processed cheese), eggs (fertile if possible). The eggs may be soft-cooked, scrambled, or raw. If you have problems with congestion, use only the yolk.

Group II Meat or Fish: Lean beef, lamb, chicken, turkey, duck, and all organ meats. If possible, obtain meats from private parties who do not use chemicals in the animal feed or sodium nitrate as a preservative. Some healthfood stores also carry naturally-raised meat. All forms of fish are good; those from the sea are richer in essential elements than the freshwater fish; however, all types of seafood (such as clams, shrimp, and crab) are highly recommended as long as their purity of source and processing is assured. Fish and seafood contain less toxic substances than meats.

Group III Nuts and Legumes: Nuts, lentils, dried peas, beans, and seeds (sunflower, sesame) may be used but with caution because they are difficult to digest and must be used as directed later in this diet.

Starches

Have only one starch at each meal because more than one leads to overeating. Health-building starches should be chosen from the following:

Whole-wheat bread made only from the most natural ingredients. Make your own or use a whole-grain bread obtained from a healthfood store. Nutritious bread is-one of the most important parts of a diet; be sure yours is the best. Aside from the staple bread, the following carbohydrates are recommended: baked potatoes, natural brown rice, unpearled barley, millet, steel-cut oats, and any products made from natural unrefined grains—for example, cornbread, wholewheat pancakes, waffles, and bran muffins.

A small amount of fat is useful in most diets. Real butter and soybean-lecithin spreads such as those found in better healthfood stores can be used. In cooking, only the following products should be used: cold-pressed oils, such as peanut, soy, safflower, sunflower, and sesame. For solid shortening, butter or the soybean spread may be used. These fats may be more expensive than those in common usage today, but they may prevent diseases that could cost a thousand times more.

Vegetables

The rest of the meal should consist of vegetables. It is best if they make up at least half the bulk of the meal. This helps to normalize body chemistry. Half the vegetables should be raw. (If you can eat something raw, don't cook it.) If at all possible, try to obtain vegetables that haven't been sprayed with pesticides or grown with chemical fertilizers. The best vegetables are those fresh from the garden—yours or a friends Canned and frozen vegetables are allowed, but they are second best. Each meal should start with a raw vegetable; this is vital. Tomatoes and/or cucumbers should not be eaten with regular meals, only with other vegetables, meat or fish, not with starches or dairy products.

Additional Instructions

Some products used in food preparation are necessary but harmful. More healthful substitutes are available and should be used. A list of these follows:

Baking Powder. Use only Royal, Rumford, or special healthfood brands containing no aluminum salts.

Table Salt. Use sea salt from healthfood stores.

Corn Starch. Arrowroot flour or rice polishings.

Chocolate. Carob candy and powder (El Molino is best).

White Sugar, Syrups. Use only turbinado, uncooked honey, sorghum, Grandma's molasses, maple syrup, and maple sugar.

Desserts. Cakes, pies, and cookies can be made from unrefined foods but should be served as the starch for the meal and not afterward, as is usually done.

Coffee, Tea. Use the alkaline teas: alfa-mint, fenugreek, shave grass, clover, rose hips, dandelion coffee.

All foods should be simply prepared. If you avoid spices, the natural flavors soon will prevail, enabling your senses to appreciate their delicate but distinctive character. Natural spices in moderation are not condemned, however.

Don't eat fruit with regular meals, only for breakfast or as a snack between meals and at bedtime.

Nuts, dried legumes, and soy beans can be used by those whose digestion allows it, but they must constitute the only starch or protein taken at that meal.

Don't under any circumstances drink fluoridated water or use it in food. Buy bottled water if necessary.

Hypoglycemia Diet

Note: This is only a guide; your doctor may not permit some of the listed items.

Upon Arising: A small bowl of yogurt and 1/2 grapefruit.

Breakfast: One egg with or without 2 slices of ham or bacon. 1/2 slice of bread only. It may be toasted with plenty of butter. Herb tea or decaffeinated coffee.

2 Hours after Breakfast: A snack of 2 shrimp, raw nuts or slices of roast beef.

Lunch: Salad (large serving of lettuce, tomato, vinegar and oil dressing). Vegetables if desired. 1/2 slice of bread or toast only, with plenty of butter. Dessert: see below list of allowable foods. Beverage.

2 Hours after Lunch: Attempt 8 ounces of milk but if you cannot tolerate milk, use water, and mix with that milk or water one teaspoon of Brewer's Yeast and one teaspoon of Veal Bone Meal. Several days a week you may alternate this with 4-6 ounces of cranberry juice with Brewer's Yeast added.

2 Hours before Dinner: A light snack of raw nuts, cheese or celery stuffed with cheese.

Dinner: Soup, if desired (not thickened with flour). Vegetables. Liberal portion of meat, fish or poultry. Beverage.

2 Hours after Dinner: Dessert: a dessert made from plain gelatin, fruit juice and sweetened with honey. May be topped with unsweetened whipped cream.

Every 2 Hours until Bed Time: A small handful of nuts or Brewer's Yeast and Bone Meal Drink.

Allowable Vegetables: Asparagus, avocados, beets, broccoli, brussel sprouts, cabbage, cauliflower, carrots, celery, cucumbers, eggplant, onions, peas, radishes, sauerkraut, squash, string beans, tomatoes and turnips.

Allouiable Fruits: Fresh and whole 1 small apple, ½ grapefruit, pineapple. If on occasion you feel you must use some canned fruits, be sure that they are unsweetened. May be cooked or raw, with or without cream, but definitely no sugar. Lettuce, mushrooms and raw nuts may be taken as freely as desired.

Allowable Juices: Any unsweetened cranberry or vegetable juice is allowable.

Allowable Beverages: Herb teas, decaffeinated coffee and coffee substitutes. Once on the road to recovery you may sweeten your drinks with Tupelo Honey if desired. Remember, use honey only in mild cases or after the initial program is relaxed.

Allowable Desserts: Homemade gelatins sweetened with fruit juice.

Avoid Absolutely: Alcoholic and soft drinks such as club soda, dry ginger ale, whiskey and liquors. Sugar, candy and other sweets such as cake, pie, pastries, sweet custards, puddings and ice cream. Caffeine—ordinary coffee, strongly brewed tea and beverages containing caffeine. Potatoes, rice, grapes, raisins, plums, figs, dates and bananas (starch and sugar). Spaghetti, macaroni, noodles, donuts, jams, jellies, marmalades (starch and sugar). Wines, cordials, cocktails and beers. (Alcohol content is a high carbohydrate).

Four Day Rotation Diet

Day One

Food Families:

Citrus:	Lemon, orange, grapefruit, lime, tangerine, kumquat, citron
Banana:	Banana, plantain, arrowroot (musa)
Palm:	Coconut, date, date sugar
Parsley:	Carrots, parsnips, celery, celery seed, celeriac, anise, dill, fennel, cumin, parsley, coriander, caraway
Beet:	Beets, spinach, Swiss chard, lamb's quarters greens
Pepper:	Black and white pepper, peppercorn
Herbs:	Nutmeg, mace
Cashew:	Cashew, pistachio, mango
Bird:	All fowl and game birds including chicken, turkey, duck, goose, guinea, pigeon, quail, pheasant, eggs

Tea:	Comfrey tea (Borage family), fennel tea
Oil:	Coconut oil, fats from any bird listed above, butter
Sweetener:	Use sparingly: Date sugar, orange honey (if honey is not used on another day of rotation), beet sugar
Juices:	Juices may be made and used without adding sweeteners from the following: Fruits: Any listed above in any combination.
Vegetables:	Any listed above in any combination desired, including fresh comfrey
Grains:	Wheat
Fish:	Salmon, tuna

Patients may wish to make their own rotation diets. The four-day diet presented here is given to show how it can be done. The basic requirement is that menus be prepared for four days so that a food on the menu on one day is not included on the menus of the three intervening days.

Day Two

Food Families

Grape:	All varieties of grapes, raisins
Pineapple:	(Juice pack, water pack, or fresh)
Rose:	Strawberry, raspberry, blackberry, dewberry, logan berry, young berry boysenberry, rose hips
Melon:	(Gourd) Watermelon, cucumber, cantaloupe, pumpkin, squash, other melons; zucchini, acorn, pumpkin, or squash seeds
Mallow:	Okra, cottonseed
Pea:	(Legume) Peas, black-eyed peas, dry beans, green beans, carob, soy beans, lentils, licorice, peanut, alfalfa
Subucaya:	Brazil nuts
Flaxseed:	Flaxseed
Mollusks:	Abalone, snail, squid, clam, mussel, oyster, scallop
Crustaceans:	Crab, crayfish, lobster, prawn, shrimp
Tea:	Alfalfa tea, fenugreek
Oil:	Soybean oil, peanut oil, cottonseed oil, butter
Sweeteners:	(Use sparingly) Carob syrup
Clover honey:	If honey is not used on another day
Juices:	Juices may be made and used without added sweeteners from the following: **Fruits or berries:** Any listed above in any combination desired.

	Vegetables: Any listed above in any combination desired including fresh alfalfa and some legumes
Fish:	Sardines, kippers, halibut
Grains:	Corn, millet
Red meat:	Beef, veal

Day Three

Food Families:

Apple:	Apple, pear, quince
Mulberry:	Mulberry, figs, breadfruit
Honeysuckle:	Elderberry
Olive:	Black or green or stuffed with pimento
Gooseberry:	Currant, gooseberry
Buckwheat:	Buckwheat
Aster:	Lettuce, chicory. endive, escarole, artichoke, dandelion, sunflower seeds, tarragon
Potato:	Potato, tomato, eggplant, peppers (red & green), chili pepper, paprika, cayenne, ground cherries
Lily (onion):	Onion, garlic, asparagus, chives, leeks
Spurge:	Tapioca
Herb:	Basil, savory, sage, oregano, horehound, catnip, spearmint, peppermint, thyme, marjoram lemon balm
Walnut:	English walnut, black walnut, pecan, hickory nut, butternut
Pedalium:	Sesame
Beech:	Chestnut
Saltwater fish:	Sea herring, anchovy, cod, sea bass, sea trout, mackerel, swordfish, flounder, sole
Fresh-water fish:	Sturgeon, herring, whitefish, bass, perch
Tea:	Kaffir tea
Oil:	Safflower oil, butter
Honey:	(Use sparingly) Buckwheat, safflower, or sage honey (honey can be used if it has not been used any other day)
Juices:	Juices may be made and used without added sweeteners from the following: **Fruits, Vegetables and herbs:** Any listed above in any combination desired
Red meat:	Lamb, mutton
Grains:	Rice, wild rice

Food Families:

Plumb:	Plum, cherry. peach, apricot, nectarine, almond, wild cherry
Blueberry:	Blueberry, huckleberry, cranberry, wintergreen
Pawpaw:	Pawpaw, papaya, papain
Mustard:	Mustard, turnip, radish, horseradish, watercress, cabbage, kraut. Chinese cabbage, broccoli, cauliflower, brussel sprouts, collards, kale, kohlrabi, rutabaga
Laurel:	Avocado. cinnamon, bay leaf, sassafras, cassia buds or bark
Sweet potato:	Sweet potatoes or yams
Grass:	Oats, barley, rye, cane, sorghum, bamboo sprouts
Orchid:	Vanilla
Protæ:	Macadamia nut
Birch:	Filberts. hazelnuts
Conifer:	Pine nut
Fungus:	Mushrooms and yeast (brewer's yeast, etc.)
Bovine:	Milk products—butter, cheese, yogurt, milk products, oleomargarine
Tea:	Sassafras tea or papaya leaf tea, lemon verbena tea
Oil:	Butter
Sweetener:	(Use sparingly) Cane, sugar, sorghum, molasses. Avocado honey if honey is not used on another day
Juices:	Juices may be made and used without added sweeteners, from the following: **Fruits and Vegtables:** listed above in any combination desired.

Appendix C
The Leaky Gut Syndrome

What is Intestinal Permeability?

The intestines are the defense barrier between what we eat and our immune and organ systems. A healthy body and mind requires the proper balance between the assimilation of critical nutrients and the exclusion of toxic substances. Any irritation to the gut lining can contribute to increased "leakiness" of the intestine, what is called "the leaky gut syndrome." When damage or injury occur to the intestinal lining, then toxic substances from our food, pollutants and toxins from the intestinal breakdown products can "leak" into the blood stream to cause a whole host of problems.

What Are The Causes Or Triggers Of The Leaky Gut Syndrome?

The following substances and conditions may lead to damage of the intestinal lining and promote the leaky gut:

1. Intestinal Infections and Overgrowths such as: Viral, bacterial, parasites and yeast.
2. Exposures to toxic substances such as: Alcohol, Anti-inflammatory medications like aspirin, advil, motrin and other similar prescription anti-inflammatory drugs, Pesticides/chemicals/free radicals and certain drugs such as antibiotics and those used in chemotherapy.
3. Mal digestion caused by: Low stomach acid, gastritis, low pancreatic digestive enzymes, lactose intolerance and gluten intolerance.
4. Food allergy causing inflammation in the intestine.
5. Certain types of surgery and long lasting or crash reducing diets

What Are The Consequences Of The Leaky Gut?

Chronic irritation to the gut lining leads to maldigestion and malabsorption of critical nutrients. These deficiencies result in a wide array of systemic problems. Furthermore, these deficiencies make the gut lining weaker and a vicious cycle is created. Continued passage of toxic substances leads to an increased burden on the liver's detoxification abilities and eventually to disease. In addition, increased passage of undigested food particles may lead to the development of food allergies. As you can see, the leaky gut can lead to far reaching problems in almost any part of the rest of the body.

What Are The Major Symptoms Of A Leaky Gut?

Fatigue and day time sleepiness, fevers, abdominal, pain/cramps, diarrhea, "toxic" feelings, shortness of breath, muscle and joint pains, food reactions and/or intolerances, abdominal bloating and gas, skin rashes, poor memory and thinking and poor exercise ability.

What Conditions and Diseases are Associated with the Leaky Gut Syndrome?

Ulcerative colitis/Crohn's Disease, Rheumatoid arthritis/Lupus, Eczema, Hives, Cystic fibrosis, liver diseases, Chronic Fatigue Syndrome, Autism, Environmental Illness, Multiple food allergies, Infectious diarrhea, Acne, Psoriasis, AIDS, Pancreas diseases, Irritable Bowel Syndrome (spastic colitis), chronic arthritis and joint pains, Attention Deficit Syndrome, Hyperactivity, chemical sensitivity and various chronic pain patterns.

How Do We Test For The Leaky Gut?

Following an overnight fast, we have you collect the first morning urine sample. Then we have you drink a premeasured solution of lactulose and mannitol (two sugar type molecules that the body usually does not absorb or utilize). After ingesting this drink, you collect all your urine in one container for the next six hours and bring this sample and the first morning sample to us, at our Center, as soon as possible. To help in diagnosing food allergies, this test is sometimes done after eating a specific food or foods that are in question, rather than after an overnight fast as previously described.

Other testing that may be needed, depending on the individual problems are: a Liver Detoxification profile, food allergy testing (elimination/challenge diet, skin testing or blood testing), stomach pH testing, breath test for bacterial overgrowth, comprehensive stool analysis, hair analysis and blood cell analysis for vitamins, minerals and toxic metals.

What Is The Treatment For Leaky Gut?

The first step in treatment is to eliminate and remove the cause or triggering mechanism. To accomplish this we: stop the suspected drug or medication, test for and remove suspected food allergies, have the patient eat organic and unpolluted food and treat any suspected infection or parasite overgrowth condition. The use of vitamins and other nutritional supplements must be tailored to the individual. Our basic, but flexible, protocol is as follows:

Phase I (First 4-6 weeks)

Springreen Intestinal Cleanser—consists of liquid caprylic acid, bentonite clay and psyllium fiber. Used mainly for the treatment of yeast overgrowth, it is also an excellent intestinal cleaner and detoxifier. Use as directed by your Center physician. May be used once or twice a day but is not to be taken with other supplements unless so directed by your physician.

Permeability Factors—Take *between* meals. Contains L-glutamine, N-acetylglucosamine, gamma-oryzanol, GLA and vitamin E. All of these are specific for healing of the intestinal lining.

Anti Oxidant Formula—1 pill two times per day with meals. Helps defend against and repair free radical damage from chemical, pollutant and toxic exposures. Also supports the liver's detoxification process. Contains vitamin A, B's, C, E, minerals like selenium and small amount of zinc, grape seed extract, green tea extract, N-acetyl Cysteine and threonic acid. We withhold anti-oxidant treatment during therapy for parasites if indicated, since antioxidants may block the effectiveness of parasite therapy.

Diet—Follow the Basic Health Maintenance Diet (See Appendix A) with special emphasis on avoidance of known food allergens and full attention to the suggested food combinations. The addition of artichoke and beets to the diet may be of beneficial help to the gut lining repair process. The addition of sulfur containing foods such as lentils, beans, garlic, onion and the vegetables cabbage, broccoli, cauliflower and brussel sprouts all help support the liver detox function.

Phase II (Next 4-6 weeks)

The **Springreen** is to be discontinued.

Permeability Factors—continued as needed up to 12 weeks.

Anti Oxidant Formula—if the desired improvement occurs it may be decreased to one a day or stay at two a day if required.

High quality, pure potency multi vitamin-mineral is added as tolerated (2-6 per day)

Acidophilus Supplement—with or without fructo-oligosaccharides (food for the good guy bacteria).

Liv-Rinse or S.A.T.—additional liver detox support.

Diet—as above, continuing the emphasis on food allergy avoidance and proper food combinations.

Phase III (Long term maintenance)

High potency multi vitaminmineral supplement recommended by your Center physician.

Blue Green Algae or **Green Vibrance**—as tolerated or indicated.

Diet—same as above with perpetual emphasis on food allergy avoidance and proper food combinations

Retesting—Retesting of intestinal permeability test 8 to 12 weeks after the above phases are completed.

Other Selected Remedies for Special Needs:

Digestive enzymes for suspected or test proven pancreatic insufficiency.

Betaine HCL or **"bitters formula"** for low stomach acidity.

Tricycline (Artemesia, Berberine and grape seed extract), and or **Gentian** (Biocidin)—to treat bacterial or parasitic overgrowth. Both are very powerful natural substances. Stool analysis often guides the choice here.

Zinc (NTF or citrate)—Recommended if lab testing reveals low zinc or it is clinically suspected. Zinc is very important to healing of inflammation and ulcers of the skin and mucosal lining anywhere.

Quercitin—to block food allergy reactions in the intestine.

Cellulose fiber or flax fiber—as alternative to the psyllium or for continued fiber supplementation.

Cat's Claw (Uncaria tomentosa)—Peruvian herb with intestinal healing properties.

Appendix D

Multiple Food Elimination Diet Part One

During the first week, most meats, fruits and vegetables can be eaten. The "allowed" and "forbidden" foods are listed further on in this diet. Keep detailed records in a food diary of exactly what you eat. Most individuals who are going to respond favorably to this diet do so about the sixth or seventh day; others respond as early as the second day or, rarely, as late as the fourteenth day.

If you or your child are better in a week or less, begin part two of this diet on day eight. Improvement noted on day two may greatly increase by day seven. The object is to see the maximum amount of improvemnet that can be noted during the first seven days.

If you want to help your entire family, urge everyone to try the diet at the same time. Typically, several family members will note improvement in how they feel or act when this is done.

If you or your child are not better within one week, recheck the diet records for the initial week to see if only the allowed foods were eaten. If you or your child repeatedly forgot and ate the wrong foods or drank the wrong beverages at school, work or at home, the item which was not deleted or omitted from the diet may be the culprit. Try Part One of the diet again, but this time try much harder to adhere strictly to the diet. It's best to do the diet only one time, but do it right. This fast, inexpensive method of food sensitivity detection can some times provide rapid, safe relief of many chronic medical and behavioral complaints.

Occasionally, a person is worse during Part One of the diet. This may be from a "clearing out effect" of prior food sensitivities or it may be that you or your child have begun to ingest an excessive amount of an unsuspected offeding food or beverage. If this happens, immediately stop the diet. A child who substitutes apple or grape juice for milk, for example, may act or behave much worse if the apple or grape juice is the cause of this child's symptoms. Retry Part One of the diet, but do not include the suspected food or beverage which you believe made your child worse.

Sometimes, a person who was not helped during the first week will dramatically improve with a more prolonged effort. If you are not helped by the first week of the diet continue Part One of the diet for two weeks. If Part One of the diet is tried and has not helped by the fourteenth day, this particular diet is probably not the answer for you or your child. Your medical problems may not be related to foods or are possibly due to other frequently eaten or craved items, ie, mushrooms, cinnamon, yeast, tobacco, molds, chemicals, etc., which were not removed from the diet.

If an infection occurs during the diet, stop the diet until you or your child is well. It is too difficult to interpret the results if it is continued during such infections.

During Part One of the diet, the following foods are omitted in all forms: Milk and dairy products (yogurt, cheese, ice cream, casein, sodium caseinate, whey), Wheat (bread, cake, cookies, baked goods), eggs, corn, sugar, chocolate (cocoa or cola), peas and goobers (peanut butter, peanuts), caffeine (coffee [including decaf], tea, colas and other caffeine rich soft drinks), citrus (orange, lemon, lime, grapefruit), food coloring, additives, preservatives, lucheon meats, sausage, ham and bacon.

If there is some question about a specific food, *do not eat it.* Also, exclude any other food or beverage that is craved in excess because such items are frequently unsuspected causes of various medical or emotional problems.

Major Caution: Do *not* eat any food you already know causes a severe allergy. This diet is to detect foods that you eat frequently but that are *not* presently recognized as a possible cause of certain medical, behavior, hyperactivity or learning problems.

Foods Allowed During Part One

Cereals/Grains: Rice—rice puffs, rice cakes. Oats—Oatmeal made with honey. Barley.

Fruits: Any fresh fruit, except citrus. Canned—if in their own juice and without artificial color, sugar, or preservatives.

Vegetables and Starches: Any fresh vegetables, except corn and peas, French fries (home made only), Potatoes.

Meats: Chicken or turkey (non-basted), Louis Rich ground turkey, Veal or beef. Pork. Lamb. Fish.

Beverages: Water (preferably spring water). Single herb or plain tea & honey. Grape juice, bottled in glass. Frozen apple juice. Pure pineapple juice (no corn surup or dextrose).

Snacks: Potato chips without addititives. Ryekrisp crackers and pure honey. Raisins (unsulfured).

Miscellaneous: Pure honey. Homemade vinegar/oil dressing. Sea salt. Olive Oil (cold pressed). Pure maple syrup. Homemade syrup.

Foods to Avoid During Part One:

Cereals/Grains: Foods containing wheat flour, (most cakes, cookies, bread, baked goods)

Fruits: Citrus—orange, lemon, lime, grapefruit.

Vegetables and Starches: Any frozen or canned vegetables, corn, peas or mixed vegetables.

Meats: Luncheon meats, wieners, bacon, artificially dyed hamburger meat, ham, dyed salmon, lobster, breaded meats, meats with stuffing.

Milk or dairy: Drinks with casein or whey. Fruit beverages, except those so stated. Kool-Aid, Coffee Rich (yellow dye), 7-UP, Squirt, Teem, colas, Dr. Pepper, ginger ale, coffee, black teas (even Decaf)—be sure to wean slowly off caffeine to prevent headaches.

Snacks: Corn chips (fritos), chocolate, cocoa, hard candy, ice cream or sherbet

Miscellaneous: Sugar, dextrose, bread, cake, cookies (except special recipes), eggs, dyed (colored) vitamins or other pills, mouthwash, toothpaste, medicines, cough syrup, etc. Jelly or jam, Jell-O, margarine or diet spreads (dyes and corn). Peanut butter, peanuts, Sorbitol (corn), cheese. All nonessential medications. All nonessential food and vitamin supplements. Red pepper (cayenne)

Be sure to read all labels before you eat anything. Refer to the last page for more details on food groups.

Part Two: The Food Challenge

During Part Two of this diet, one food is reintroduced into the diet, in excess, each day in the following manner:

On day eight add .... **Milk.**
On day nine add .... **Wheat.**
On day ten add .... **Sugar.**
On day eleven add .... **Eggs.**
On day twelve add .... **Cocoa.**
On day thirteen add .... **Food Coloring.**
On day fourteen add ...... **Corn.**
On day fifteen add .... **Preservatives.**
On day sixteen add .... **Citrus fruits and juices.**
On day seventeen add .... **Peanut Butter.**
On day eighteen add ...... **Coffee or Tea (for adults).**

Keep detailed records of how you or your child feels at the beginning and the end of each day, and observe carefully for one hour after a food is tried or eaten again. Start with a teaspoon or ½ cup of the test food item and double the amount eaten every few hours, so that by the end of the day a "normal" amount has been ingested.

Do any symptoms suddenly reappear? If you want to know even

more about what each food does when it is eaten again, do the following (or have your child do the following):

1. Write or draw. Is there a change or deterioration from before a meal to twenty minutes after the tested item is eaten? If so, the item(s) ingested could affect your child's school work.

2. Take the pulse before and after eating a food item. If it increases by twenty to forty points after eating a particular food, this may be an indication of a sensitivity to that ingested item.

3. If you or your child have asthma, use a Pocket Peak Flow Meter before and twenty minutes after each tested food. If the reading on the guage drops 15%, or fifty or so points, that food or beverage could be the cause of wheezing or asthma symptoms. Ask your Center physician for the hand out "The Big Five" for more information on how to perform items one thorough three above.

If there are no symptoms during that day, during the night or the next morning before breakfast, the food tested the day before is probably all right and may be eaten when desired or, preferably, as part of a rotation diet. If the test food causes symptoms, stop eating it in all forms (see end of this appendix) until you can obtain advice from your Center physician. *Do not give your child another test food until the symptoms from the previous food test have subsided.* You may have to push back the above schedule of that day to test a food if he reacts. This is perfectly OK. Usually, however, you will notice that a symptom(s) caused by a food occurs within one hour. However, symptoms such as canker sores, bedwetting, tight or painful joints, ear fluid, and bowel problems that are food related, tend to be delayed reactions occuring several hours or sometimes several days later.

If symptoms persist, you may use Alka-Seltzer Antacid Formula without aspirin (Alka-Seltzer Gold) or Alka-Aid (can be purchased from a health food store) to help alleviate them. Dose is one tablet for age six to twelve and two tablets for those over twelve. Don't use this if you or your child has liver or kidney disease. Your usual prescribed allergy medications can be taken if needed for symptom control.

Note: If one of the listed foods causes a reaction which is not helped by Alka-Seltzer Gold or Alka-Aid and/or that lasts over twenty-four hours, DO NOT TRY to check the response to the next test food item until the reaction has entirely subsided.

Watch closely to see what happens each day. One food might cause a stuffy nose, the next, no reaction at all. Some reactions occur immediately, others in several hours. Once again, if a food obviously causes serious symptoms, it should not be tried. NEVER TEST ANY FOOD WITH-

OUT YOUR DOCTOR'S ADVICE IF IT CAUSED SERIOUS MEDICAL PROB-
LEMS IN THE PAST. For example, if eggs or peanuts caused immediate
throat swelling or fish caused severe asthma, it is unsafe to try even a tiny
bit of these foods.

If you are uncertain whether a food causes symptoms or not,
discontinue it until the other foods have been checked. Then give your
child the suspected food again at a five day interval, ie., Tuesday and
Saturday. See if symptoms recur each time and stop when you confirmed
a food reaction.

You may add back food and vitamin supplements one at a time in
the above fashion to determine if they are causing any symptoms or
reactions. Furthermore, it is wise to retest all supplements in this fashion
every six months to make sure a sensitivity has not developed to that
supplement. Stop them all for a week and add them back one new one
each day.

Once you have determined which foods are tolerated and which
foods give symptoms, it is best to avoid the symptomatic foods for three
to six months and then retry them to see if they still cause symptoms. All
other "safe" foods should be eaten in a rotation manner as described in
the Appendix B "Rotation Diet." This will hopefully prevent the development of other and new food sensitivities from developing.

Specific Details of Part Two: Food Challenge

Day 8, The day you add Milk: Give you or your child lots of milk,
cottage cheese and whipped cream sweetened with pure maple syrup or
honey. No butter, margarine or yellow cheese unless you are absolutely
certain they contain no yellow dyes. Remember to make sure any and all
symptoms provoked by milk are totally resolved before proceeding to
the next food.

Day 9, The day you add Wheat: Add triscuits or pure wheat cereal.
If your child had trouble from milk, be sure *not* to give milk products.
Use Italian bread or kosher bread because these should not contain milk
(casein or whey), but always read labels to be sure. You may bake your
own bread if you wish, but you must not use eggs, milk, or sugar.
Remember, the child can eat no dairy products or drink any milk if these
seemed to cause problems. Remember to make sure any and all
symptoms provoked by wheat are totally resolved before proceeding to
the next food.

Day 10, The day you add Sugar: Whole sugar cubes are eaten and
granulated sugar is added to the allowed foods. If milk or wheat caused
trouble, they must be avoided or you can't tell if sugar is tolerated. Many

children react within one hour after four to eight sugar cubes. Remember to make sure any and all symptoms provoked by sugar are totally resolved before proceeding to the next food.

Day 11, The day you add Eggs: Give eggs in the usual forms, cooked or as eggnog or custard (as long as dairy is tolerated). Remember, again, no wheat, milk or sugar can be consumed if any of these caused problems. Be sure to skip this food challenge if you already know egg is a problem. Remember to make sure any and all symptoms provoked by egg are totally resolved before proceeding to the next food.

Day 12, The day you add Cocoa: Give dark chocolate with water, cocoa (pure Hershey's cocoa powder) and honey or pure maple syrup. No candy bars are allowed because most contain milk and corn. Remember, no milk, wheat, sugar, dyes or eggs are allowed if any of these caused symptoms. Remember to make sure any and all symptoms provoked by cocoa are totally resolved before proceeding to the next food.

Day 13, The day you add Food Coloring: Give Jell-O, jelly or artificially colored fruit beverage (soda pop, Kool-Aid), popsicles or cereal. Try to give lots of yellow, purple and red items because the patient might react to only one of these colors. Remember to avoid milk, wheat, cola or sugar in all forms if any of these were a problem. If sugar caused symptoms, use honey or pure maple syrup, as a sweetener or add food coloring to plain pure gelatin. If milk, wheat, or sugar were tolerated, they may be eaten. Remember to make sure any and all symptoms provoked by food coloring are totally resolved before proceeding to the next food.

Day 14, The day you add Corn: Give corn, corn meal, corn flakes, and plain popcorn. Popcorn can be made with salt. If milk, wheat, sugar, dyes, eggs, or chocolate caused trouble, you can't give them on the day you give corn. If you do, and your child is worse, you won't be able to tell which is at fault. Do not use butter on popcorn if your child has a milk sensitivity. Remember to make sure any and all symptoms provoked by corn are totally resolved before proceeding to the next food.

Day 15, The day you add Preservatives: Give foods which contain preservatives or food additives. Read every label. In particular, eat luncheon meat, bologna, hot dogs, bread, baked goods, or soups which contain many preservatives and additives. Remember to make sure any and all symptoms provoked by preservatives are totally resolved before proceeding to the next food.

Day 16, The day you add Citrus: Give large amounts of lemons, limes, grapefruit or oranges as fresh fruit or in juice. Avoid artificial dyes if food colors were a problem.

436

Day 17, The day you add Peanut Butter: Give lots of peanut butter or peanuts. Test for this only if it's a favorite food. Use RyeKrisp if no wheat is allowed. Use pure peanut butter without preservatives (Smuckers or other natural brands).

Day 18, The day you add Coffee/Tea: For adults and older adolescents who consume coffee or tea. Go back to the number of cups of coffe/tea or other caffeinated drinks per day you were consuming prior to starting this diet. You may not be able to drink as much if symptoms are rapid and extreme, ie headache.

Special Tips for the Multiple Elimination/Challenge Diet

The "allowed" foods may be selected, combined and eaten in any quantity. If you are suspicious of a food, start with a small amount and gradually increase it during the day if no symptoms manifest. For a beverage, you may mix the allowed fruits in the blender with spring water and honey or pure maple syrup.

You or your child's medications may be taken during the diet. If improvement is seen, you may find that certain medicines such as antihistamines are needed less often by the end of the first week. Try to use only white pills (crushed for small children and placed in applesauce or potatoes) or colorless liquids. Most liquid medications contain corn, sugar, artificial flavors and artificial dyes which may cause symptoms in many children. Check with our Center or your or your child's physician about any questions you may have regarding this.

Once you determine which foods cause specific symptoms, you must discuss these foods with your Center physician. Some foods cannot be omitted for indefinite periods of time if proper nutrition is to be maintained.

Do not try the diet when you or your child has an infection or is receiving antibiotics which contain dyes, sugar, flavoring, or corn. Holidays are also not a good time to start this diet.

Although symptoms from a single food vary, food sensitivities are often evident in several family members. One child might have headaches, another a stuffy, congested nose, a third family member may be hyperactivity and another child might wet the bed. The same food, ie., milk, may be a problem for several generations of a family. For this reason, make cooking easier by placing the entire family on the diet. A fringe benefit may be that you relieve some "emotional" or "learn-to-live-with-it" health problems caused by certain foods or beverages in several family members.

If your child refuses the diet, try offering rewards. Promise a gala party if there is no cheating and if it is obvious that the child is truly trying very hard to cooperate in every way. The party should take place *after* both parts of the diet are completed. At that time, give your child the foods which caused the symptoms providing they were not severe and incapacitating. This will be a double check confirming the effect of these foods on your child. Alka-Aid (from health food store) will prevent or stop reactions in many children in ten to fifteen minutes depending upon whether it is given before or after a problem food is eaten.

Alternatively, you may offer a reward at the end of each completed day, ie. a hobby item (new stamp, coin, fishing lure, etc) and then an additional gift at the end of the week. Younger children often respond well to a gold star chart. Make a chart with a space for each meal of every day of the week. Give a star for every meal successfully completed. You might even suggest that for every x number of stars (two, three, etc.) the child earns a special treat—a trip to the park, a small toy, etc. Be sure to let the child in advance know what are the goals and then help him to stick to them. In the end, you must realize, that if your child does not want to go on this diet, he or she won't. Hopefully you can convince them to at least meet you half way.

If your child has asthma, add the test food back into the diet with extreme care. It is possible that an unsuspected food could precipitate a sudden severe asthma attack. Have asthma medications on hand during Part Two of the diet and use the *Pocket Peak Flow Meter* to help find out exactly what is causing your child to wheeze. Ask your Center Physicain for the hand out "The Big Five."

You may have some difficulty finding suitable substitute foods during your elimination and challenge phases of this diet at conventional grocery stores. If so, try your local health food or gourmet stores for various foods and food products. It is also helpful to plan your diet for the whole time and then purchase exactly what is needed for each day; this way you won't get caught short at the last minute looking for a particular food item to be added or substituted.

Admittedly, this diet is not the easiest to follow; it requires patience and discipline. However, once hidden food sensitivities are discovered, you can take the first step to free yourself or your child from symptoms and difficulties that have, up to now, been only partially or even ineffectively treated. Do the best you can, never give up and the desired results will follow.

The following books provide more information and recipes to help you with the elimination diet:

Eating Alive, John Matsen, N.D. $16.95
Detecting Your Hidden Allergies, William Crook, M.D. $10.95 (pb)

Food Allergies, How To Tell If You Have Them, What to do About Them If You Do, N. Orenstein, Ph.D. $9.95

These books can all be provided to you by your Center physician.

Table of Food Ingredients

The following table lists those foods which fall into the major categories eliminated from the diet. Any thing listed in the category should be evaluated to determine whether it contains some or all of the major listed item.

ARTIFICIAL SWEETENERS
aspartame
NutraSweet
saccharine

SUGAR
brown sugar
candy
cake
corn syrup
soft drinks
succanat
glucose
sucrose
fructose
dextrose

CORN
alcohol-most
bacon
bread products
candies
corn batters
corn breads
corn flakes
other corn cereals
corn muffins
corn oil
corn starches
cured meats (ham, sausage, bologna)

COCOA
cakes
candies
chocolate cereals
chocolate & cola drinks
frosting
pastries
pies

CITRUS
grapefruit
lemons
limes
oranges
citrus beverages

WHEAT
bagels
beer
biscuits
bran
bread (wheat, white, rye. pumpernickel)
bulgur
cakes
cereals (most)
commercial gravy
cookies
cous-cous
crackers

dextrin
dextrose
envelope and stamp adhesive
fresh/frozen corn
fructose
hominy grits
ice cream
jelly
ketchup
maize
mazola oil
mixed vegetable oil
modified food starch
mustard
pastries
peanut butter with corn syrup
popcorn
salad dressings
sherbet
toothpaste
tortillas
zein

doughnuts
farina
flour (wheat, graham. white,
    high gluten, enriched, unbl.)
french toast
matzos
meats containing fillers
    (meat loat; hotdogs,
    bologna, luncheon meats)
muffins
noodles
pancakes
pastries
prepared batters/mixes
rolls
semolina
soups (noodles, dumplings,
    thickened with wheat flour)
soy sauce
tabouli
wheat cereals
wheat germ

EGGS
battered (fried) foods
bread
cakes (including all cake
    mixes)
candy
casseroles
cookies
custard
doughnuts
eggs in any form
egg salad
egg sauces
French toast
fritters
hollandaise sauce
ice cream
mayonnaise

DAIRY
butter
biscuits
cakes
candy
chocolate
cookies
cottage cheese
crackers
cream soups
doughnuts
ice cream
luncheon meats
milk (whole, skim,
    evaporated, goat's,
    condensed. instant,
    nonfat, dry)
pastries

440

meringues
noodles
omelets
pancakes
pasta
pies
prepared mixes and frozen dinners
salad dressings
sherbet
souffles
tartar sauce
waffles
Read labels for egg
derived ingredients—albumin

ARTIFICIAL PRESERVATIVES
sodium benzoate
(benzoic acid)
BHA
BHT
MSG
Metabisulfite (sulfites)
   sulfites are not always
   listed in ingredients,
   foods possibly containing
   sulfites:
beer
wine
any alcoholic beverage
soft drinks
cider vinegar
shrimp (esp. frozen)
soy protein
avocado dips
potato chips
french fries
dried potatoes
cake mixes
processed fruits (canned,
   juices, frozen,

yogurt
Read labels for milk
derived ingredients—
   casein, lactoalbumin,
whey

SEASONINGS
Don't pick up
anything
and shake it on your
food until you read
the label

ARTIFICIAL COLORING
There are many colorings
Yellow dye #5 is most trouble
causing and is found in:
butterscotch chips
cake mixes
candy drops and
hard candies
certain breakfast cereals
certain candy coatings
certain instant and
regular pudding
colored marshmallows
chocolate chips
commercial frostings
commercial gingerbread
commercial pies
flavored carbonated beverages
flavored drink mixes
ready-to-eat canned puddings
refrigerated rolls and
quick breads

YEAST
baker's yeast
brewer's yeast

bottled. dried, jam)
fruit drinks
lemon juice concentrates
many medications
salad bars at restaurants

condiments that contain
vinegar (mustard, ketchup,
  relish, horseradish, pickles,
  mayonnaise)
dried fruit
fermented foods
  (miso soup, soy sauce)
grapes
nutritional yeast
peanuts
sauerkraut
vinegar

Yeast products may occasionally cause trouble but were not specificallyaddressed during the elimination and challenge phases. If you suspect they may be a problem or wish to see if they are, just eliminate the above foods in the yeast category and add them back as described.

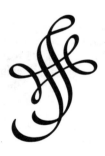